Till Death Us Do Part

A Vet's Life

Till Death Us Do Part.

A Vet's Life

Richard Holden

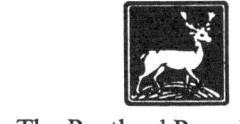

The Pentland Press Limited
Edinburgh • Cambridge • Durham

© Richard Holden 1995

First published in 1995 by
The Pentland Press Ltd.
1 Hutton Close
South Church
Bishop Auckland
Durham

All rights reserved.
Unauthorised duplication
contravenes existing laws.

British Library Cataloguing in Publication Data.
A catalogue record for this book is available
from the British Library.

ISBN 1 85821 240 5

Essex County Library

Typeset by CBS, Felixstowe, Suffolk
Printed and bound by Antony Rowe Ltd., Chippenham

In Memoriam
Hugh McKean, MRCVS,
age thirty-one years,
killed in a car crash
27 February 1961

ACKNOWLEDGEMENTS

To Mr J A Wight OBE FRCVS, DVSc
(James Herriot)
for sending quotations to me

To Mrs Barbara Bainbridge for, again,
typing out my manuscript.

FOREWORD

by

Mr J B Johnson, BVSc, DVSc, MRCVS,
Senior Vice-President of The Royal College of Veterinary Surgeons

Mr Richard Holden (the pen-name of Mr Roger B. Hornby) qualified as a veterinary surgeon earlier this century, and now is a living tribute to the healthy lifestyle of the profession. He gained his working experience in Lancashire and he evokes nostalgic memories of the unspoilt Lancashire countryside free of heavy traffic and motorways. His capture of the dialect and colloquial language of the farmers and stockmen is instructive and charmingly expresses so vividly life as it existed some fifty years ago.

This is the second book which Richard Holden has written and we are indebted to him for accurately retaining the memory of what veterinary practice was like in those days of hardship during the war and the enormous risks which veterinary surgeons took with their own safety in dedication to further scientific knowledge whilst helping animals and their owners. Old husbandry methods and the way in which disease problems were handled in those days are poignantly described and we owe a great deal to Richard for reminding us of those primitive yet exciting days in the life of such a dedicated professional man.

I hope that Richard Holden's book – timely as it is with the approach of the 21st century and the 150th anniversary of the granting of the Royal College of Veterinary Surgeons Charter – will provide encouragement to young members of the profession faced with problems of animal welfare.

Though the story is written during the war it demonstrates the sheer enjoyment and deep pain of a large animal practitioner dedicated to his work.

1942

Little snowflakes began to fall as Richard was driving down Beech Hill in the semi-darkness of late afternoon in that bitter January of the third year of the war. He thought to himself, it looks as though we are going to have snow again from January to March for the third year running, so he was glad when he reached Cross Street and drove the car into the garage. He appreciated the warmth when he walked into the kitchen, closed the door and switched on the light. Jim and Ming, together by the stove, looked at him sleepily as he took off his hat, leather driving gloves, overcoat and leather jerkin. He was kicking off his wellingtons when from upstairs Flora called, 'Richard, there are no more messages. Come up and have a cup of tea; I've just brewed it.'

'OK. I'll be up in a jiffy.'

He locked the door and went upstairs to the lounge.

'Was it WVS work today, Flora?' he asked as he took his cup of tea.

'Yes, but I was back at half past three because Marjorie had to go early – it didn't matter because there were eleven women there.'

'And what were you all doing?'

'Packing up gifts for the services. Some were doing the woollens – mittens, gloves, socks, scarves, balaclavas and long stockings for the Navy – they want them for the submarines and minesweepers.'

'I bet they do – I'm cold in the car, they must be perished with freezing sea water and spray everywhere.'

'They want them urgently. We get some nice letters back from the ships, but they like the fags more. That's what I've been doing, writing the addresses on the packs of cigarettes. There are six tins of fifty in a pack, all makes: Woodbines; Players; Senior Service; Churchman; Gold Flake and . . .'

The phone rang and when Richard picked up the receiver a breathless voice said, 'Mr Holden, wilta cum to Higher Syke reet away? We've a cow in t' tank.'

'Yes, that's Bill Wallbanks?'

'Aye, I'm his lad George.'

'Right, George, we will want a three legs and a block with an endless chain.'

'We hev 'em at farm, builders are there.'

'That's handy, and some strong planks, and four or five men to help.'

'Aye, mi Dad will 'ev gitten 'em. Tha' won't be long, will ya, Mr Holden, because cow were only bought today.'

'No, I'm setting off now, George.' He replaced the receiver.

'And what was all that about?' asked Flora.

'A cow has fallen into the tank at Higher Syke, and will have to be got out. It will be a dirty, cold, stinking job so I want all my old gear. Will you get them while I go and fill up the car with the lifting tackle?'

'Yes, I'll bring them here and you can change in front of the fire – at least you will set off warm.'

Later, when he had changed into the old clothes, Flora laughed and said, 'Well, you look a proper scarecrow, especially wearing the deerstalker.'

'Thanks a lot – listen, I will probably be two hours, and he's not on the phone, so ring anything that is that way to Catley Post Office. I'll call there on the way back.'

'Yes, love, I'll do that,' and she gave him a kiss.

The light, powdery snow was falling steadily, swirled about by the icy wind, and was slowly freezing onto everything, making the road very slippery. With the scarcely adequate light from the cowled headlamps, Richard made slow progress on the long drive to Higher Syke, but at last he saw the gate posts in the dry stone wall which marked the entrance to the field across which the unmetalled track led to the farm. As he drove in he saw the track had disappeared, buried by the snow, so he stopped the car, wondering how he could find the buildings in the snow-filled blackness. At that moment a Shire horse and rider appeared, and when he wound down the car window a voice shouted for Richard to follow. He did so quickly because the horse and rider almost vanished into the swirling snow, glad that Bill Wallbank had sent a guide for him, but sorry for the rider who must have been almost frozen stiff. When a yellow glow became visible, Richard drove up to it, and saw that oil lamps were illuminating a group of men near to the shippon wall. I must explain that these hill farm houses and buildings were entirely built of stone; most were 150 years old and some very much older. The buildings were two storeys high, the first floor being the hay loft, and the ground floor, the shippons in which the cattle were tied up. Under the building a cellar or tank was always constructed into which drained all the urine and semi-liquid excrement from the cattle, horses and even pigs. An eight-inch diameter pipe, closed by a hand-operated valve, led from the base of the tank to a suitable place lower down the hillside. Here in the back end of the year or in spring-time the muck carts were filled with the liquid which was then spread onto the pastures.

As Richard got out of the car the intense cold of the wind almost made him gasp, but the men seemed oblivious of it as they stood round the eight by six feet hole from which a ladder protruded, and over which the three legs were positioned; but the snowfall had almost ceased.

'Good evening, Mr Holden,' said Bill Wallbank. 'Hes ta gitten lifting tackle?'

'Yes, it's in the back of the car. Have you caught the cow?'

'Aye, we hev 'er fast. Frank, git tackle froe't car.' Frank moved at once, and Richard took his place. He switched on his torch and, shining it down the hole, saw young Bill Wallbank standing on the ladder. He was out of reach of the high curved horns of the big Ayrshire cow whose head, neck and upper back were above the fluid level. The halter holding the cow was tied to the ladder.

'Bill, first we want the belly band round the cow, so lower it down now. Frank, you go and stand on the ladder ready to let the halter loose, and young Bill can get the band under the cow.'

This was done by using a draining rod which had a hook on one end which caught the rope, and it and the band were dragged under the cow. The metal Ds on each end of the belly band were hooked onto each end of the steel bar, which was in turn attached to the hook on the endless chain of the block, this hanging down from the centre of the three legs.

'Reet, lads, let's get pulling.'

'No, wait a minute, Bill, we want the breast piece and the breeching on next.'

'Nay, we don't need 'em; band ull hold 'er. Frank, thee come up an Bill stand on t' ladder, and keep cow's head this way. Now, pull.'

They did, and as the chain came round down through the liquid and then up out of the tank the stinking filth dripped and splashed all over them, but they kept pulling and slowly the cow was raised a foot or so out of the liquid. Then suddenly she reared up, plunged forward and with a mighty splash dived out of the belly band, swimming round the tank dragging Bill behind her.

Amid curses and recriminations, Bill shouted, 'The silly devil, hang on t' cow, lad; Frank, thee go down and ge us belly band.'

A louder voice shouted, 'Put those lights out,' and the snow-covered figure of the local bobby wheeling his bike appeared – Harry Mather.

'We're not putting bloody lights out, it's an emergency. We've got to get cow out, and neither you nor your damned Hitler ull stop us. We can't do t' job in t' dark.'

Tempers cooled when Harry said he would help, and now Richard took charge. The cow was brought to the foot of the ladder; the belly band was replaced under her and hooked onto the bar. Then the breastpiece, the breeching, the straps and the crupper piece were all attached to the bar, into which the hook was fixed.

'Bill, call your lad up or he'll catch his death of cold.'

'Bill thee git t' halter to Frank and come up, git them clothes off and go and hev a 'ot bath.'

Though the snow had stopped the wind was strong and Bill must have been very cold as he emerged from the hole and ran off towards the house, leaving an incredible stench behind him.

'Reet, let's have another go. Are you ready, Frank?'

'Aye.'

'Nay, wait a minute, you lot,' and Mrs Wallbank appeared carrying a big wicker basket.

'You must have a warm drink,' and she put on the window sill some pint mugs, two bottles of whisky, and a big kettle. She poured whisky into each mug, poured in the hot water, and gave one to each man, including young Frank and George.

The toddy was eagerly drunk, and Richard felt it warming his stomach.

'Thanks, lass,' said Bill to his wife, 'now, come on, let's be doing.'

Richard was the fourth man on the chain and as it passed through his gloved hands he was quickly splattered with the muck which was dropping onto them, and the smell was appalling. Light snow started to fall again but, puffing and cursing, they kept on pulling.

'Here she comes!' someone shouted as Frank's and the cow's heads appeared above ground level. Everybody pulled faster, and steadily the cow came up.

'Get the planks ready!' shouted Richard. 'Keep pulling, now shove 'em over the hole quick!'

This was done and the cow lowered until she was standing on the planks, with George now holding her head. Everybody took a breather, the mugs were passed round, and their contents quickly drunk. Richard could feel the perspiration running down his back under his clothes, though his face and feet were frozen.

'Reet, hang onto her, George, while we get this gear off her.'

Richard said, 'We'll want some buckets of hot water, sacks and string.' As the cow was led into the shippon he went to the car to get two bottles of stimulant medicine. In the warm, steamy shippon Richard held the cow's horns while she was drenched with the medicine. Bill came in with a whisky bottle which was one-third full.

'Gi' her that, it ull do her more good than us,' he said. 'It's all that's left.'

The cow was now washed down with hot water and roughly dried, then covered in straw over which sacks were placed, and all were tied on with string. She was given a bucket of water to drink, and an armful of good hay was thrown to her.

'That's it,' said Bill. 'Go t' t' house, all of yer, wife's got tea ready.'

Divesting themselves of their stinking, sodden top clothes and kicking off their footwear, they walked onto the flagged floor of the kitchen, at one end of which a large wood fire was brightly burning. At the big stone slopstone they all washed their hands with carbolic soap, and then sat down round the long table. Slices of home-baked bread and a block of freshly churned butter were in front of them, and Mrs Wallbank and Ruth the daughter gave each man a large plate of fried eggs and home cured bacon. Mugs were filled with hot milky tea, and they all ate and drank eagerly.

'Well, Bill, tell me: how did all this start?'

'It wor like this, I bought her this morning at th' auction, 'cos wi' this weather good cows were going cheap. Chris Robson comes about four and backs up t'ut shippon door, and then as he drops back board, cow which hed gitten loose, charged onto it and it came down wi' a hell of a crash, and as cow landed on t' flagstone, the whole bloody lot disappeared. If Chris had gone in an all, there would have been hell to pay.'

'I bet there would! Anyway, I must be off.'

As Richard stood up, he realised he was a little drunk.

'Bill, that was strong whisky you gave us.'

'Nay, it weren't, dus ta know, eight of us have supped three and a half bottles. Anyway off ta' goes, I'll clean thi tackle, and bring it soon. Oh, and tek some sacks to sit on. Thanks, Mr Holden.'

'And thank you for tea, Mrs Wallbank. Goodnight all! Harry, do you want a lift to Catley?'

'Yes, please.'

'Aye, tha' go wi' him; we'll bring thi bike tomorrow somehow, and George, tha tek 'em to the road.'

There were no messages at the Post Office. It was a tired Richard who, having pulled off his wellingtons, was standing in the kitchen at Cross Street taking off his top coat when Flora came into the room and, laughing, said, 'Good Lord, what a sight you look!'

'Why? What's the matter?'

'Just look at yourself in the mirror.'

The dirty deerstalker crowned a muck-smeared, flushed face.

'Um, I'm not very attractive, am I?'

'Not at the moment. I don't know which smells worse, you or the whisky!'

The severe frost continued, with little thawing in the daytime, but even so Richard worked every day though it took much longer to do country visits. After occasional falls of snow, he had to dig the car out of drifts, so in spite of the petrol rationing he often took an alternative and longer route to a farm rather than risk getting stuck. As the days went by he noticed that he never really got warm except in bed. After a supper of hot bread and milk sweetened with part sugar and part saccharine, Richard and Flora would have a hot drink, toast themselves in front of the lounge fire, and then run into the smaller bedroom and get into bed as quickly as possible. The milk they used for cooking was reconstituted powdered milk which had now appeared in the shops, much to Flora's relief.

Though the cold irritated Richard and aggravated his chapped hands and sore arms, it did not depress him, but the war news did, as things seemed to be getting worse day by day. Both he and Flora were very despondent when on a late January day Jean phoned to say that Flora's cousin Ben Lawson had been killed while serving in the RAF in the battle against the Japanese for Singapore. Richard sensed that something dreadful had happened when he received a message at Leach House in Middleton asking him to go home at once, as it was urgent. He drove as quickly as he dared and rushed into the house by the front door. Marjorie shouted from the office, 'Richard, Flora is upstairs!'

'Whatever is wrong, Marjorie?' he asked as he kicked off his rubber boots, but he ran up the stairs so quickly he did not hear her reply. In the lounge, he found Flora sitting on the settee with her head in her hands. As she raised it, she revealed a tear-streaked face and reddened eyes.

'Darling, whatever has happened?'

'Oh Richard, cousin Ben's been killed, poor Auntie Margaret,' and she began to cry again. Richard sat down beside her and, putting his arms round her, drew her close to him. He kissed her gently, and said,

'I'm dreadfully sorry for you, love, and for all of us, especially the Lawsons; what with Mark's blindness and now this. I feel so damned helpless and useless. What do you want to do, Flora?'

'I really feel I should go to Holme today.'

'But have you had any lunch?'

'No, but I've had a cup of tea; anyway I'm not hungry, I want to go and get the train.'

'Very well, if I take you to the station now you can catch that 11:30 train.'

When Flora had gone he drove out of the station along Dock Road and Wharfe Street, then onto the East Promenade and stopped the car.

Seawards, the meeting of the grey sea and leaden sky was hidden by a fog bank, and frozen snow and ice marked the high tide level on the sand – an arctic scene of bitter cold, matching Richard's downhearted, sombre mood. The news of Ben's death had made him miserable, yet annoyed with himself that since Christmas he had almost forgotten the war owing to working so hard under such cold, difficult and even dangerous conditions. In that moment the name 'Frank Bradshaw' flashed through his brain, and he felt a cold prickling sensation on his neck; his legs trembled, and a wave of intense sadness broke over him. 'Oh no, please God, not Frank as well,' he said, and recalled his uneasiness on New Year's Eve; tears came to his eyes and he began to cry silently. Ben had been a pleasant acquaintance, but Frank had inextricably been a part of half of his life to date. He found a handkerchief, blew his nose and drove back to the surgery, disturbed to realise that he was just as fey as his mother had been; and that each incident was correct in predicting death.

At the station at 9:30 that night, a weary Flora got into the car. After a brief kiss, he asked,

'And how did you find them, Flora?'

'All devastated by the news, Aunty Marge worst of all. She looked a distraught little old lady – my heart ached for her. Uncle Jack was his usual grave and courteous self and thanked me and Jean for going to see them. Jack and Brenda came home about four, the boss in the Town Hall giving them compassionate leave, and Mary, also having got it, came in just before I left. She looked worn out, because the battery she is with had been in action against the German bombers last night.'

'Do they know what happened?'

'No, not yet.'

'It is tragic for them, but I'm glad you're back. Let's get home.'

When they walked into the surgery John, who was polishing the floor, got up and said,

'Mr Holden, your Ming is acting proper funny; she keeps getting up, running on a bit and getting down again, and looking round at herself. She was a bit like it when you were doing surgery tonight, but she's been worse this last hour.'

'Thanks, John, for telling me. I had forgotten about her, though there is a note on the calendar. You've done enough for tonight, get away off home, and be careful on your bike, it's freezing hard.'

'OK, Mr Holden, TTFN,' and off he went.

When they had eaten supper, Richard carried Ming into the surgery, and while Flora held her, he gently examined her.

'It's strange, but with my little finger I can feel a kitten, but I don't know whether it's the head or tail end. Move your hands forward while I examine her tummy.'

'Can you make out what is wrong?'

'Not definitely, but there is a big lump just in front of the pelvis, and a kitten in front of it. She will never pass that lump, it is a monstrosity of some sort.'

'So what are you going to do?'

'A caesarian straight away. Everything is sterile in the sterilizer, I boiled it up when I was doing surgery.'

'Very well, and the anaesthetic?'

'That will be ether oxygen; it will be safer for the kittens than Nembutal.'

And so the operation was performed, and the big lump proved to be 'Siamese twins': two kittens joined back to back, neither with an abdominal wall; but there was also one live white kitten. Flora cleaned the mucus from its mouth, wiped it dry and put it in a cardboard box which was warm, being on top of the central heating radiator. Richard said that he was not going to let Ming go through this again, and did an ovaro-hysterectomy, then quickly sutured the peritoneum and muscle, and finally the skin. Ming was put into a basket near the radiator, and when they had cleaned up the operation table, they went into the kitchen and made supper.

'Gosh, it's been a long day, Flora, you must be tired.'

'I am a bit, but I'm glad that's over; I think she will be round from the anaesthetic soon, and then she can have her kitten.'

'I'm sorry there was only one kitten, but I'm definitely going to keep her, she will be company for Ming.'

They both ate ravenously, and when they had finished found that Ming was conscious, so they put the kitten onto a teat, and shut the lid of the basket.

The old saying, 'As the days grow longer, so the cold gets stronger,' was very true this year. Though no snow had fallen during the night, it was bitterly cold when George Dobson of East View Catley rang at 7 a.m., and Richard was soon on his way to a heifer which was having difficulty in calving. Outside the Borough boundary the untreated road was very slippery, and as he drove slowly towards the brightening east, the fields, hedges and trees were revealed sparkling with ice and white with the frost. When he arrived at the farm George came out of the shippon.

'Mornin', Mr Holden, by gum it's a cold 'un, and t' heifer's getten out in t' neet an' oo's down t' field near t' fence o' t' airfield.'

'Really, well, we had better get to her quickly or this cold will kill her.'

'Ee, it won't kill 'er, but it's killing me carrying all t' water to t' stock, 'cos the troughs are frozen solid. T' horse and cart are ready, I'll get 'em.'

Richard put his equipment in the cart and climbed up beside George who, on leaving the yard, drove down a long field up to some buildings.

'That's box she's getten out of,' said George, and Richard, looking at the ramshackle place, was not surprised. They soon reached the heifer which was down and would not get up. As Richard took off his top clothes he felt the cold penetrate to his skin. George spread straw and sacks behind the beast and Richard, after spreading antiseptic cream thickly on his arms, knelt down and examined her. It was a breach presentation, and as the calf was big he had to lie flat on his stomach so that he could get the nearest leg into the correct position, while George knelt behind him pulling on the rope. Suddenly a voice shouted,

'Do you want any help, Mr Dobson?'

Looking up, they saw two airmen watching them through the fence.

'Aye, we do that, come and gi' us a pound.'

They did, but even with their help, it was at least quarter of an hour later before the calf was delivered alive. Richard was frozen to the marrow and shivering.

'Here, dry thi' arms an git thi clothes on quick afore thi catches thi death of cold.'

As Richard did so, George thanked the two men, one of whom said,

'I wouldn't have his job for all the tea in China.'

'Aye, mebbe tha' wouldn't, but we couldna' do bout him. Off you go now but call at farm when tha's time,' and climbing into the cart he asked Richard to give him the calf. When it was safely in the cart, Richard punched the heifer until she got up, and she followed them to the buildings.

He was so cold he felt dazed as George ushered him into the kitchen and told him to sit by the fire. Mrs Dobson gave him a pint mug of steaming coffee and chicory.

'Here, luv, drink this; we can't hev thee getten badly.'

With the hot drink, and the warmth from the fire, life came back to his fingers and feet, and soon he was in agony from the tingling sensation. He drank the rest of his coffee and realised that it was strongly laced with rum, but accepted and drank some more because it was warming the whole of his body.

He was a bit tight after drinking it on an empty stomach, but when he arrived at Cross Street, Flora forgave him, and was pleased that Mrs Dobson had looked after him so well. In the evening paper that day it reported there had been 37 degrees of frost in the previous night; no wonder he had been so cold at East View.

Next morning, while in the office, Richard saw a Bishop's van stop at the front door, and Tom got out; Richard went to meet him.

'Good morning, Tom, and how are you?'

'I'm very well, Richard, and you look pretty fit yourself.'

'Yes, in spite of the cold we are both well, and how is Joan?'

'Really blooming; I'll let you into a secret, Richard, she is expecting.'

'Oh, when? I must tell Flora.'

'July's the date, but I can't stand here chatting all day, because I'm driving the delivery van because the driver is off ill. What I want you to do is see one of the horses – the big one, it's lame. Will you go this morning?'

'Of course I will, Tom.'

'Right, cheerio, then,' and off he went. When Flora came into the office she asked, 'Who was that?'

'Tommy Bishop, he wants me to see a horse this morning, but he also had some important news.'

'What was that?'

'Joan is expecting a baby in July.'

'Really, how nice for them.' The acid tone of Flora's reply made Richard realise that the baby in question was still a sore point with his wife, but he just replied, 'I'll be off now, here's my list of visits.'

After treating a scouring cow at the Home Farm, he went next to Tithebarn because it was rarely Tom Hoggarth needed his cows seen.

'Good morning, Tom. Now, what have you got wrong?'

'Two things, Mr Holden; come with me.' Richard followed him up the warm shippon.

'This un, calved three days ago, and a took calf off last neet. Now that reet front tit milks very slow like, can'ta do owt for it?'

Richard squeezed out a stream of milk, and then very slowly the teat refilled.

'You've got a chambered teat here, a bit blocked probably by skin. I may be able to move it; will you hold her nose, Tom?'

'Aye.'

Richard washed the teat with diluted Dettol, and then took a corkscrew instrument from his little steriliser, and carefully threaded it through the teat orifice. On pushing it up the teat, it met resistance, so he twisted the instrument round.

'Now, hold tight, Tom.'

'Aye, I've gitten her nose.'

Richard smartly pulled the instrument down and was pleased to feel the teat fill with milk, so he extracted the instrument and pulled four good squirts of milk from the teat. 'There, try that now, Tom.' Tom got a bucket and quickly milked the two front quarters.

'That's a good do, Mr Holden; now t'other thing is wil'ta gimme a packet of them mastitis powders for one wi' specks in 'er milk. I squirt a bit on t' floor and tha' can see 'em.'

'You don't want to do that, Tom, you'll spread the germ to other cows. Milk it into a tin and pour it down the drain.'

'Nay, I'll gi' it to a calf.'

'If you do you'll give it the scour.'

'Reet, it 'ull go down t' sough.'

'Good, then here are the powders, and cheerio, Tom.'

Richard met Edward when he walked into the stables at the Ropery bakery.

'Good morning, Mr Holden, it's the big 'un that's lame.'

'Yes, I know; Mr Bishop told me; lead him out, will you.'

'I'll try, but he is very lame.' He did, and the horse was hopping lame near fore. Richard felt down the leg but found nothing unusual until he reached the hoof which felt warm. He gently tapped the hoof, which the horse snatched away.

'That's tender, Edward, I'll go and get a twitch.'

When this was applied to the animal's nose, Edward held it. Richard picked up the foot and, tapping at the sole, found the most tender area in front of the frog. He scraped the sole with a foot knife, and found a dark mark in the white horn.

'It's a pricked foot, Edward. I'll open it, so keep that twitch tight.'

Using the searcher, he soon cut through the sole and liberated the pus. He then injected anti-tetanus toxoid into the horse's neck.

'That's it, take the twitch off. Twice a day soak the foot in warm disinfectant, and then tie it in a clean dry sack. I'll tell Bob Towers to come in two days' time and put a tin plate on under the shoe. She should be ready for work in three or four days.'

'These nails are a devil, Mr Holden. Since Christmas, I've twice found them in the frog.'

'Yes, it's getting worse with people starting their fires with wood with nails in it, and then they throw the ashes and nails onto the road. I had a puncture with one not long ago. There is not much you can do, but look at every foot every day.'

'I'll do that, Mr Holden, and I've another. She is out at the moment, but she is quidding a bit.'

'I'll make a note to rasp her teeth soon.'

At lunch time Flora was quiet, not her usual self at all.

'Is anything wrong, love?' he asked.

'No, but I am depressed, that's all.'

'Well, you must be after Ben's death, and the cold and the rationing.'

'It's not only that. Why, now even Joan Bishop is having a baby. Why don't I? What's wrong with me? Tell me that. It's seven months since we saw the specialist, and nothing has happened except I've gone five weeks twice, and there's Liz Meadows with two children and Isabel Lord's got one. And then mother makes me mad, asking don't we want any children in that tone of voice that suggests I sleep in the attic and you in the bloody garage – it all gets me down,' and she started to cry.

Richard pushed away his plate, and put his arms round her.

'Come on, Flora, there is no call for tears. I'm certain it will come right in time. Let's give it a few more months and if nothing happens I'll get an appointment with the Professor of Gynaecology at Liverpool, because having studied at Liverpool for four years I will get some preferential treatment.'

'Will you really? I think it's a good idea, Richard; you see, I'll be thirty next year, and after that it all gets more difficult, so I want a baby before then.'

'And so do I. Come and finish your lunch. I don't want to get anybody's back up about the etiquette for this, so I'll ask Bill McConnell the correct way to go about it.'

'Not just at the moment, Richard, let's wait till Whitsuntide.'

'Oh, I will, and whenever you say I will go and see him.'

The weather did not change, some days with flurries of snow, and severe night frost – even forty degrees of frost were recorded. The ice and snow had accumulated on the copper telephone wires until they were as thick as one's arm, and, stretched by the weight of ice, hung down almost to ground level between the posts on Beech Hill. Along the Droughton Road, sand, ashes and even clinker were spread on the roads to make them passable for both horse and motor traffic. When Richard called to pay Bob Towers for attending to Tommy Bishop's horse, he found Bob's father standing at the anvil making a shoe.

'It's nice to see you, Mr Towers,' said Richard.

'Aye, and the same to thee; it's a good bit sin I laid eyes on thee.'

'Well, you know, being so busy, doesn't give me time to call in here.'

'Ee, I know that. We're so busy, it's like the first war wi' folk waiting tilt last minute to hev their horses shod, but I'm too old at seventy-six to be working from eight in t' mornin till six at neet.'

Bob shouted across the smithy, 'Don't tha' believe all he tells yer, Mr Holden, it's nine o'clock afore he shows up here. It's me and apprentice as is here afore eight, and anyway he don't do any nailing on, he only meks shoes.'

'Aye,' said Albert, 'and tha'll go a damn long way afore tha'll see any better.'

'That's reet,' said Bob, 'but we tap 'em and then screw in t' frost nails to give t' horses a grip.'

Richard was sorry to leave the warmth of the forge, but pleased that Bob and Albert were doing well with the increased number of horses being used, owing to the severe petrol rationing. And rarely a day passed without him seeing a horse somewhere. When Arthur Gardner from Dunthwaite Farm Underly rang up wanting a visit to a horse, Richard asked at once if any other vet had been treating it.

'Yes, but I've finished with him, and Bill Bainbridge frae Duckworth Hall told me to ring you.'

Arthur Gardner was a very well known Shire horse breeder, so Richard was pleased to go to the farm, and meet him.

'Yes, that's it, Mr Holden, he's been treating it for a fortnight and it's worse. He lost a colt for me last back end so I've paid Kennedy up, I'm fed up with him. Come on and have a look at th' horse.'

It was an eighteen-hands Shire, steel grey, a magnificent specimen.

'Here he is, he can't go across yard wi'out falling about.'

'Is he eating and drinking?'

'Aye, but not like he should do.'

Richard's examination rapidly dissipated the euphoria of having obtained a new client. The first heart sound was muffled, the second almost inaudible, and the heart was beating about ninety times a minute.

'How did this start?'

'Well, he had a chill like, and were breathing bad, so we were giving him electuary, and holding his head over boiling water wi' medicine in it, so he could breathe it in. He seemed to get a lot better, and then began to blow badly after a bit of work. Kennedy kept giving me powders for him, but he wouldn't eat them.'

'Mr Gardner, I have got to tell you, your horse has got advanced heart disease, and unless that heart-beat can be brought down from ninety to thirty beats a minute, it can drop dead at any time.'

'Hell, is it as bad as that?'

'Yes; now we can do one of two things: treat him and risk him dropping dead any time, or send for Bob Whiteside because there is still plenty of meat on him. What do you want me to do?'

'You treat him.'

'Right, quietly turn him round while I get what I want from the car.'

Richard passed the stomach tube, and put a funnel in the end and then poured in a quart of water containing thirty grammes of Pulv. digitalis. After removing the tube, he found some digitalis hyperdermic tablets in his bag, made a solution containing one gramme, and injected it subcutaneously.

'I can't do more now but I will come back tonight to repeat the treatment. The drug I have given him will slow down the heart rate.'

'Well, I must say I'm right glad to see some medicine got into him.'

'Very well, I'll be here tonight.'

When he arrived at the farm at five o'clock his first question was,

'Is he still alive?'

'Yes, Mr Holden.'

'Very well, I'll just listen to his heart.'

It was still beating just as rapidly, and Richard came quickly out of the stall.

'It's not slowed down at all, Mr Gardner, so I am going to repeat the treatment, but if there is no change by morning, then it will be hopeless, and not worth going on treating him.'

At that moment the horse fell sideways and downwards with a crash, as dead as a doornail.

'I'm glad tha' wasn't standing in t' stall, Mr Holden,' said Arthur.

'So am I, and though I was expecting this, I am sorry he's died.'
'So am I, but tha' did all tha' could.'
'Is he insured?'
'Yes, I told th' agent he were ill.'
'Then I'll have to do a post mortem at Whiteside's. Will you ask Bob to let me know when he has got him at Southall.'
'Yes, I'll do that. Goodnight.'

It was two days later when Richard arrived at the Old Mill in Southall and walked into the shed where the carcases were cut up. There were a lot of dead sheep stacked up outside and a few cattle carcases were lying there. Inside he found Bill McDonald examining a cow slaughtered under the TB order.

'Mac, what a nice surprise! Why, it must be three years since we last met; how are you all at Corchester?'

'Oh! You don't know then that the Major has retired?'

'No, I didn't, when was it?'

'The 31st December last year; he divided the practice in half at Hartford, and I'm buying the southern half.'

'Where are you living, then?'

'Here in Southall, over a surgery I've made near the Farmer's Supply Stores. I don't think Bert Woods likes it.'

Bob broke in. 'Th' horse is ready now, Mr Holden.'

They both watched as the butcher extracted the lungs from the chest cavity with difficulty, because they were attached in places to the chest wall, and especially around the heart, which was very flabby. When the pericardium was cut open fluid flowed out, and the heart muscle was pale.

'In my opinion that's a case of heart failure following pericarditis and myocarditis, what do you think, Mac?'

'I agree with you. No treatment could have saved that one. You know, they couldn't save Elizabeth, Johnny's wife; she died of cancer last year. Then in November Tony who was in the RAF was lost on a bombing raid over Germany. I wasn't surprised when the Major retired to live at his sister's near Troon; he'd had a hell of a twelve months.'

'I didn't know that, I am really sorry for him, for he was such a great help to me.'

'Yes, and to me as well. But I must be off; if you're this way, give me a ring – it's 143.'

Richard realised that in concentrating all his time and energy on making his practice a success he had ignored the existence of his many professional friends, but they continued to appear from the past. One morning, after he had been to Old Hall Farm at Markhey to cleanse a cow, he went to Droughton to Uncle Tom's to see a horse which had been down. It had severe deep lacerations of both knees and superficial skin abrasions around the eyes and hocks. The knees were swollen, and serum was weeping from the raw areas, which contained grit picked up from the road surface. When Auntie Nellie had heated the kaolin poultice Richard applied it on lint to both knees and bandaged it in position. He then gave the horse a dose of sulphanilamide by stomach tube, followed by an injection of tetanus anti toxin. He asked about Frank, and Tom said he was well, but his letters came intermittently. Richard left the poultice with them and gave instructions for it to be applied twice daily until he came again. He then went on his regular visit to the steel works at Marshgate, where three more Shires had been bought. Tommy Atherton was obviously very proud when he led them out one by one for Richard to examine.

He was driving back through Droughton at lunch time when he had to stop in Bridge Street. Looking across the narrow street he saw Joan Matthews waiting in the queue at the bus stop. Recognition was immediate and mutual; they both waved to each other at the same moment. Richard felt his heart beating quickly as he smiled at her, but the policeman on point duty directed the traffic to move on and Richard turned left to Standfordgate, then pulled into the side of the road and stopped the car. His thoughts were in a whirl. Should he go back and take her home to Weston? What would he say to her? Why did he feel like this when it was seven years since he last saw her? He was very bewildered by the strength of his feelings for her, and was astounded when he realised that he loved her just as intensely, with that deep longing, as he had years ago. Quickly he pulled himself together, saying, 'Look, you fool, it was your own fault that you had to jilt her; you can't go back now, you've made your bed, so you must lie on it.' But that little voice somewhere inside his brain said, 'You're a liar; own up, you know you will always love her to the end of your life.' He drove off home humming the song he had heard first on the gramophone at Joan's – 'Love walked in' by Gershwin.

It was already dark and freezing when Richard had to go to Brow Farm, Ashfield, on an evening early in February to a cow which could not calve. Ashfield was the name of the large village which had grown up around the Mear and Willand collieries, about three miles from Marshgate. The village was drab and dirty, with coal dust everywhere which blew off the big motor lorries which drove from the pits down the main street continually every day. From the Mear pit, coal was transported on a narrow gauge railway to the new gas works, not far from the steel works. This railway ran through a cutting for most of its length of 1½ miles and Brow Farm lay on the opposite side of it, away from the main road. When Richard drove up the track to the farm, the dull light from his shaded headlights revealed that ahead the track was obliterated by snow. He drove on slowly until he was certain he was near the cutting. He stopped the car and, leaving the sidelights on, decided to carry his bag and overall and walk to the bridge over the cutting. Using his shaded torch he walked in that direction, conscious only of the quietness and the intense blackness of the night. Without warning he fell into the cutting. Holding onto his bag and overall probably slowed down the speed of his descent, but may have increased the amount of powdered snow which fell on top of him. In panic he let his bag and overall fall to his feet and, reaching up through the snow, pushed it away from his head and felt for the top of the cutting. He could not reach it, and more snow came down which he cleared away from his face, but it penetrated into his overcoat and up his sleeves and was intensely cold. He stopped trying to scramble out, and began to think what he should do next. Looking up he could see a few stars, so he knew he would not suffocate. He decided to feel in his obstetric bag for two chisels, a hammer and some hooks, then to hammer the chisels into the wall one above the other and, standing on these, to use the hooks to help him climb out. His relief was enormous when he heard a voice in the distance shouting,

'Where arta, Mr Holden?'

He kept shouting, 'Over here in the cutting!' until a light shone down and Stan Earnshaw said,

'What the 'ell arta doing down theer, tha' knows where t' bridge is?'

'I fell in before I found it. Help me out, quick, I'm freezing to death.'

'Reet, I'll drop rope down; grab 'old and I'll pull thee out.'

'Drop it down, and I'll tie my bag and overall on first.' In spite of being partly smothered by the snow he managed to do it and, getting a good hold of the rope, said,

'Pull up, Stan, go on,' and so he reached the surface, wet and freezing.

'By gum, Stan, I can't thank you enough for getting me out of there.'

'It's nowt. Gimme thi' bag and follow me.'

They quickly crossed the bridge and reached the shippon, and Richard was grateful for the warmth when they went inside. Working together, they soon delivered a live calf. Later, in the house, Stan asked, 'Why did ta' leave thi' lights on t' car?'

'Because I thought it would make it easier to find my way back to it.'

'It's lucky for thee tha' left 'em on, cos when I looked out and saw 'em, I thought, he'll soon be here. So when tha' hadn't come up in a few minutes I thought to missel, yon silly devil's fallen in t' cutting, so a got rope and torch and came looking for yer.'

'It was a life saver, it was that, and thanks for the tea, Mrs Earnshaw, and thanks again, Stan.'

'Aye, but I'll see thee back t'ut car, tha's not first un to get in there.'

In the kitchen at Cross Street, he was taking off his partly frozen overcoat and his wet jacket when Flora came downstairs.

'Will you bring me a shirt and pullover? I've got very wet and cold at Earnshaw's.'

When she brought them, he told her what had happened, and then they went upstairs to have some supper.

'There are no more messages then.'

'No, there has been enough for one night.'

'Any news on the wireless?'

Her reply left him speechless.

'Yes, it's been announced that three German battleships have sailed up the Channel, and the Navy couldn't stop them.'

Next morning at Brook Farm, Walter Scott's remarks accurately reflected Richard's thoughts about the ships' escape.

'Aye, it's bad the devils got away; nowt's going reet at moment, but I believe Churchill – we'll beat the bastards in the end.'

'Walter, those are my feelings exactly,' and somehow he felt a little better. He inspected two more herds and then went home for breakfast, where Flora told him that the news was that the army was retreating in Africa after heavy fighting. After they had eaten he went to the newsagent's in Victoria Street and bought two large maps of the war zones. These he fastened to the wall of the lounge and, taking a greater interest in the war, began to mark the positions of the various armies on them at weekly intervals, those of the Allies in red, the enemy in black. It was but a fortnight later when he had to colour Malaya, and then the city of Singapore, black when they fell to the Japanese. That night he and Flora together listened to Mr Churchill speaking to the nation on the wireless, but what they heard did nothing to raise their spirits out of the depression into which they had sunk. Among the troops captured by the Japanese were many men from the locally recruited regiment and in Sandhaven the one topic of conversation was what would be their fate at the hands of their brutal conquerors.

On Sunday, though St. Luke's Church was filled to capacity, it was still cold. The Vicar, the Revd Evans, wearing a long black woollen cloak, began the service with the hymn 'Oh God, our help in ages past' which was sung with great feeling. After the three Collects, he recited the prayer used in storms at sea, and some people in the congregation were crying. 'Onward Christian Soldiers' was the closing hymn, followed by the first verse of the National Anthem heartily sung to the thunderous accompaniment of the organ played by Mr Tomlinson. Outside they chatted to their friends Dick and Betty Heyes, and to the Bishops; Dick it was who spoke for all of them when he said, 'Well, I've been really down in the dumps all of this week, but I feel a lot better now.'

In the bitterly cold weather which continued into March, Richard began to carry out at least one herd inspection every day after the afternoon milking was finished, to try and reduce the number of herds outstanding. He arrived at Cross Roads Farm in Wyreham before milking had ended. Bill Harrison said,

'Will ta do small shippon fost and by then we'll hev finished in 'ere, and I can gi' thee a hand wi' one or two ockard devils?'

'Yes, I'll do that, Bill, because I want to get on; I've my surgery at six o'clock.'

Having examined the fourteen cows in the small shippon, Richard came out to find Bill ready.

'Mek a start at this end, Mr Holden, will ta?' Progressing up the shippon he looked at each cow in turn and examined her udder. When they had got to the stall containing cows numbered 27 and 28, Bill said,

'Tha wait till I get this un by its nose, or it will punch thee.'

When Bill had got No 27 firmly by its nose, Richard pushed No 28 over and took a step forwards in between the two animals. At that moment No 28, a big shorthorn, twisted her rear end towards Richard and kicked with all her power, hitting him on the inside of the left thigh and making him lose his footing and fall back on to the path.

'Oh hell, my bloody leg!' he yelled. Bill reached him in a split second and dragged him up to the shippon wall clear of the cows.

'Ar ter al reet, she hasn't broken it, has she?'

'No, she hasn't,' said Richard, almost crying with pain.

'Don't thee move,' said Bill, 'I'll be back in a tick.'

Soon he came clattering back with some whisky in a mug which he made Richard drink. After a minute or two, Bill helped him up, saying,

'I'll get thee to thi' car.'

'No, Bill, I'll finish these last three.'

'Wilta? Then I'll let this 'un out and tha can feel this devil. I've never known her kick before.' So the herd inspection was concluded.

On arriving home Richard's leg was extremely painful and he walked slowly into the kitchen. Flora, dishing up the meal, looked round and cried,

'Richard, what's the matter with you?'

'I've been kicked by a cow at Bill Harrison's. Will you go and get me another pair of trousers, these are filthy.'

He took off his rubber boots and then his trousers and saw inside his left thigh a blood blister about eight inches long and three inches wide, blackish-blue in colour. Flora, returning, took one look and said, 'I'm getting Dr Bill at once,' and rushed through to phone him.

He came in a short while and very gently examined the area. He felt for a pulse in the artery near Richard's ankle and then said,

'I am certain you have been lucky in that your femur is not damaged, nor your femoral artery. This is a venous haematoma which I am going to bandage to try and prevent it swelling more. It will be absorbed in four to six weeks but I would not like to predict what the long term effects on the artery will be. Here are four aspirin compound tablets, take two now and then at nine o'clock. This phenobarbitone tablet take with a warm drink half an hour before you go to bed.'

'Thank you very much, Bill, I'll do that and let you know how I get on.'

Flora, who had been very pleased to get a small tin of corned beef, was very disappointed that the appetising hot-pot had to be eaten half cold. After finishing surgery, Richard spent the evening wrapped in an eiderdown lying on the settee, saying that the milk samples would have to wait until tomorrow. In three days' time the leg was far less painful, but Bill rebandaged it and said he was pleased that no sign of infection was present and that the haematoma was smaller.

Richard was thankful that his leg was so much better when, a week later, on the first frost-free morning for months, the first ewe was brought in a trailer into the yard at Cross Street. He was able to kneel behind the ewe and soon delivered live twins.

'It's nice to see the little beggars, but I don't know when I'll be able to let the ewes and lambs out. There's nowt to eat yet, though the weather's milder,' said Bob Barker.

'I'm glad they are alive, and that it's not last week, because then I couldn't have knelt down.'

'Oh, why not?'

'I got a hell of a clout on my leg from a cow at Bill Harrison's.'

'Thee be careful lad, we don't want you laid up.'

'OK, Bob, I'll try, off you go.'

By the last week of March the days were spring-like, warm and sunny, and the flowers began to show in the gardens and hedge bottoms, all helping to cheer people up.

But though the retreat of the army in Africa continued it was offset by the increasing bombing of Germany by the RAF. The defence of Moscow and Leningrad by the Russians evoked a grudging admiration from Richard who hated both Fascists and Communists. But the war against them was making more work for Richard, with more home-produced meat being needed. Tom Bolton asked him if he would castrate a boar for him. Richard agreed and told him to starve it overnight and that he would need four men to help, a good strong rope, a fire made, and last of all a good very strong table.

Tom said he had one which Tom Hardman the pork butcher used. Richard said that would do fine and that he would be at Blacklands Farm at 10 o'clock two days later. Most farmers in Ryton reared pigs, so there was no shortage of help when Richard arrived. They were quizzing Tom.

'What's th' idea of heving him cut?'

'Tha' knows he'll be worth more – the meat won't be tainted.'

'I bet beggar will be damned tough.'

'Maybe, but Ministry want 'em as heavy as we con mek 'em, and who'll be able to tell when meat's in a pork pie?'

'I bet I could.'

'What's it matter, let's get on.'

Richard made his instruments ready, and put his searing irons in the fire which was glowing red in an old bucket. Four men carrying a section of corrugated iron sheeting jammed the boar against the wall of the sty, while one of the men put a twitch rope on the boar's upper jaw and pulled it tight. The boar struggled mightily, shaking the man back and forth, but he held on to the twitch while the others dropped the iron sheet, and pushed and dragged the boar to the tress, as the table was called. Its top was a six-inch thick plank of elm, and the legs four-inch square beech. Two strong ropes, each with a loop at one end, were under the table.

'Now one on each ear and leg and keep twitch tight. All together now, lift!' shouted Tom. The boar squealing at the top of its voice was almost deafening them.

'Hell, Tom, he's a noisy bugger.'

'Tha'd be too if tha' were in his place,' was the amusing reply. The boar laid on his side was tied firmly onto the tress.

'Now, let him have a breather, ease that twitch a bit,' said Richard. The boar stopped squealing long enough for him to listen to its heart-beat through his stethoscope.

'His heart is OK, but there is always slight risk from the anaesthetic; are you prepared to take it?'

'Aye, Mr Holden.'

'Very well, you can be the anaesthetist.'

'Nay, I can't do that.'

'Yes, you can; I'll show you and besides he is your boar.'

'All reet, then.'

George, Tom's son, was holding the twitch rope,

'Loosen that twitch, George, and Tom, hold his ears while I put this mask on.'

When it was in place Richard poured in the chloroform and the two men hung on until the boar ceased struggling.

'Right, you two. George, every now and then just touch the boar's eye gently like that; you see, he just felt that, don't let it go away and Tom, you just watch that he is breathing nice and regularly like he is now.'

When he had washed the scrotum with Dettol he made an incision and squeezed out the testicle. He then put a spring steel clamp on the spermatic cord and, squeezing it tightly, closed it, cut away the testicle with the hot iron and seared the stump. He slowly released the clamp and, as there was no bleeding, let the cord retract.

'How's he doing, Tom?' said Richard, taking a quick look.

'Reet gradely.'

The operation was quickly repeated on the other testicle and the wounds dusted with sterile sulphanilamide powder.

'Quick, off with the mask and twitch; now carry him back into the sty.'

With much grunting and some ribald remarks, he was carried there and the ropes removed.

As the boar was rapidly recovering consciousness, the tress was tilted and he slid onto a bed of straw. Carrying the tress, they quickly got out of the sty and bolted the door.

'When con I gi 'im his grub?'

'Probably in an hour, Tom, when he is on his feet and back to normal, and while he is eating dust the wounds once a day with this powder, and keep his bed clean.'

When Richard had cooled the irons in the trough and was drinking the tea Tom brought out for him, he asked,

'Wilt do two more for me in a bit?'

'Yes, just let me know a day or two before.'

Within a few weeks he had operated on nine boars in the district and was back at Tom's farm for the third time, operating on a big old boar, when it stopped breathing. Richard pulled off the mask and the two men rhythmically compressed the boar's chest giving artificial respiration but all to no avail and Richard could detect no heart sounds.

'He's gone, Tom; I'm sorry about that.'
'What's happened to him?'
'His heart's packed up. Did you breed him?'
'No, I wanted a good Large White so I bought him from Poolside. Tom Parkinson bred him.'
'His heart sounded normal when I listened to it, so it could be his age or he could have had Diamonds at some time and that would weaken his heart. What will you do with him?'
'I'll get Whiteside to tek 'im.'
'Then will you tell him I want to see the pluck, heart and all.'
'Aye, I'll do that, Mr Holden; I'll tell him to let you know.'

And so the work increased, and he also made more visits to the herds under the Panel Scheme, finding two cows with Johne's disease – a Friesian and a Jersey – after examining stained films of faecal material under the microscope at the surgery. There Marjorie and John spent a lot of time dispensing just to keep Richard's car full of all the medicines he needed every day and to replenish those sold in the surgery. At one time he had tried to carry almost everything a client might ask for, but now had with him only those remedies which were more specific for the various conditions he met with most often. In the car in 8, 10, 20 and 28 fluid ounces capacity bottles were:

Astringent medicines for cattle and calves; medicines for colic, fever, garget, wooden tongue and mastitis; stimulants and sedatives: all packed in a wooden crate which was divided into twelve compartments. In another crate were white and black liniment; garget oil; wound lotion; anti fly oil; also bottles of calcium, magnesium and dextrose for use intravenously in cattle. In a big leather suitcase were packets of powders; appetiser for cattle; alterative for horses; cooling; red drench; cleansing drench; phenothiazine; sulphanilamide, plus boxes of ringworm dressing; teat ointment; canker and thrush dressing; cough electuary; and specifics for lamb dysentery and pulpy kidney; and swine erysipelas serum.

They had almost used up their stock of cough electuary, and had no black treacle with which to make it. When John went to Field's the grocers to get some tins, George told him that it was now rationed and that he could not let him have any. Richard had to write to the Ministry of Food to obtain a permit allowing him to purchase 7 lbs of black treacle. When he told Flora she was pleased. 'I'll be able to use some for making parkin.'

'But I'll need it for the surgery.'

'I don't care, when I need it I'll take a quarter of a pound. You don't seem to realise that everything we want is rationed or on coupons, and then it's difficult to find. The only things you can be sure to get are the weekly rations and God knows they're little enough.'

'I know that; everything is getting worse, what with the Army getting beaten in Africa and withdrawing in Burma, and the Japs in Rangoon. It means everything I want is in short supply or on permit as well.'

'Well I've made up my mind,' said Flora. 'From now on whether it's over or under the counter, if you're offered anything, you take it.'

'But you know I don't like doing it – it's illegal.'

'To hell with it being illegal; they are not going to prosecute you for a few bloody currants or half a dozen eggs. It's the black marketeers selling stuff by the hundredweight they are after, and Betty Heyes told me confidentially that Dick gets eggs and a chicken every now and then at George Bamber's.'

'What at Higher Conden Hall?'

'Yes.'

'That confirms the rumour I've heard that they are selling chickens and killing three pigs on a licence for one – that one goes to the Ministry and the other two are quietly sold. I am beginning to see that I'll have to try and get stuff when it's available, both for us and for the practice.'

'That's more like it. Anyway they always say, "God helps them that help themselves", so I've asked Liz Meadows to get Bill to leave us some manure and then John and I can get digging.'

'But I won't be able to dig, my leg's not right yet.'

'I know that – that's why I said John can, I'll pay him half a crown each time and Dick Hoggarth said he can get seeds and plants when I want them.'

When George Duke arrived to take the books as it was the end of the financial year, he admired the way the garden was being made ready for the spring sowing. His report showed that further progress was being made in increasing the turnover of the practice and in reducing the mortgage.

On a Saturday afternoon early in April, Richard, sitting in the office, was writing the heading of the columns in the new expenses book when the door bell rang. At the door he found a lady dressed in black, and a RAF officer who was carrying something wrapped in a blanket. He said,

'Good afternoon, I see from your notice that it is not the time for your surgery, but could you please see to this dog which is ill, I do apologise that we are out of hours.'

'As it is an emergency, do come in, both of you.'

The man put the bundle on the surgery table and said, 'This is Mrs Benson, I am Wing Commander Townley-Turner. Over the last few days, I have been very busy, and it was only at lunchtime today that I discovered that Angus has not eaten for at least two days, and has been vomiting.'

Richard could smell whisky on the officer's breath, and sensed he was in a rather emotional state. Flora came in as Richard opened the blanket, and there was an Aberdeen terrier looking very ill. Flora had to hold the dog on its feet as Richard's examination was made, and it revealed a foreign body in the dog's bowel.

'Wing Commander, your dog has a foreign body in its bowel and needs an immediate operation. I'll be frank with you, his chances of coming through it are very poor.'

'Mr Holden, will you please operate at once. We'll wait for him.'

'No, I don't want you to wait, because the operation will take some time, and then I want to watch over his recovery, and give him further treatment. Will you please sign this consent form and give me your telephone number.'

'Yes, it's Shipton 432; ask for me and they will put your call through to me – I'll be waiting for it.'

Flora led the couple to the front door and when she returned she asked,

'Is Angus as bad as that, Richard? The woman started crying as they went to the car.'

'Yes, he is; I'll be really pleased if he comes through it.'

After a small dose of Pentothal had been given intravenously, the anaesthetic was switched to ether and oxygen. When Richard opened the abdomen, he told Flora to leave the mask off, and bring a piece of raw potato as thick as a fountain pen. When she came back he had got the bowel outside the abdomen and packed off with swabs. It was blackish purple in colour and Richard decided to cut away the three inches of small bowel with the foreign body inside it. After putting bowel forceps at each end of the dead area, he cut it out and, picking the cylinder of potato out of the Dettol solution, pushed it into each piece of the bowel until they were touching. After sewing the bowel and the mesentery carefully, he dusted it with sterile sulphanilamide powder and pushed it back into the abdomen, quickly sewing up the incision.

'That's great, Flora; just hold his foreleg and I'll inject 20 c.c. of glucose saline.'

When this was done, the dog was wrapped in the blanket and a hot water bottle was placed against it. After the ropes had been taken off his legs, he was carefully placed on the floor.

'So far so good, but I'm not going to ring them yet; first we'll inject 50 c.c. of glucose saline subcutaneously.'

When he had done this the dog had a faint corneal reflex, but a very weak pulse at the femoral artery.

'I'll ring them at five o'clock if he lives till then.'

At five o'clock the dog was still alive so Richard phoned the news to the Wing Commander. In less than an hour the couple were back at the surgery and the piece of hard grey rubber which had been the foreign body was shown to them.

'Do you want to see him?'

'Oh yes, and we'll take him back with us to look after him.'

'Look, you can't do that,' said Richard. 'He is too ill to move yet.'

'Oh yes, I can, because he is Mrs Benson's dog.'

'But if you do move him, I am certain that you will destroy whatever chance he has of recovering.'

They took Angus with them. Richard looked at Flora.

'I wonder why the hell they won't take my advice. It makes me damned annoyed to do all that work, and they persist in wrecking it.'

'Oh come on, after all it is their dog. Let's have tea and get the surgery over.'

It was almost eight o'clock when the door bell rang, and Flora let the couple into the surgery again.

'We've brought him back, because he was making funny noises as he was breathing.' When Richard opened the blanket the dog was dead.

'I am sorry but it is too late to do anything; he is dead.'

The woman, crying loudly, ran out of the room, so Flora followed her, and put her arms round her.

'This is most distressing, Mr Holden. You see, Angus was the mascot of Flight Lieutenant Benson, Betty's husband, and he was shot down in flames in a raid over Germany early on Thursday morning. Having lost both of them she will be inconsolable, so I'll take her home at once. Don't send the account to her, send it to me – you see he was my brother-in-law.' The voice trembled as these last words were said, then very firmly he continued, 'Thank you very much, Mr Holden, for all you have done.' and, gathering up the dog in the blanket, he marched out of the surgery followed by Betty.

The RAF came into the picture again, when on a lovely spring morning Richard had made six farm visits by midday. He was driving to the last one at East View at Catley when he came up behind one of the sixty feet long vehicles of the RAF. He pulled out and as the road was clear ahead, he began to accelerate past it. At that moment a lorry appeared coming towards him, so he pressed hard on the accelerator pedal, but quickly realised that the car's response was sluggish. He was approaching on his right one of the entrances to the airfield, so he drew in there and stopped the car. He quickly got out when he saw the lorry was one of Bob Whiteside's, and waved the driver to stop. Syd leant out of the cab and shouted,

'As ta brocken down, Mr Holden?'

'No, Syd. What I wanted to know was what Bob found in a boar of Tom Bolton's the other day.'

'Nowt save its heart were as big as a bucket and all flabby like.'

'Thanks, that's all I wanted.'

On leaving the farm to go home he tried the car's acceleration twice and found that it was poor each time. He had not been able to accelerate hard on icy roads for the last three months, but now he needed to do so. He went straight to the garage and Gordon told him the car should be decarbonised and the valves ground in.

'How long have you had it now, Richard?'

'Just twelve months.'

'And what mileage have you got on the clock?'

'19,184.'

'Hum, it's done very well for you, running on the rubbish they call petrol.' So for two days Richard had to use Gordon's old Hillman Minx.

When he went to collect his car, Gordon said, 'I've been out in it, and it's going very well but for how long I wouldn't like to say. Now, at the moment very good low-mileage cars are coming on the second-hand market because their owners can't get any petrol for them. It crossed my mind that one of them would make a good replacement for your Austin, which isn't really made to stand up to the hammer you give it.'

'Do you think they would be a better proposition?'

'I think they would, having been made of the best of materials before the war started.'

'Right then, I'll be glad if you'd do that – but nothing too expensive – I don't want a Rolls Royce! By the way, how is Pat?'

'Oh, she's very well. She's the accountant to both businesses – fairly full time job.'

'Just like Flora – I keep her nose on the grindstone.'

'I'll tell her that next time I see her.'

'You dare and you'll lose a good customer! Cheerio, Gordon.'

Next week Richard went to New Laund Farm, Shipton, a dairy farm run by Mrs Noblett and her son Harry who was a bit simple. They were both very pleasant, and what Harry lacked in intelligence he made up for in strength. When her husband had died suddenly eight years earlier, Mrs Noblett with great courage decided to run the farm, helped with advice from her brother-in-law Fred who lived at Highgate in Ryton the next village on the Droughton road. He it was who on her behalf interviewed then hired Dick Banks.

He was a good stockman, but rather deaf, and lived with his wife in the farm cottage. Each year the milking herd had been increased, and the land was now in good heart.

'Good morning, Mrs Noblett, how are you?'

'Very well, thank you, Mr Holden. The three bull calves are in the small shippon, and there are some heifers which want extra setts taking off.'

'I'll do them, come on, Harry.' They went into the small shippon and walked up to the first bull calf. Richard told Harry to nose it, and then shouted at Dick to push its tail straight up. With the burdizzo forceps he crushed the animal's spermatic cords, and repeated the operation on the other two bulls. He then began to examine the heifers, and with Harry holding the nose and Dick the tail, any little extra teats were crushed with the small burdizzo forceps, and then cut off with scissors. He had just cut off a little teat from one heifer when Mrs Noblett said,

'Mr Holden, will you look under that one – it's got an angleberry growing.'

Richard did not notice that Harry had let go of its nose and that Dick had lowered its tail, because he was bent down trying to see the size of the growth. In a flash the heifer kicked him on the right side of his face just in front of his ear. He staggered back, holding his face, and shouted,

'Why the hell did you let her go?'

Harry grinned and Dick looked blank. Mrs Noblett, to defuse an explosive situation, said,

'Come across to the house, Mr Holden, and wash your face, and I'll make you a cup of tea.'

By this time his face was swollen, discoloured and aching intensely. He washed and dried it very gently and drank his tea. Feeling less dizzy, he went back to the shippon, and with the heifer well held and its hind legs hobbled, he tied a rubber ligature round the neck of the growth.

When he walked back into the surgery, Flora took one look at him and exclaimed, 'Good God, Richard, now what's happened to you?'

'A heifer kicked me; will you ring Dr Bill and make an appointment for me to see him urgently.'

Bill took Richard to the hospital and X-ray photographs were taken. Later the radiologist said,

'You have been very lucky, Mr Holden, there are no fractures. You know often the vertical ramus shatters with this type of blow.'

Flora was worried. 'Richard, do you know why you are getting hurt like this, your leg and now your face?'

'No, I don't know; it could be I am slower with being tired, but this accident wouldn't have happened if that idiot Harry hadn't let go; I suppose I shouldn't say that, he can't help being a bit mental.' It took a long time for the swelling to go down, and when it did, Richard could feel a depression in the bone which made up the wall of the joint, and it was permanent.

The discomfort the injury caused made Richard depressed, and this deepened when he read of the heavy fighting in North Africa, followed by the bombing of Mandalay by the Japanese. As he moved the lines on his maps, he saw how everywhere the British were losing ground to their enemies. With his depression increasing, so did his bad temper, and little things began to annoy him. A good example of this happened on the day when he found that his stock jar of obstetric cream was almost empty. He went to Field's the grocers, and on entering the shop, walked up to the counter and said to George,

'I want a 7 lb tin of soft soap.'

'Mr Holden, you must know by now that I can't let you have that.'

'Why ever not, George?'

'Because it's on coupons now.'

'Look, George, I've been getting these tins from you for years, and I want one now urgently; I can't do my damned job without soft soap.'

'Mr Holden, I know you are a good customer, but I can't let you or anyone else have it without coupons.'

'Well what am I supposed to do? Write to the Food Ministry and be without it for weeks, all due to your obeying every bloody tin pot rule that's made.'

'Yes, you'll jolly well have to, and as soon as you bring your permit you can have some. Don't be offensive, this job's not easy with everybody grumbling at me all the time because what they want is not available.'

'All right, damn it,' said Richard and slammed out of the shop in a temper.

Back at the surgery he found he had very little leg dressing which had a soap base. Looking in a cupboard in the kitchen he found a partly used tin of soft soap.

He shouted, 'Flora, I'm taking this tin of soft soap.'

She came into the kitchen and said, 'Why?'

'Because I must make some more cream to use on my arms when I'm calving cows.'

'All right, take it then, and you can replace it when you get some more.'

'Don't be damned silly, I can't replace it when George Fields won't let me have any without a permit, and I need all I can get.'

'I'm not being damned silly, you fool, what have I and John got to wash the floors with? You can order two more stones of the stuff straight away and then there will be enough for all of us.'

'All right, calm down.'

'Calm down, I like your cheek! It's you who's in a bloody temper at the slightest thing and smoking your silly head off. I don't know what's got into you lately.'

'I'm sorry, love, I don't know either, but I'll try and not smoke so much and I'll write now to the Food Office in Manchester.'

'You do and don't forget the black treacle.'

He did and it was over two weeks before the permits came. George Fields put four seven-pound tins of soft soap into one cardboard box, and the two seven-pound tins of treacle into another, and carried each to Richard's car.

'I've put them into these boxes to stop passers-by seeing them, and saying I am letting you have more than I should; you know the saying – what the eye doesn't see, the heart doesn't grieve over.'

'Yes, that's true; thanks a lot, George.'

He then went into the toffee shop next door, and bought a half a pound of Nuttalls Mintoes and a block of Cadbury's Chocolate. He ate these during the day in an attempt to reduce the amount of tobacco and cigarettes he smoked.

About two weeks earlier, the news reader on the radio had announced that on the previous night enemy planes had bombed a town in East Anglia, and that damage and casualties had occurred. In the post was a typewritten envelope bearing the postmark 'Norwich'. Richard felt uneasy as he opened it, but was pleasantly surprised to find that it was from Mary, his sister, who after giving their address had written:

Dear Richard,

Just to let you know that we are both well, as we were nowhere near the bombing because this bungalow is two miles from the city centre. Occasionally father's heart bothers him when he has done too much gardening.

    Hope you are well,
    Mary

'Just read that letter, Flora, it takes the prize for being short and to the point. It's just like the radio news.'

'True, she could not say much less, but at least they are unharmed, and your father is managing.'

'I agree but, reading between the lines, it seems he jolly well has to.'

The lambing season was over and had been a good one. With the cows being out at grass Richard was busy rushing to the usual crop of staggers cases. As well as cattle there was the horse work, castrations and dockings, and the endless cases of injury, greasy legs and lameness; in the treatment of some of the last he had to take Bob Towers, the shoeing smith, with him. The new stallion got some very good foals, and to Richard's relief no deformed ones which could not be born – this now was a thing of the past. He had to foal two mares in June; both cases were malpresentations, which he easily corrected. One day when he went to Dobson's at East View to cleanse a cow, he was surprised to see an army of service men and civilians working at the airfield. They were extending the runway almost to the Goswick – Wellington Road.

'I bet you're glad that they decided to extend it to the south and not up here.'

'I am that; if they had come this way, I'd have had no farm left. The lads tell me it's because they are getting these big Lancaster bombers here, and the Yanks may be coming with theirs an' all.'

'By Jove, Catley's going to be a different place when that lot get here.'

'I'll tell thee something, Mr Holden, Catley's like a football match most nights, what with Air Force men, and civilian workers and girls. The Manor Inn is sold out of beer by nine o'clock.'

'That won't please the locals.'

'Mebbe not, but they've just got to put up with it, like they have with the RAF police having to come and stop fights and thieving. But the lads have to have a bit of life, when you think that some from here didn't come back from that thousand bomber raid on Cologne.'

'Well, you always lose some when you are fighting but I must say I was really cheered up by the news; it's time we started paying them back in their own coin.'

'Aye, it is that, and most folks say the same.'

Tom Collinson at Park Hall Farm, which was the other side of the ploughed up nine-hole golf course, was the owner of a herd of pedigree Friesians. This he started before the war when his father died and he cleared out all the cross-bred shorthorns and Ayrshires. He restocked by buying tuberculin tested pedigree cattle from a Friesian breeder in Cheshire. He had had a Grammar School education, always spoke quietly and to the point, and worked hard. He ran the farm most efficiently with the help of Victor who was a very good stockman, and three other men.

Richard took the message that he had a cow off colour, and went straight to the farm. Victor met him in the yard, and led him into the road shippon which was empty except for one cow, a good looking animal. Above her was a nameplate: 'Foxland Princess'.

'This is her, Mr Holden; she's one of our show cows, and a wonderful milker. She were down on her milk last neet but this morning she's hardly given a drop, and hasn't eaten owt.'

'Right, I'll have a look at her,' and Richard found that the cow's temperature was over 104° F and her pulse rate was 100 per minute. There was little sound to be heard in her rumen, and only a little dung behind her.

'Has she been grunting, Victor?'

'No, she's just gone quiet, not doing owt really.' Richard examined her udder which was normal, and her mouth but there was no abnormality there.

'Well, Mr Holden, what's wrong with her?'

Richard turned to see Tom walking up the shippon.

'She has a septic focus somewhere in her body, and it's pushed her temperature over 104. How long has she been calved?'

'Near on five week,' said Victor.

'That's right,' said Tom, 'and she was giving just on six gallons a day.'

Though the cow was breathing faster than normal, Richard found nothing wrong with her lungs, so he asked for a bucket of water. Having soaped his arm he examined her per rectum and found that the uterus was normal in its non-gravid state; there was no discharge from it.

'Will you bring a strong fencing post?'

Victor brought one, and it was placed under the cow's belly with Tom holding it on one side, and Victor on the other. Richard listened to the cow's chest through the stethoscope and then said, 'Lift.' They tried to lift the cow on the post; she was uneasy, but did not grunt.

'She did not like that, Mr Holden.'

'She didn't, but there was no grunting which confirms my belief that the septic area is in her guts, so I am going to treat her with sulphanilamide and a laxative.'

This was done, but when Richard examined her again in the evening, her temperature was only slightly down, and she was ignoring some freshly cut grass which was in front of her.

'There's no change, Tom, so keep on drenching her and I'll be here in the morning.'

Still there was no change.

'How long is this going on for?'

'I don't know, there is very little change in her condition, and she is still very feverish.'

'I can see that,' said Tom. 'You see, Mr Holden, she was in good condition and she was milking so well. Now her flesh is swaling away, but she would still make a good carcase.'

'But Tom, she will be a fevered carcase and will be condemned.'

'I'll have to risk that, but if she isn't on the mend in the morning she goes to

Droughton abattoir straight away.' And so next morning Tom phoned to say that she was no different and he had sent for Robson to take her in. Richard said he would write a note for the abattoir manager, Tommy Noblett, to tell him the drugs she had had, and would Robson collect it from the surgery.

'I want to see her opened to see exactly what is wrong.'

'Aye, you do that and let me know,' said Tom.

He rang the abattoir at eleven o'clock and Tom Noblett told Richard that the cow had arrived. He drove there quickly and at the far end of the killing floor hanging from an overhead rail was the cow which had been shot, her back end slightly raised. Tommy Rainford the butcher had laid back the skin, cut away the udder and legs below the knees and hocks. He now raised the carcase, and was cutting open the abdomen when Mr White the meat inspector came up.

'Good morning, Mr Holden, thanks for your note. What have you found?'

'Nothing yet, but it should be something in her bowels.'

Tommy pulled out the paunch, but the other stomachs did not follow though he pulled on them.

'Cut right round the skirt, Tom, and then pull the lot out,' said Charlie White, and when this was done the three men could see that the second and third stomachs and the skirt were all joined together. The meat inspector had begun to cut the stomachs loose when a greenish pus began to run out of the mass.

'There is it, Mr Holden; Charlie, you can finish dressing it but it is condemned. Do you think the owner will want to see it?'

'Definitely, I'll go and ring him from the office.'

Richard informed him that the cow was condemned, but Tom said he didn't believe it. He was coming over at once and would Richard wait for him. One of the girls in the office brought Richard a cup of tea, and as he was drinking it he recalled when he was seeing practice being told he would see this condition sometimes at a post mortem.

'Yes, Mr Collinson, there has been a local peritonitis, and an abscess has formed between this second stomach and the skirt. I'll show you.' The inspector cut the liver and skirt away and was freeing the stomach when more pus ran out.

'There's the abscess, that's why the carcase is condemned. Also it's fevered; you can see it's wet and dripping onto the floor.'

'It's a bad do,' said Tom. 'She was one of my best cows, and in good flesh.'

'Yes, you've been unlucky. Usually it's just a mass of gristle, so we just throw the skirt and stomach away.'

'Yes, it's bad luck, but I must go and get on,' said Richard.

'So must I,' said Tom, 'and thank you for waiting, Mr Holden,' and the three men went their separate ways. As he drove back to Sandhaven, Richard wondered if he had lost a good client, because Tom was annoyed at getting nothing for a show cow worth well over £100. Only time would tell.

At the surgery Richard found Marjorie waiting for him to arrive because Flora had gone to Field's where they had some tinned fruit. Richard was halfway through his lunch when Flora came home successful, having got a tin of peaches.

'Hello, love, I'm sorry I wasn't in, but Betty Hayes told me to go and queue at Field's because they had got some tinned fruit, and then I had to queue to get some fish for tea. I've been over an hour waiting and, you know, everybody was fed up and grousing about shortages. Even Cyril Melling, the fisherman, was telling everybody to bring newspapers with them to wrap their fish in, because there's no wrapping paper now.'

'If paper is getting as short as that I had better order some more billheads. What won't we be able to get next?'

'I don't know; I've hardly enough fat to fry the fish in for our dinner tonight, though I save every bit of fat I can.'

'Did you get some fish heads for the cats?'

'Yes, Melling always lets me have some; if he didn't, some days I wouldn't have much to give them, and Bumble eats as much as Ming now. Tommy's different; he'll eat anything.'

'I'm not surprised Bumble eats so much, she is a big cat for her age; the next thing she will be calling, and we will have to put her in a cage for a week and she won't like that.'

That evening the fish meal was good, and they both enjoyed it, but the news was bad; Tobruk had fallen and the army was being pushed back towards Egypt by the Germans after hard fighting.

'Do you think we will lose Egypt next?' asked Flora.

'Good Lord, I hope not. Look here on the map – if the Jerries reach the Suez Canal they will cut our lifeline to the Empire – to India, Singapore, Burma, even Australia.'

'I think it must be disheartening for Churchill, having got supplies to Malta last month after so many attempts; this now makes all that effort wasted.'

'No, I don't agree, I think the army will stand and fight on the border of Egypt, and I only hope Harry and Frank will be safe.'

'So do I,' said Flora; but only Harry survived and they received news of Frank's death two days later. Richard shivered as though with cold for a moment when Flora told him the news, and he realised that his dreadful presentiment on New Year's Eve had been correct. All he said was, 'Poor Auntie Nellie and Uncle Tom – Frank was their only child.' Flora was in tears.

Next morning, after treating a cow at Ivy Farm in Teston, Richard went on to Droughton and spent half an hour with his aunt and uncle trying to comfort them in their distress, even though he was as dejected as they were, having lost Frank, the last real friend of his childhood and youth. Later, Mary spent part of her leave at Cross Street, and when she had gone back to her unit Flora said, 'You know, Richard, the light in our Mary's life seems to have gone out, she was so despondent.'

Richard replied, 'Well, after Mark, Ben and now Frank, aren't we all? It just goes from bad to worse.'

Some days later he went to the Home Farm and opened a cow's blocked teat, and then diagnosed four cows to be pregnant out of the six examined.

Bill Griffin, the Manager, told Richard that the Colonel wanted to see him because one of his dogs was ill, so would he go on up to the Hall. The animal was Heather, an eight-year-old black retriever bitch. The Colonel told Richard that she had been in season six weeks before, but during the last fortnight had eaten less food, and was drinking a lot of water. When the gamekeeper had gone to her kennel that morning he had found she had a reddish brown discharge from the vulva.

'You know, Mr Holden, she's very like my manager's bitch was, which you operated on a year ago.'

After examining Heather, Richard said,

'Yes, it's the same condition, Colonel, it's a pyometra, but luckily the neck of the uterus has opened allowing the pus to escape.'

'Will it have to be the same treatment – an operation?'

'Yes, it's the only specific treatment.'

'When can you do it?'

'I think this afternoon. I will telephone you at lunchtime when I will know how much more work there is still to be done.'

There were only two visits to be done, so on Richard's instructions the bitch was brought to the surgery; the Colonel signed the consent form, and asked Richard to inform him as soon as the operation had been done, because she was his favourite gun dog.

With Flora helping, Richard anaesthetised the bitch with Nembutal given intravenously, and after shaving her abdomen and using 50% Dettol and water as a skin disinfectant he rapidly opened the abdomen. The uterus was very large, and he had to make a bigger incision than usual to get it to the outside of the abdomen. Soon it was excised, the intestines and the wound were dusted with sterile sulphanilamide, and the incision was sutured. They then bandaged the wound using a four-inch bandage and then covered this with Elastoplast going right round her body. They wrapped her in a blanket, and put her on a carpet on the floor with two hot water bottles near her.

Richard phoned the Colonel and told him that the operation had been done and the condition of the bitch was good, also that as soon as she was fully conscious he could take her home. She recovered from the anaesthetic by six o'clock and at eight was trying to get to her feet. Richard decided to let her go home, and soon the Colonel and Bill Griffin carried her out to the Colonel's shooting brake – a big Morris Isis. Richard gave him strict instructions to keep the bitch quiet and not to give her a lot to eat.

As they were having their evening meal they discussed the operation.

'I hope we don't have trouble with her, Flora. It's a big wound, and the way she was flopping about makes me worried that the sutures may give way.'

'But though she is a big bitch, you very carefully sutured that wound. I don't think you need worry about it, Richard.'

Flora was wrong. On the third morning, in response to an urgent message, Richard went to the Hall. His worse fears were confirmed when he saw that the bandage round the bitch was wet and stained reddish-brown, but she was lively and wagging her tail.

Later at the surgery he anaesthetised her and, on removing the bandages found that the sutures had given way and that there was a three-inch long hole, through which mesentery and a loop of small intestine were protruding.

'By jove, Flora, am I glad we put plenty of Elastoplast round her.'

'So am I, we would have been worried if her guts had fallen out; it would have to be the Colonel's bitch, wouldn't it?'

'Yes, don't I know it!'

With great care he disinfected all exposed tissues using more sulphanilamide and then scraped the muscle edges raw, and after dusting more powder into the wound sutured the different layers. Again she was firmly bandaged, and when this was changed four days later, there was a lump about the size of a thimble in the middle of the wound. By the time the sutures were removed on the eighth day it was the size of a small hen's egg.

'What is the swelling, Mr Holden?'

'It is a small rupture or hernia, caused by some stitches giving way, due to her being so boisterous.'

'She has always been like that, but I have tried my best to keep her quiet this week. Will it hurt her?'

'I don't think it ever will, because it is hard and is probably filled with fatty mesentery.'

Richard was a bit embarrassed because the bitch had this hernia, but it did not bother her, and she regularly went with the Colonel when he was shooting, although after a year he pensioned her off.

Richard drove along High Street and as he turned into Victoria Road, there was a loud bang. The car lurched to the left and mounted the pavement. Though he had jammed on the foot brake the car had stopped only inches from the window of the newsagent's shop, and a yard or so from a woman who was pushing a pram, who had stopped dead. Richard jumped out and said,

'I'm terribly sorry if the car scared you, but I could do nothing, it all happened in a flash.'

'Oh, I'm all right, but for a moment I was proper frightened.'

Richard turned and could see that the near side front tyre had burst. Charlie Robinson came out of the shop.

'Hello, it's you, is it Mr Holden? I wondered what the hell that bang was; I'm glad you didn't smash my window.'

'I am too, Charlie, will you phone Gordon at Dock Garage to come at once, please.'

Gordon soon arrived and put on the spare wheel.

'I'll repair the inner tube and then put a gaiter inside the tyre. You know, you'll have to get a permit to get some more, because there is a gaiter in one of the tyres at the back; I'll be calling you 'The Bishop' soon if this goes on.'

'That's one way of looking at it. I've applied for a permit, but it's not come yet. I'll let you have it as soon as it arrives. By the way, any sign of another car?'

'Yes probably a Morris 1000; I'll let you know soon.'

'Oh good, I hope it is very soon. Cheerio.'

On the Saturday evening Jack Clough phoned and asked if he could come and see Richard about a project the NFU had in mind. Richard told him to come at seven o'clock, and was curious to know what the project was. Later when Tom Collinson and Bill Griffin along with Jack walked into the surgery all was revealed. Bill was the spokesman,

'We don't want to waste time in this good weather, so I'll come straight to the point. The Government want local events to begin again, so our local branch of the NFU is planning to revive our one-day cattle show on August Monday. Now what we would like you to do is to be the third judge in the cattle classes. Really an impartial final opinion if the other two judges can't agree, and of course we want you to be the vet to the show, Mr Holden. Now, will you do that for us?'

'Gentlemen, it is very nice of you to ask me, and I'll try and do what you say. Being the vet to the show will be a pleasure.'

'That's great; it's all settled then. Thanks, Mr Holden, we will let you know the details when the committee has got them arranged.'

With that they left, and Flora too was curious to know what was going on.

'What did they want, Richard?' He told her.

'It's nice of them to ask you, but what will you wear?'

'My ginger jacket and fawn trousers.'

'You can't, Richard, they're absolutely threadbare. You've had them since before we were married, they must be seven years old.'

'Oh, then I could wear my dark suit.'

'You will not, that's as old as the hills, and you'll look daft at an agricultural show dressed up like a tailor's dummy.'

'Thanks, that is a nice thing to say.'

'No, don't take it that way, I'm not trying to be rude; I'm only saying you'll have to get a new suit.'

'If that's what you want, Flora, I'll go to Hill's on Monday morning.'

The result of that visit to the tailor was one light brown suit in a tweed with a herringbone pattern, which used up all the clothing coupons he had; Flora, feeling sorry for him, bought him a shirt to match.

The amount of Elastoplast which had been used on the Colonel's dog had reduced

Richard's stock to two tins, so he went on Monday to the chemist's and Jim Lord was pleased to see him.

'Hello, Richard, nice to see you. How are things?'

'Not too good, really, we are just getting over my cousin Frank Bradshaw's death. He was killed near Tobruk last month; he was in the Royal Artillery.'

'I'm sorry to hear that. Aren't they the coal merchants in Droughton?'

'Yes, it's my Uncle Tom's business. I don't know what they will do now, because he expected Frank to run the business when the war was over.'

'There's no sign of that yet, what with Burma lost and the Germans almost in Egypt, and everything rationed or hard to get; it's a lot worse than last year.'

'I'm sure it is; now I want four blocks of camphor, a dozen tins of two-inch, and a dozen of four-inch Elastoplast, four one-pound tins of antiphlogistine, six toilet rolls and some saccharine tablets.'

'Right, there's the antiphlogistine and the camphor. I can let you have half a dozen of each size of Elastoplast, but only two toilet rolls; and there are the tablets.'

'But I want more than two rolls, Jim.'

'I dare say you do, but they are in very short supply. I've only a dozen rolls in the shop.'

'Well, whatever next?'

'I don't know; George Fields was in the other day and was saying that the rationing is getting tighter, and he has less stuff to sell, and his customers sometimes get damned rude. How's your Flora?'

'She's very well, thanks. By the way, what about James Edward and Isabel?'

'They're both blooming; you know, it was the best move I've ever made coming here, she's never looked back.'

'I'm really glad she's so well, so I'll say cheerio.'

Richard, having put his purchases in the car, went back to the surgery. Flora was pleased with the saccharine tablets, because she wanted to make rhubarb jam from a plant in the garden which was growing very well. The result of Flora's and John's hard work in the spring, digging in the manure which Bill Meadows had brought, was shown in the straight lines of healthy looking vegetables in the plot – potatoes, cabbages, carrots, runner beans, onions, lettuce and radishes. Flora and Richard were both very pleased it was a success.

At the evening surgery Mrs Robson was very apologetic.

'I'm sorry to have to bring my Mitzi back again, but 'er's got real bad. George ses she looks moth eaten'

Richard smiled at what he thought was an accurate clinical description. The dachshund had no hair on her ears or down her forelegs and had lost some from her hind legs. The hairless skin was slate grey in colour, and covered with little scabs. The surgery card showed that this was the third visit since March for this condition which the sulphur tar dressing relieved but did not cure.

'I'm sorry she's bad again, but I think I may be able to cure her this time.'

'I hope tha con, Mr Holden.'

'I want you to use this new dressing, it's called Ascabiol; I've used it on a sheep dog and it's cleared up very quickly. Just follow the instructions, and don't let her lick it off – just put a muzzle on her for an hour or so after you've dressed her.'

'I'll do that, she's ever so good, tha' knows. How much is it?'

'Nothing – it's my way of paying George for the help he's given me; he'd never take anything, you know. I want to see her again in a fortnight.'

After Frank's death Richard made a point of listening to the news on the wireless every night, and, having a great admiration for Mr Churchill, was glad his government survived the censure motion in the House of Commons.

When Gordon Hindle was pumping petrol into the tank of his car, Richard and he were talking about the war and Richard said how pleased he was that the government had not fallen recently.

'By God so was I,' said Gordon. 'You know, if he were kicked out who could take his place? I can't think of any of them who could lead like he does, and in spite of being an old chap he can still get a move on – it's not taken him long to sack all the desert generals, and get these new ones, Alexander and Montgomery.'

'I hope they'll fare better than the others did and we get some good news soon.'

'Aye, we damn well need some for a change, but I'm certain he's building up stocks ready to attack, because we've never been busier making parts for ships, and engines.'

'Well, we'll hope for the best.'

The best came in the news from the Market Café that Joan Bishop had given birth to a baby boy weighing 8lbs 2oz. Flora was quite excited.

'After all, Richard, they have been married twelve years and it's their first baby. Mabel Bishop said Tommy had been worried stiff about Joan these last two months and has had Dr Bill going to see her once a week, and then after all she only went into the Memorial Hospital at half past seven this morning and even Mr Graham was there when it was born before ten o'clock with no trouble at all. Would you believe it?'

'Oh yes, and it's nice to get some cheering news for a change; I bet Tommy's pleased as punch.'

'Oh, Mabel said he was cock-a-hoop.'

'So would I be if it happened to me. Anyway there's a chance for us; do you think we should see Mr Graham again?'

'I don't think just yet, Richard; let's wait a bit longer.'

'Whatever you say, love.' When Flora came home after visiting Joan in the hospital she was rather quiet, forcing Richard to conclude that her worries had returned and that she was envious of Joan's good fortune.

When Mrs Robson came into the surgery with her dachshund, she said it was a miracle. The dog had stopped scratching, and the hair was just beginning to grow.

Richard gave her another bottle of Ascabiol and told her to continue the treatment. At last he was doing something positive to repay George.

August Bank Holiday morning dawned grey with the odd shower of rain. Richard got up early and before breakfast went off to do two visits and some repeat visits, so that he could be at the Show at 8.30 a.m. Wearing his new brown suit he was standing behind Mrs Laycarte-Porter when before a good crowd of people she declared it open. Soon the judging of cattle and horses was taking place in the roped-off rings. Jem Stuart and Joe Fowler were the judges for the horse classes, from Shires to children's ponies. In the cattle ring were Jack Clough, Tom Collinson, and Richard – the latter not for long, because soon he had to go to a cow which could not calve at Rose Farm at Shipton. All the way there he was in a line of army vehicles, in many of which were American servicemen. The wagons went onto the airfield which was next door to the farm.

'I'm sorry I'm late in getting here, Harold, but I've been held up by all these trucks. Where are they coming from?'

'From the camp two miles up the road; they have a railhead there, and take stuff there from Sandhaven docks.'

'They are Americans, aren't they?'

'Aye, they are, they began coming here in March, though some were over Catley way last year.'

'Are there a lot of them?'

'Thousands, I should say; all in t'camp the've built on Fred Noblett's land – tha' knows the've taken a lot of Highgate land.'

'Yes, there are changes and shortages everywhere.'

'Aye, too many for my liking.'

Between them they soon calved the cow, after Richard had corrected the malpresentation, and the calf was alive in spite of the delay.

Back at the Show he met Flora and they went to the refreshment tent. There was only tea and pies, and a lot of banter about the latter from folk sitting on benches at the long trestle table.

'Pies are good.'

'Better than shepherd's pie down at Tom Bolton's.'

'Get on wi' yer, he never med any.'

'I know he didn't, you don't use pigs fries in 'em. Aye they're all reet are these, I wonder what's in 'em?'

'If tha knew, tha wouldn't eat 'em.'

'Don't be daft, all meats inspected at th' abattoir. I bet they're Walter Haslem's; he meks best in t' town.'

'Nay, Frank Wood's are better; his taste of pork, these don't.'

'Why should they when these are meat pies, you can put owt in 'em.'

'All reet, but I've enjoyed 'em; let's get back to the ring.'

Richard left Flora at this, and went back to the surgery, where Bill Meadows from Whingate had left a message with Marjorie for Richard to go to his farm as soon as possible.

'Didn't he say what was wrong?'

'No, he didn't.'

'Is there anything else to visit?'

'No, Mr Holden.'

'Then I'll go straight there,' and as he drove to Pickhill he wondered why Bill had been so secretive. He soon found out; when he drove into the farmyard, Bill came out of the house and straight across to the car.

'I'm glad you've come so quickly, Richard, because I'm sure my herd's in trouble.'

'What's happened, Bill?'

'As it was fine when I got back from the show, I went and had a look at my dry cows, and my in-calf heifers. One of them cows has picked – she weren't due till October – and another of 'em is beginning to bag up.'

'Where are they?'

'I've driven the cow into the little barn, but t'others are still in the field. I didn't know what to do, but as luck would have it the heifers are in the long paddock.'

'Did you find the calf?'

'Aye, it's in a bag in the barn.'

'Come on, let's go and have a look at them.'

After filling a bucket with water and adding disinfectant, Richard examined the cow, and looked at the yellowish grey patches on the cleansing, which was hanging from her. He then tipped the pink, almost hairless, foetus out of the bag.

'Bill, I am certain this is contagious abortion, but I'll take a blood sample and swabs from the cow, and take the stomach out of the calf, and send the lot to the lab for confirmation.'

'What the hell am I going to do, Richard? I've never bought owt unless it's been blood tested; where's it damn well come from?'

'I don't know – when did you buy any cow last?'

'Near enough three years ago.'

'That's that ruled out. What about your neighbours?'

'Next door there's George Bolton.'

'Of course there is; and he's in beef and swill feeds pigs.'

'That's right, and Wyresham side there's Bill Gregson at Corner Farm, he milks about forty and gets replacements from his brothers at North Farm. There's a double fence to keep cows out of the drainage ditch, I can't see it coming from there, and the railway cutting is my north boundary.'

'I'll take your word for it that it has not come from there. Now, there are two other ways, either indirect contact with an infected cow, through its discharges; or from boots, clothes, straw or brushes from cattle wagons.'

'I don't use cattle wagons.'

'I didn't think you did, so that leaves only an indirect contact with an infected cow or calf or cleansing.'

'Richard, I'm baffled. There hasn't been any contact; it's not like five year ago when I bought two heifers that had it.'

'I'd like to know where it has come from, and then we could stop it breaking out again.'

'Aye, so would I.'

'Right then, scrub your hands and boots in this disinfectant and put a sack soaked in it across the doorway, and use one lot of brushes for here, and get your George to bring his horse box and take the heifers to his place.'

'I'll do that right away.'

'Bill, remember that field is badly infected, so don't let anyone in or out without disinfecting themselves, and no other cattle have got to go near it. I'll get off now with these samples. I'll be in touch as soon as I get the results,' and after scrubbing with disinfectant he left.

The laboratory report was positive for the germ brucella abortus bovis, so Richard went to the farm and with Bill went into the house, where Liz gave them mugs of tea.

'Bill, I've got the lab. report and I'm sorry to say it is contagious abortion.'

'Aye, I thought it was.'

'Now she picked in the field, so the other five probably will have got the infection so they stay isolated there. When did you turn out?'

'Near the middle of April, just about four months ago.'

'I think we must take it that infection happened about then, that they were all exposed to it, so we will have to blood test the lot. How many have you?'

'Thirty-seven without that six.'

'If they are clear on the test, I'd pack the six off straightaway; but if many have it you'll have to decide what to do. Now, when can I blood test them?'

'Would Sunday morning at half past nine be right for you?'

'Yes, that will do fine.'

'Good. Now, while you are here, would you take that cleansing from that cow.'

After putting plenty of cream on his arms Richard tried to remove it, but it proved impossible, so he disinfected himself and got fully dressed again.

Sunday was a lovely day, but as there were only Bill and Richard to do the test they were too busy to notice it. Bill's cowman was ill at home, so Liz wrote out the labels which identified each tube. Soon after eleven o'clock they had finished and were sitting in the farmhouse kitchen drinking tea, when Richard asked,

'Do you know what's wrong with Bert?'

'No, the doctor doesn't seem to; you see Bert had this do of pneumonia back in February and was off work three weeks and he's not been really well since then. Every now and then he is ill for a few days. It's a shame because he's a good worker and conscientious. He will be in in the morning probably.'

'He is having a rough time. Anyway, many thanks for the tea, Liz, and I'll be off.'

The test results showed three positive cases and five doubtful, which was not as bad as Richard had feared.

'What do you think I should do, Richard?'

'Get rid of the three positives at once because, you see, this is often the course of events, you get one or two aborting this year and if you don't get rid of them they leave so many germs about it goes through most of the herd next year. We call it an abortion storm. It happened two years ago in Birton. He said it almost made him bankrupt.'

'I know that; it was at Walter Lee's.'

'How did you find out, Bill?'

'He told me; he's a relative of mine by marriage; you'll learn we are all related one way or another round here.'

'Then the positives go; mark the doubtfuls so you can identify them and keep an eye on them, watch out for bagging up or passing slime; they don't all bag up before they abort.'

'I've started ploughing up that field.'

'Good, and get a certificate with any you buy to show they have recently passed the test. Oh, and don't forget about Johne's disease when you are buying.'

'No, I won't that. When will they want testing again?'

'In three months time, and really clean and disinfect that little barn when it's empty.'

'I will, Richard, at once before we start harvest, because if we have another bad winter, the heifers will have to be tied up in there.'

Richard was thrilled with the news of the big attack on the French Coast, but this was tempered the next day by the news of heavy losses on both sides. The news reader said it was only a raid, and not the start of the Second Front, the pros and cons for which were being widely debated. Recently there was more war news, which made people hope that the Allies were getting ready to take the initiative, because the Russians were having a very bad time, being pushed back steadily by the German armies.

In spite of the news, the lovely weather made Richard work harder. He had many cases of August bag and was selling a lot of his udder ointment. Outbreaks of swine erysipelas made him use many bottles of serum of the 250 c.c. size. There were blessings too in the shape of the cabbages, carrots, lettuce, early potatoes and radishes which Flora brought in from the garden. She swapped sage and thyme for shallots with Dick Hogarth and went to the allotments and exchanged runner beans for cauliflowers which she had not grown.

When Richard was getting petrol Gordon came out of the garage and said, 'I've got that car for you, Richard, and I'm just giving it a service.'

'That's great; let me have a look at it.'

He was pleased to see FYE 180, a smart-looking dark blue Morris 1000. The boot was of a fair size, big enough to take his overalls and rubber boots and some heavy equipment.

'I like the look of it, Gordon.'

'Yes, it's smart and when I drove it, it was quite nippy.'

'Where has it come from? I don't know that FYE registration.'

'It's come from London, and it's been used very little, there's only 4000 on the clock, you can see that from the tyres, they are like new, and it's economical on petrol.'

'It's almost too good to be true. Thanks, Gordon, when can I have it?'

'Tomorrow. I'll have everything in order, but you'll have to see the insurance chap for the substitution.'

'I'll do that, I won't forget.'

Two days later when Richard went to Whyngate to cleanse a cow, it proved to be one of the four which had been left after the two positives had been sent for slaughter. He managed to loosen some of the afterbirth, but could not remove it, so he put four Entozon bougies into the uterus, hoping these new pessaries would kill off a lot of the infection.

'How far was she off her time, Bill?'

'Only a fortnight; she was due early in September. That's her calf in the little pen. It's small but it's doing well.'

'Was she one of the doubtfuls?'

'Yes, she was.'

'And where did she calve?'

'In here. When I saw her making a bag I brought her in straight away. I didn't want her to muck up the long pasture with the other three in there.'

'Good, keep her here, Bill, because she'll keep discharging and it will probably be very yellow from these new pessaries. I'll test her again in a fortnight.'

'She'll still be here. I like your car, Richard, where did you get it from?'

'Gordon Hindle got it for me. It's come from London and I'm very pleased with it.'

At Middleton he was sent on to George Whiteside's at Seedhill to a sow which couldn't farrow.

'Will you bring a sack and some straw, George, my knees are killing me.'

'Aye, I will that.'

After getting prepared, Richard knelt down and began to explore the sow.

'I bet it's a big un holding everything up; she does bring good pigs.'

'No, you're wrong, George. It's something I've not met before in a sow – a twisted womb – and God knows I've farrowed a lot of sows this last few years.'

'Con ta do owt?'

'Yes, we want some help and more straw.'

'I'll gi' mi lads a shout; they're opening up big wheat field.'

He arrived back carrying the straw and accompanied by his two sons, young strong men.

'We'll have enough power now, what hev we ter do?'

'Turn her over, and when the lads have got hold of a bottom leg each, lift and push her over as quick as you can, and George, you turn her head with her body.'

'Reet, one, two, three, over er goes.'

On the third attempt the vagina opened, and Richard quickly pulled out two dead piglets and then seven live ones.

'That's a good do, Mr Holden, I'm glad tha got here quick.'

Richard got to his feet and his knees hurt.

'I'll give her this injection, and in a few minutes I'll see if she has finished.'

'Aye, but thou hasn't, I want two litters cut.'

The sow had finished and Richard soon castrated the eight-week-old weaners, with George holding the piglets, whose wounds were dusted with sulphanilamide powder, while the boys caught them.

'That's it, George, put them on straw bedding, not on those wood chippings you get from the saw mill.'

'I'll do that, Mr Holden.'

The news on the wireless that lunch time was of the death of the Duke of Kent, killed while flying on active service in the RAF. Flora was really upset when it was announced that his baby son was only two months old.

'I know it's tragic, Flora, but so it was for us when Ben was killed at Singapore. We are all in it together; you remember how near even the King and Queen came to being killed when the Jerries bombed Buckingham Palace, and we were less than twenty yards from that bomb in George Street.'

'I know the news is never good, and somehow we've got used to it, but when it's something like this it makes your heart ache.'

'I know, love, now come on and have your lunch,' but Flora ate very little.

That evening Tommy Knowles who was the assistant to the absent R.N.R. Townsend of Wilton asked Richard to go as a second opinion to see some yearling cattle which he thought might be being poisoned by effluent from Droughton gas works, which ran into a stream which flowed through the field where they were grazing.

The meeting at the field was arranged for eleven o'clock the next day. The cattle belonged to a client of Tommy's who had rented the grazing for the summer. When Richard arrived Tommy and Bert Earnshaw the farmer took him to another heifer which they had just found dead. There was froth around its nostrils and it was in good condition.

'How many have died, Tommy?'

'Three now.'

'Aye, and I'm going to sue the gas works; the water in that brook stinks of gas tar, that's what's poisoning them,' said Mr Earnshaw.

'Have they had any cake?'

'No,' said Tommy, 'and I tested the first two for anthrax and they were negative, and this looks the same.'

'Maybe,' said Richard, 'but I will still test this carcase.'

It was negative, so it was decided to do a post mortem at once while the carcase was still fresh. Richard got his post mortem equipment from the car, while Bert brought a bucket of water from the brook, and Dettol was added to the water. After cutting back the skin from the chest and abdomen, Richard opened the latter, quickly cut the stomachs free and pulled them out. He opened the rumen and they all sniffed, but could not detect a smell of tar, and the chewed-up grass was quite normal, as were the liver and kidneys. He now cut through the skirt, and cut out the heart and lungs; the latter were enlarged and when he cut into them frothy fluid oozed out.

'Is it fog fever?' asked Tom.

'I don't think so, this pasture has not a lot of grass on it. I'm going to open the trachea and the bronchi next.'

Here he found slightly blood-stained froth.

'Tom, have you got a magnifying glass in your car?'

'Yes, I have.'

'Would you bring it, please, and some microscope slides.'

When he came back, he smeared some of the froth onto one slide and put another on top of it to make a thin film.

'Will you have a good look at it with the glass, Tom, while I wash my gloves and overall?'

Tom did and suddenly said, 'Well I'm blessed; there are lung worms on this slide.'

'Let me have a look.' That look confirmed the diagnosis that the cause of death was husk or verminous bronchitis. 'Would you like to see them, Mr Earnshaw?'

'Nay, I haven't mi glasses wi' mi; so it's no good me having a look.'

Richard said to Tom, 'How long have they been coughing?'

'Do you know, Mr Earnshaw?'

'Nay, I don't, I just walked into the field and counted them, that were all I did and they looked all reet.'

'Let's go and have a closer look at them.'

When the remaining nine were driven into a corner of the field, some coughed, and two were breathing rapidly.

'Tom, they must be put onto dry feed at home at once, and dosed with husk medicine. Those two want an intratracheal injection to help to move the worms.'

'I'll get 'em moved home this afternoon and Mr Knowles can doctor them.' said Bert. 'And thank you, Mr Holden. I'd a bin a damn fool suing gas works, when it's husk and nowt to do with them.' After he had paid Richard his fee, the two vets walked back to their cars.

'Thanks a lot for coming, Richard, I didn't know they were coughing and Bob Whiteside on the phone said he thought it was fog fever.'

'Tom, my advice is, after you've excluded anthrax always do a PM if possible or get Bob to do it, you nearly always find the cause.'

'I will next time, Richard, believe me.'

At Wyreham Post Office there was a message for him to go to a cow which couldn't calve at Moss End, Ryton. Mr Birtwell, very obviously annoyed, said, 'Hello, Mr Holden, I thought tha hadn't gitten me message, I sent for thee at eleven o'clock and I were going to send again.'

'I'm sorry I'm late, Tom, but I have been delayed in Droughton trying to find out why three yearlings had died – it took longer than I expected.'

They walked across to a box.

'She's in here, she's a full pedigree tha knows. She touched eight gallon last time, and is mi best milker, she's worth every penny I paid for her.'

The very big fit Friesian cow had a huge udder, from the teats of which milk was dripping and regularly she strained very hard.

Richard liked Tom Birtwell. He was an efficient and progressive farmer, and when he whistled two men came at once. Everything was ready so Richard poured the Dettol into the water, washed his arms and hands, dried them and thickly smeared them with his obstetric cream. On examining the cow, he found one fore leg was back, and when he tried to reach it she strained powerfully.

'By jove, she's fit; have you been steaming her up, Tom?'

'Aye, course I hev. I want her to gi' as much as last lactation, they can't milk off nowt, and she's a week o'er her time.'

'Well, she's put plenty of meat on her back, but more on the calf – it's a big one, so I'll give her an anaesthetic to stop her straining so hard.'

He gave her an epidural anaesthetic, injecting the local anaesthetic called Parsetic very slowly. After 6 c.c. the tail stopped moving, but he had to give her 12 c.c. before she stopped straining. Richard rarely used this type of anaesthesia except in difficult cases.

'Now, that should make it a bit easier.'

He soon got a rope round the leg below the knee, and brought the leg forwards until he could reach the foot, which he pulled upwards and forwards till it lay beside the other in the vagina. The hoof was almost as big as his fist.

'Tom, I've got the leg up which was causing all the trouble, but it must be a big bull calf because its hoof is as big almost as my hand.'

'Mebee, it's as big as that, but we three 'al shift it, you'll see.'

'Will you give me three ropes from the bucket, Tom?'

He put one over the calf's poll and round through its mouth, and also one on each leg.

'Now, Tom, you've got the head; pull hard.' Tom did so. 'That's enough, leave off.'

Richard, feeling round the calf, realised that with its head on its legs in the correct position it was very big to come through the cow's pelvis.

'It's very big and it's alive; now, pull one leg and the head together.' They did and both parts moved towards him. 'Now pull the other leg.'

The man pulled powerfully but nothing happened and then suddenly it jerked forwards but the head had gone back.

'Damn it, the head's gone back. Let's try all together. Tom pull first, now all of you.'

The head slowly came into the vagina.

'Pull the legs harder, hold that head Tom.'

The feet showed briefly at the vulva, but in spite of all their efforts, it would not come any further.

'Let's have a breather, and tie a milking stool leg to each rope.' This done they pulled with all their strength.

'What the hell's holding it?' asked Tom.

'Nothing but its size, it's so big, but I want to have another feel round, after I've put some Lux into her. It's very slippery stuff, and it will help.'

After he had inserted the Lux, he pushed the calf back and felt all round the base of the neck and the shoulders.

'Tom, it's so big I'm certain I'll have to cut a leg off it, and then it should come so long as it doesn't get stuck at the hips.'

'Nay, let's hev another go afore tha' does that.'

They all pulled and the calf moved slightly towards them, and then the cow lay down and would not get up in spite of Tom hitting her with a strap.

'The lazy devil; why won't she get up?'

'Because of the pressure of the calf on the nerves in her back legs. Put a strong halter on her and tie her to that ring, and let's have some more bedding. Now, there are three things we can do; first one is I take a leg off the calf, the second is a caesarean operation, or we send her straight away to the abattoir.'

'Nay, I'm not hevin 'er killed and what's this caesarean?'

'The calf is taken out through the cow's side. The operation is done occasionally but less than half recover.'

'That's no go then. I want to keep her, she's a full pedigree, get damned leg off.'

'All right then, Tom, let's be doing.'

After twenty minutes kneeling, and once having to lie flat on his stomach, Richard, using his embryotomy knife, cut the leg free, and asked them to pull on that rope steadily. The leg slid out of the cow's passage onto the straw.

'That's a big 'un, Mr Holden.'

'It is, Tom. Now give me more Lux and then we'll try again.'

Though the cow's pelvis was wide, they had to pull very hard, and slowly the leg, the head, then the chest appeared as the cow rolled onto her side.

'Now move round, and pull down towards her feet.'

'We're pulling all reet,' said Tom; the three men were grunting, and their faces were red, and wet with sweat from their exertions.

Richard put his arms round the calf's chest and slowly moved it round. Suddenly with a rush it came, knocking Richard backwards, and the three men fell in a heap onto the straw. The afterbirth came out after the calf.

'Thank God for that,' said Tom. 'It is a big devil. I wish it had bin a heifer; it would a come easier.'

'It would that,' said Richard, putting pessaries into the cow's uterus, after which he wearily got to his feet, conscious that his knees were sore.

'Let her head go, come on and push her up.' When they got her sat up, her head flopped round onto her chest. 'Now she's got milk fever, I'll get two bottles and inject her.' This he did, injecting the solution slowly intravenously, after which she lifted her head, belched noisily, and moved her legs to get comfortable.

Tom hit her with his cap, shouting, 'Come on, git up wi' yer,' but she would not.

'Let her have a rest, Tom; give her a drink and some grass and try her in an hour. If I don't hear from you at four o'clock, I'll know she's got up, and only take a drop of milk off her tonight.'

'Aye, I'll do that; now, come on and have a cup of tea.'

'Thanks very much, Tom, but it's almost half past one. I must go.' He stopped at Ryton Post Office and telephoned Flora, who told him to come home for his lunch at once.

When he sat down at the kitchen table, he shivered and felt ill, but as Flora didn't notice it he ate the vegetable soup and thick chunks of fresh bread she had made. This was followed by an egg salad which he enjoyed. Flora answered the phone, and Richard had to go to a sow farrowing at Alan William's farm in George's Lane at Pelham. In this area Williams and Bob Hall were the only pig breeders. There were a lot of small holders many of whom owing to physical disabilities only did a part-time job, but also kept pigs. These were fed on swill, waste food which they collected from the hotels and boarding houses in Mereside. The farms varied from the efficiently run with good buildings, to the worst, with ramshackle buildings made of salvaged timber and corrugated iron sheets; with very poor means for food preparation or storage and inadequate disposal of effluent and manure. There were two poultry farms in the area run by Tom Walker and Jim Jemson and they also kept pigs. Apart from the two breeders they all bought weaners or store pigs for fattening at Droughton or Southall Auction Markets. This practice caused diseases of pigs to be widespread, especially swine fever and scour, with resultant losses which sometimes were so great that a farmer would go bankrupt and do a moonlight flit, which was to move during the night, leaving no forwarding address and paying nobody, including the vet! The roads in the area were poor, pot-holed, and rutted in summer and so muddy and flooded in wet weather as to be almost impassable.

Alan Williams was a judge of large white pigs at local agricultural shows, an extrovert who greeted Richard cheerfully, and it was not long before the latter had delivered the sow of many live and one or two dead piglets. On rising to his feet, he limped towards the door.

'Has ta gitten a bad leg, Mr Holden?'

'No, Alan, it's just that I have been doing a lot of kneeling and my knees have got very sore. Cobblestones are the very devil.'

'Tha reet, we've teken all mine out, an' t' pens hev bin concreted.'

'Yes, you've made a good job of your buildings and you do keep them so clean. I wish some of the others round here would do the same.'

'Aye, I do too, some are real mucky buggers. Council should stop 'em keeping pigs. Tha knows mi lad and missel hev spent hours mekin things better, but that's bin stopped wi' t' war, cement's as scarce as gold dust.'

'I'll tell you what, Alan, if I find a bag of either I'll bring you some.'

'Tha do lad, but bring gold dust fost.'

At evening surgery Richard was limping and when the last client had gone Flora asked,

'You're not well again tonight, are you, love?'

'No, I feel as though I've got a bad cold starting again.'

'Right then, have your bath, and off to bed you go.'

'I will; it will be nice just to lie down.'

He awoke after midnight feeling very thirsty, and he was sweating profusely. So he moved carefully to get up, but Flora was instantly awake.

'Where are you going?'

'To the bathroom for a drink of water.'

'Leave your pyjamas there, they are wet through, and get another pair out of the airing cupboard.'

'I will that, and will you get me some aspirin comp. tablets from the surgery, I'll take a couple now.'

He did and soon went to sleep again. The phone rang just after six o'clock, a cow down with milk fever at Duckworth Hall.

'You're not going, Richard; ring Tommy Knowles, he's always making use of you.'

'I can't ask him to go to Bill Bainbridge. He came to me because he was fed up with Knowles.'

'How do you feel?'

'As though I have been through the mangle. Make me up a cup of tea, love, and I'll take two more tablets. At least the sweating's stopped, and it's a lovely morning.'

When he was kneeling beside the cow giving her the treatment for milk fever his knees were less painful. The cow soon got to her feet, and Bill, always the gentleman, with Emma at his heels, saw Richard to his car.

'Thanks for getting here so quick, Mr Holden.'

'It's a pleasure. Cheerio, Bill.'

Richard, feeling more cheerful, drove home quickly. He enjoyed his breakfast, and after it took another tablet, continuing to do so for two more days; but though he was feeling better, his indigestion returned.

Later in the week at Uncle Tom's stable, he had to treat a horse which had a swollen sheath; Richard did not know the man who led out the horse and applied the twitch, but he had the water, soap and towel ready. The swelling of the sheath in horses, especially geldings, was caused by the accumulation of smegma inside the prepuce – it was a brown waxy material which sometimes was very foul smelling and difficult to remove. In this case he found it easy, and after syringing warm diluted Dettol into the sheath, he applied plenty of obstetric cream to the horse's penis and prepuce. He had just finished when Uncle Tom arrived.

'Hello, Uncle, how are you?'

'Nay so bad, Richard. I wanted to catch thee 'cos I wanted to tell thee mysel that I've sold business to Tommy Turner, we've bin friends for years, tha' knows.'

'What's suddenly decided you to sell out?'

'Well, now there's only Nellie and me, and 'er's not too good, so we'll go to Coleford to be near her brother Frank. Turner's in t' coal business like me and he hes two lads to think about. A bit sin I saw him, and told him I wanted to sell and he jumped at chance of buying. He'll tek oer on t' fost of September, and wants thee to be his vet and he'll be ringing if he gets any trouble.'

'That's a nice surprise, thanks very much, Uncle.'

'It's nowt; now come on and hev a proper wash and a cup of tea.'

For some time Richard sat and chatted, but finally rose to his feet, and said, 'Thank you very much for the tea and cake, Auntie. I do hope you will like living in Coleford, and you will let me have your new address when you've got settled.'

'Aye, I will that, and tha con come and see us when tha's going to Holme with the missus; it's not out thi way.'

Richard said, 'I'll do that,' and kissed her and then he shook hands with his uncle.

He felt near to tears as he drove away, knowing that a bond which bound him to his family and which stretched from his childhood to that very moment was about to break. He had not heard from his father and sister for months, and now his uncle and aunt would be gone in a few days; but he did not mention his dejection to Flora, as another event dispersed it. This was Rommel's attack on the Eighth Army, which caused heavy fighting and many casualties on both sides before the battle was won and the Germans withdrew. Richard thought it strange that he had no premonitions of trouble, and was hoping nothing would occur.

It didn't; weeks later a letter from Alresford informed them that Captain Harry had been awarded the Military Cross.

'Richard, do you know it's September 3rd today? That's the start of the fourth year of the war. Do you remember how frightened I was when it started?'

'Yes I do; you thought Hitler would do to us in a few days what he was doing to Poland; and then you got really worked up when he blitzed Holland and Belgium.'

'Oh, I was; I never thought he wouldn't blitz us and then invade.'

'Neither did I when France fell. It was a real miracle the army escaped, and then the RAF stopped him coming.'

'We were lucky then, but there's still no end in sight.'

'I know; I wish there were. I'll get the phone.'

He put down his breakfast cup and it was Tom Priestly at Beech Tree on the line, in a hurry as usual because he had a cow down trying to calve. When Richard arrived John and one of the men were waiting in the box with everything ready. He was injecting the cow for milk fever when Tom rushed in.

'Hello, Mr Holden, con ta finish it as quick as tha con, I want calf alive.'

'Tom, I can't give the injection any faster or it will kill the cow.'

'I know that, but let's get on. John, bring t' water here.'

The cow was recovering rapidly. Richard said, 'Push her onto her brisket and wedge that bale behind her.'

He found that the head of the calf was turned back to its side.

'What's wrong wi 'er, Mr Holden?'

'Calf's head's turned back, but it's coming forward easily – it's not a big calf.'

'Is it wick?'

'Yes and kicking.'

With the ropes attached to it, it was soon delivered, but Tom disappeared.

'John, tell your dad to let the calf have a drink off her now, but don't take much off her tonight.' Richard gave the cow a clout with his overall and the cow got to her feet.

Tom came in. 'Is it a heifer?'

'Yes. I wondered where you'd got to.'

'Gerrin on wi t' harvest. It's a real good 'un. We've getten thirty-six hundredweight to the acre i' one field. It's most I've ever getten. Come on, you two, tek bucket out, let's be doing.'

What a complex character Tom was, Richard thought. He was rarely polite and never friendly; endowed with too much energy, he was a slave driver and a bully at times. He had one object in life and that was making money and getting a discount on everything he bought, even from Richard's account. To Tom farming was strictly business, not a way of life to be enjoyed, and other farmers were beginning to be like him.

From there he went on to Higher Conden Hall. George Bamber had a cow with peracute mastitis and a very high temperature.

George's son John helped Richard pass the stomach tube to administer a loading dose of sulphanilamide and a double dose of fever medicine. He then emptied the yellow secretion from the quarter and infused it with a solution of Soluseptasine.

'Where's your dad, John?'

'He's busy in t' barn; he's getten a licence to kill a pig and that's what they're on wi'.'

'Then I won't disturb him, but you tell him this cow is very ill and I'll be back tonight to dose it again; give it plenty of water to drink.'

'Reet, I'll tell him, Mr Holden.'

Richard expected to be back there in the late afternoon, but he was busy all day and after evening surgery went to the docks to treat a horse with spasmodic colic.

There were more messages at the surgery, so he drove quickly the ten miles to Conden Hall. As he got out of the car he could hear a pig squealing, so he walked across to the barn and was trying to open the small door when a voice shouted, 'Who's theer?'

'Holden the vet.'

George opened the door and in the lamp-light, Richard could see some half pigs hanging from a rail. George stepped out and closed the door.

'Tha' hes n't sin owt, has ta, Mr Holden?'

'Of course I haven't, George.'

'Tha sees, it's like this. I git a licence to kill a pig and I does and chap what's bought it comes and teks all of it away. I cleans floor and then I does another, so if police come there's no'but one dead pig on t' shop.'

'So that's how you work it, George; it's very clever but one day you will get caught. By the way, who takes the pig?'

'Well, fost un's mine, so half's going into our larder for salting and t'other half to Ministry. T'others go to folk who keep the boarding houses in Mereside. They hev to hev summat to feed theer lodgers wi'. Let's see what cow's doing.'

Because she was responding to treatment and her temperature was lower, Richard was repeating the treatment, when a car drove into the yard and stopped.

'Are yer in t' shippon, George?'

'Aye, is that thee, Harry?'

Harry Ball came in.

'Hello, Mr Holden, I thowt it were thy car, but I didn't think tha would be tekin pigs round t' country in t' dark.'

'I'm not, Harry. I've come back to George's cow because it was very ill this morning and I'm giving it another dose of medicine.'

'I'll go and tek mi pig then, George.'

'Tha do; our John ull gi thee thine – it's a good 'un. Yon chap hesn't bin for fost yet. I'll be suited when thine's gone and theer's only one dead un on t' place.'

They walked into the yard and Harry, having opened the door of his car, lifted out a wicker skip which was full of dressed chickens and handed it to George.

Richard said, 'I'll look in again tomorrow. Goodnight, both of you,' but George said, 'Here y'ar, Mr Holden, thee tek it,' and handed a plump bird to Richard.

'It's for seeing tut' cow, 'ers a grand un, tha's done well to git her round.'

'Thanks very much, George, it's very kind of you.'

When he arrived home with the bird Flora was very pleased and gave him a smacking kiss.

'Where did you get it?'

'George Bamber gave it to me for treating his cow; it's on the mend.'

'And how do you feel tonight?'

'Much better than I have for a week or two.'

Later their love-making was vigorous and after, Flora murmured, 'That was lovely; you're back to your old self, thank God.' Richard was puzzled.

The next evening John was doing the routine cleaning of the waiting room and surgery when the door bell rang and Joan and Tommy Bishop walked in.

'Hello, John, is Mr Holden in?'

'Aye, he is, I'll tell him you're here.'

John went to the foot of the stairs and gave Richard the message. He called down, 'Come on up, you two.'

When they walked into the lounge, Flora said, 'What a nice surprise to see you. Do sit down, and how are you, Joan?'

'Oh I'm very well and so is Tommy. How nice your lounge looks, have you been decorating?'

'Not me this time; it was Richard and Dick Hogarth. You see, Dick somewhere got hold of some distemper and asked us if we could make use of it. We got a tin of white for the ceiling and two tins of cream for the walls. I must say it has made it much brighter.'

'You were lucky to get any,' said Tommy. 'I wonder if he has any left, you know, our house could do with some decorating. I'm hoping to get some white paint for the bakery – I've applied for some because the Sanitary Inspector said the mixing room must be done. What will you have?'

'Like Flora, please Richard, a whisky and a drop of water.'

Richard had given Joan a sweet sherry and now poured one for himself. Tom, seeing they all had a drink, said,

'Now, the reason we've come, is to ask you to be godparents to our Thomas John.'

'Oh, what a lovely thought,' said Flora. 'Of course we will, won't we, Richard?'

'Most definitely and here's a toast for good health and a long life to your son and heir.' They all drank to his health.

'Is the christening this coming Sunday?'

'Yes, immediately after morning service.'

'Then I hope nobody has a cow in a fit or a mare foaling at twelve o'clock on Sunday, because I don't want to miss it,' said Richard. He was prevented from attending the service at 10.30 a.m. but, wearing his brown suit, he went into St. Luke's just before midday, to find Flora who was dressed in her powder blue costume talking to the Reverend Tom. He greeted Richard and led them to the font which was at the back of the church and where Joan, who was holding the baby, Tommy and many of their friends had assembled.

In the service which followed, both godparents were unprepared for the large part they had to play; nevertheless Flora was in her element holding the baby, until the vicar gently took him from her and after announcing his name carefully dipped him into the water. Flora brushed away a tear and when Richard held her arm he discovered that she was trembling. On leaving the church, they and other friends of the Bishops went to their house on Wyreham Road. At short notice from Richard, Mr Isaacs the jeweller, had obtained a second-hand plain silver christening mug, polished it and put it in a blue silk-lined presentation box. Richard and Flora gave the mug and a copy of the Book of Common Prayer signed by both of them to Joan and Tom, who were both almost overcome with emotion when they expressed their thanks for these gifts for their baby son. After toasts had been drunk to the baby's health, all the guests enjoyed the buffet lunch which was excellent in spite of rationing. That evening Flora, who was jealous of Joan's radiant happiness, became tearful because she was childless and at the end of what had been a very happy day they were both dejected and Richard felt he was a failure. After much talking, many bitter words had been exchanged and they decided to see Dr Bill again about their infertility problem.

During the year Flora had collected every jam jar she could find and kept them in the upstairs room in the stable block. The harvest was wonderful and she now used the jars, filling them with preserves: rhubarb; plum and apple; blackcurrant; bramble and apple jam; and apple jelly and red currant sauce. Mint sauce, pickled walnuts and chutney were also made. So now whenever Richard was in Mereside he went to Howard's the general dealers and bought jam jars for Flora and graduated medicine bottles of any size for use in the practice. At the surgery these were all put into a large zinc bath and left to soak in the diluted disinfectant. Later John washed them in clean water and sorted the bottles into groups all of the same size. Richard did this because they were easily obtainable and very much cheaper than new bottles – four dozen 10 oz graduated medicine bottles had now risen to 9s.9d. in price and they could easily use all these in one morning in the dispensary; also new bottles were becoming more difficult to obtain.

When he blood tested the cow at Whyngate, the sample proved positive for contagious abortion, so the animal was slaughtered immediately and the calf was sold. Bill did not say much about his financial loss, but Richard was concerned at the continual slaughter of cows, sale of calves and loss of milk. Yet as more cows were calving to time, Richard decided his advice was correct and when Bill asked, 'What do we do next?' Richard replied, 'The same as before, complete cleansing and disinfection of everything; all manure and straw to be burnt and another herd blood test in November.' He secretly hoped that there would be no more reactors.

Towards the end of the month outbreaks of husk occurred all over the practice and the most difficult to deal with was in eighteen in-calf Friesian heifers at John Tomlinson's School Farm at Mereside. He had sold his herd of shorthorns and Ayrshires and had restocked with Friesians over the last eighteen months. Richard injected them all intratracheally, on two occasions a week apart, and they were dosed regularly with husk medicine, but in spite of all his efforts one heifer died and three were a long time in recovering. At the Colonel's Home Farm it was the yearling heifers which were affected and three died in the first few days. This was the second outbreak he had had in a few years in spite of ploughing up the fields where the disease first appeared and growing grain there, while the young stock were put onto new leys. There were other outbreaks; in one at Harry Helm's, Reedley Lodge at Wyresham, two animals died, and Eric Vickers at Pleasant View in Shipton also lost two. These losses occurred after vigorous and continuous treatment of all the affected cattle, the segregation of young stock from the adult herd and the ploughing of contaminated fields. He began to doubt the usefulness of his own medicine and obtained two gallons of Antifilarine from Willows, Francis, Butler and Thompson Ltd, the wholesale chemists in London, but the medicine proved no more effective than his own. Richard also sold an inhalant which contained creosoti, camphor and Ol. eucalypti for use in bronchitis, strangles in horses and catarrh, sales of which increased a lot as farmers found it useful in treating husk.

'We have an appointment with Bill at quarter past seven tonight, you haven't forgotten, have you, Richard?'

'No I haven't, Flora, I saw it in my diary a couple of days ago, so surgery finishes tonight on the stroke of seven.'

Everything went smoothly until a few minutes before that hour when the door bell rang and in walked Mrs Robson with Mitzi.

'Hello, Mrs Robson, nice to see you; is anything wrong?'

'Nay there's nowt wrong, it's just I want some medicine for them tapeworms our Mitzi has; I brought her wi' me so tha could see what a lovely coat she's getten.'

Flora bent down and ran her hands over the shining tan coat of the dog.

'Yes, she is lovely now.'

'Aye oo is, George is real suited wi' er.'

'Here is the medicine, Mrs Robson. It's one dose of Tenaline; give it to her four hours after she has had her food. Goodnight to you, I must go.'

Flora quickly ushered her out and in five minutes they were on their way to the doctor's house, leaving John to clean the surgery. The housekeeper, Mrs Lucas, opened the door of Bill's lovely Regency house.

'Good evening, do come in both of you. Doctor will only be a few minutes, so please sit down in here,' and she indicated the dining room, the door of which was open.

'Thank you,' said Flora. 'Is Fiona still here?'

'No she's not; she was over for a month in the summer and then went back. She's been living in Birmingham with her husband and the children since last year.'

'So that's why she has not been in the café for a bit.'

Bill opened the consulting room door and said, 'Will you come in, please.'

As they sat down, Bill looked at them and smiled. 'I must say you are the healthiest looking couple I've had in the surgery tonight.'

'Maybe we are,' said Richard, 'but we've come because we still haven't got a child – Mr Graham's treatment last year has proved ineffective.'

The doctor referred to his notes and then said, 'When I saw that you had made an appointment, I had a word with Mr Graham and he said that in his opinion another D & C is not indicated.'

'But surely there is something which can be done to help me, Bill,' said Flora. Richard was saddened when he heard the exasperated, almost desperate, note in Flora's pleading.

'Oh yes, there is, Flora. I asked Mr Graham what other operative procedure could be performed and he said that he would like another opinion because you are a difficult case – you are two very healthy people. Now, he knows the head of the Department of Obstetrics and Gynaecology at Liverpool University; you went to Liverpool, didn't you, Richard?'

'Yes, I did.'

'Shall I arrange a consultation, then?'

'Yes, please do,' said Flora, looking at Richard who nodded his head in agreement.

'I'll let Graham know that at once and also that you went to Liverpool – it should speed things up – and I'll let you know the date as soon as I get it.'

Bill now dropped his professional manner and as a friend poured out sherry for the three of them while grumbling that the price of good sherry had now risen to 7s.6d. a bottle. They had a nice half hour chatting together. Later that evening on the wireless the news reader announced that the King had conferred the George Cross on the island of Malta, 'that unsinkable aircraft carrier anchored in the Mediterranean', to quote Churchill's words.

Richard, who knew André Cassar, a Maltese who had qualified as a veterinary surgeon at Liverpool, had a great admiration for the Islanders. They had been bombed relentlessly by the Italians and the Germans and had faced starvation at times. They had suffered greatly in loss of life and material damage, but they had not been conquered. Richard, looking at his war maps later, saw that no changes need be made, because the German advance was still stopped at Stalingrad in Russia and also at the Egyptian border, and wondered aloud when they would be forced back over the way they had come.

'Not for a hell of a long time,' said Flora the unintentional pessimist.

With the coming of October Richard did not feel too well at times, but never mentioned it to Flora, because the practice was busy. He was very pleased one day when Bill Bainbridge rang him and asked him to go to Churchlands Farm in Underly village.

'I'm asking you to go, Mr Holden, because he's not on the telephone and I've recommended you.'

'Thank you very much, Bill, I'll go today.'

When he arrived, Stan Rainford came out of the barn and Richard thought that they must both be about the same age.

'I'm Mr Holden the vet. Bill Bainbridge told me to come, Mr Rainford.'

'Aye, that's reet.'

'Now, you've not had another vet treating this animal, have you?'

'No I haven't; you see I came here last Michaelmas and I've had very little trouble. I had a good cow held her cleansing about Eastertime and Mr Wilson got it out but she died three days later. I've paid him, but I've not had anybody else on t' shop.'

'Good, let's have a look at her.'

The first calved heifer had wooden tongue; it was swollen, hard, and obviously making eating very difficult.

'This is a bad case, you know, so I'm going to lance her tongue and rub in some crystals and I'll give you a fortnight's supply of medicine.'

Richard quickly did this, rubbing the blue-black crystals of Iodum resub. into the tongue.

'By the way, where do you graze your heifers?'

'They've bin on some stubbles which had bin undersown with grass and clover.'

'Well, have a good look at the others, because stubble seems to bring on wooden tongue. If she's not better when you've used the medicine, let me know.'

'I will that, thank you, Mr Holden, and tha's to go into Bainbridge's.'

'I will. Cheerio.'

Bill Bainbridge only wanted two packets of mastitis powders because he had found a cow with specks in her milk.

Tom Walsh at Further Marsh Farm, Ryton was a cattle dealer, but milked thirty cows and had a favourite Jersey as the house cow. Tom was in his early fifties, portly, and always wore gold rimmed spectacles, a black bowler and a black suit. He looked like a parson, except for his heavy, well polished brown boots and gold watch chain.

'Mr Holden, I've just found my Jersey cow dead.'

'Bad luck, Tom; was she all right when you milked this morning?'

'Aye, but she gave a bit less at six o'clock; she was normal like and we've drunk her milk at breakfast time.'

'I'll be along then to take a sample soon.'

'You do, I'll wait for thee.'

It was about half past nine when Richard got to Further Marsh, and the dead Jersey was lying in her stall as though asleep.

'Looks as though her heart just stopped.'

'It does, but I'll examine a blood smear straight away.'

Having taken it, he carried it and his microscope into the farm kitchen and set up the microscope on the table. Mrs Walsh and the two children came into the room.

'Good morning, Mrs Walsh, you don't mind me using the table, do you?'

'Of course not, Mr Holden; we all want to know what Alice died of.'

When Richard focused the one twelfth objective lens through the immersion oil onto the blue stained blood film he was surprised to see the black rods of the Bacillus anthacis appear.

'Good gracious, Tom, it's anthrax that has killed her.'

'Oh Mr Holden, will us and the children be all right?' asked Mrs Walsh.

'I think you definitely will be, but of course if you felt ill suddenly in the next day or so you must go to the doctor at once.'

'What do I do now?' asked Tom.

'Tell the village bobby at once and I'll inform the Ministry at Droughton. I'll just go back and take another blood smear and a swab and fill that ear with cotton wool soaked in antiseptic, and that's it until the Ministry inspector arrives.'

Though the case was confirmed as one of anthrax, neither Tom nor his family took any harm from having drunk the milk from the cow which died of anthrax two hours later.

George Duke arrived on the following Monday to do the half-yearly audit, he and his assistant working in the office all day.

On Tuesday morning George came alone to see Richard at nine o'clock.

'Good morning, George; now, what is wrong? you had me worried when you left that message that you wanted to see me.'

'There's nothing wrong; your profit margin is good and you are still slowly reducing capital owed, but your bad debts have gone up almost 8%.'

'Yes, Flora had noticed that we were sending out more accounts rendered.'

'That's the problem that has to be attended to because you are losing not only your fees, but all the other costs as well, so that for every pound owed to you you're losing another pound in petrol, oil, tyres, depreciation and all the other overheads.'

'What do you think I should do, George?'

'Go and ask them for the money and if they don't pay get Tommy to put them in court; a lot will pay when they get a solicitor's letter, they don't want the scandal of their neighbours knowing they are bad payers. If in spite of a court appearance they still don't pay, I will write the amount and expenses off, and you cross them off your books; they are no use to you.'

'I'll do that if you'll give me a list of the overdue ones, and the ones I think are bad I'll give to Tommy.' (In three months Richard had collected half the money, but he lost three clients, one having moved out of the district and two who had not paid in spite of everything – he told them to get another vet to do their work.

Flora said she was glad that now she and Marjorie were not using so many stamps and bill heads for nothing. John King, of Duke, Son and King, Solicitors, appeared for Richard in court and soon a friendship was formed which lasted for many years and much money was recovered.

'Knowles, 2 Grange Cottages, Pickhill, a cow to cleanse.' Richard looked at the entry in the day book and said to Flora, 'I don't know that name, did he say if he was a new client?'

'No, he didn't, Richard, he gave the message by telephone, he didn't hesitate.'

'Well, I'll soon find out.'

As Richard walked up the path to the cottage, Bert, Bill Meadows' cowman came to meet him.

'Good morning, Bert, I was wondering who this Mr Knowles was; where's the cow?'

'Follow me, Mr Holden. Few folk know mi name's Knowles, I allus git Bert, you see.'

In the small shippon at the end of the long garden Richard looked at the cow's cleansing and was immediately suspicious.

'She didn't calve to time, did she, Bert?'

'No 'er bagged up quick, she were a fortneet off, but calf's wick and I've med it suck one quarter she's a bit wrong in, so wilta look at it?'

Richard soaked his hands and arms in the diluted Dettol and then spread on them his obstetric cream. Very slowly he managed to free some of the afterbirth from the uterine wall. Noticing that there was cow dung in the next stall, Richard asked, 'How many cows do you keep, Bert?'

'Two, but I've just sold one off-fat, so I'll hev to get one that's due for t' New Year. That 'un that's just gone were two week afore 'er time in February and held 'er cleansing three days, but oo milked well.'

'Wasn't that when you became ill?'

'Aye, I started wi' a bad cold, sweating like and it turned to pneumonia. I 'ed a real rough do, off work six weeks I were.'

Richard could not remove the afterbirth, and so put pessaries into the uterus. When he turned away from the cow he noticed how his wellingtons were soiled with the yellowish-brown discharge from the cow and the penny dropped. Bert would never have thought of disinfecting his clothes and boots after attending to the cow in February and so had taken the abortion germ to Whyngate Farm; the mystery was solved.

'You haven't been to Whyngate this week, have you, Bert?'

'Nay, I've bin 'ere; wife's not well and at start of week I weren't too good.'

'Bert, pick is very infectious, so before you go to Whyngate you must scrub your leggings and boots with disinfectant and soak your hands, and after milking her as well. Have you any disinfectant?'

'Aye, I 'ev some Condy's fluid.'

'That's no good, here's a bottle of Toxenol, use eight tablespoons to a gallon of water – it's on the label; when she drops that cleansing burn it and the straw and wash the cow's tail and legs and udder with disinfectant; you understand, don't you?'

'Aye, I'll do as tha says.'

'And here are the powders for that udder, give two for a start and then one three times a day. I hope your wife's better soon. Goodbye.'

At lunchtime at the surgery, he put his calving overall to soak in strong disinfectant, carefully scrubbed his wellingtons and wondered how to stop infection getting to Whyngate again. He must see Bill as soon as possible. 'Come and have your lunch or it will be cold!' shouted Flora from the kitchen. Richard went in at once.

'I'm sorry, I meant to come straight in, but I had to disinfectant my overall. I've been to a very dirty case.'

'I didn't mean to shout,' said Flora, 'but you know it's hard work trying to keep food warm and the allocation of fuel is only half what we applied for.'

'Only half? Good Lord, how are we going to keep this place warm?'

'I don't know, but I've turned the radiators off in the hall and waiting room already. I think you'll have to keep your eyes open for coke or logs, even slack like you got from Uncle Tom.'

'I will, and next time I go to Turner's, I'll try and get some slack. What will be in short supply or unobtainable next?'

'I wish I knew. George Field's shop is almost empty, there's only dried egg and dried milk on view, but he says he's going to get this Spam soon – it's American meat – it should be a help if only at Christmas.'

After lunch Richard lit a cigarette, looked at his working book and said to Flora, 'This is where I am going now,' and gave her the paper with the list of farms on it. 'You can get me at Bill Meadows'.'

The cow at Meatham Lodge had a very bad foul in the foot.

'Well, Brian, this is a bad one; her foot's as big as my head.'

'Aye, I know, it weren't doing so well wi' bran poultices, so George Bamber at Carden Hall gave me some stuff to paint on it but it's made it worse.'

'What was the stuff?'

'I'll bring t' bottle,' said Brian. He returned with a dirty dust-covered bottle and Richard could just read the faded label which said:

ANTIM CHLOR LIQ
POISON
SHEPHERDS, VET CHEMISTS, GARDEN STREET
DROUGHTON

'I thought it would be that stuff. I can't for the life of me understand why you use it, it would burn away bone never mind flesh.'

'Well tha know's 'ow it is, Mr Holden, most of us hev our remedies, which we try first and then we send for thee.'

'I know, Brian. Come on, let's have a man holding her nose and two with that leg over a pole.'

When that was done, and the dried-on bran from the poultice had been washed away with disinfectant Richard could see a lump of green foul-smelling dead tissue at least two fingers wide between the swollen claws. With a sterile curette he scraped away most of this, then covered the area with Iodoform ointment and bandaged it, finally putting the foot into a dry sack and tying twine round it to keep it in place.

'Right, let it down. Now, Brian, put plenty of straw for her to stand on to keep that foot dry and give her these powders. I'll come again and see her on Friday.'

'In t' afternoon, I hev to go to th' auction a Friday morn.'

Richard made a note in his book and set off for Lane Ends Farm at Mereside. Joe Townley was a typical 'John Bull', physically a big man, with a red face, loud voice and always smiling. This was very deceptive, because the smile hid a vicious temper. It was said that he would be smiling when he cut somebody's throat.

Today he was at his most courteous, efficient, best, and Richard quickly examined the cow which was not eating.

'She's just stuffed herself with food, Joe, that's all that's wrong.'

'I thought as much, she's the greediest devil I've ever had.'

'There's also some slow fever, so that's the opening drench and the powders to follow three times a day. Give her less hay and proven when you are foddering for the next couple of days.'

As Richard turned away to go, Joe's father Bill walked into the shippon. He was a tall, well built man, with thick grey hair crowned by a battered grey trilby hat and he was wearing a union flannel shirt, dark blue suit and black boots. Thus dressed, and with his solemn face, he looked out of place in the shippon.

He spoke with a slightly cultured accent. 'Good afternoon, Mr Holden, nothing serious I hope?'

'No, Mr Townley, she has a touch of slow fever and has overeaten.'

'I am pleased to hear that. I'll leave you and Joe to it then.'

When he had gone, Richard said, 'It's nice to meet your dad, Joe, he is always so pleasant.'

'No, he isn't,' snapped Joe, 'not when he's had a drink or two – he's a devil; when I was a kid he'd get drunk on a Saturday neet and punch lot of us out of the house, mi mother as well.'

'I would never have believed that of him.'

'No, appearances are deceptive.' Richard said nothing but smiled as he left, thinking that Joe had just described himself correctly.

While he was driving to Whyngate, Richard was thinking out the best way he could tell Bill to take more precautions against infection being introduced into the herd, without betraying what he knew professionally about Bert's cows.

'Hello, Richard, I think you know by instinct the time Liz brews up in an afternoon; come on in and have a mug.'

'Thanks, Bill. I must say I'm ready for one, it's cold today with this north wind.'

Richard followed him into the farm kitchen and they all sat down round the table.

'It's nice to see you, Liz, and how are the children?'

'Like potatoes now, getting bigger every day.'

'I suppose that's an earthy way of putting it,' and they all laughed, 'but I've called in because I've been thinking, Bill, that you will have to take more precautions against infection getting into your herd; you know, like you had to when Harry Allen had foot and mouth last year.'

'What? a trough full of disinfectant at the gate and anybody that wants to come in to scrub his boots?'

'Yes, because even these two chaps you hire at haytime and harvest could bring infection in on their hands or boots and it could get to the cows if they are helping you to tie them up.'

'But they don't keep cattle.'

'Maybe they don't, but you don't know where they go at night or weekends, and what about Bert, does he?'

'Now you mention it, he has one or two cows.'

'In that case I would get him some rubber wellingtons which can be properly disinfected, unlike boots and sacking leggings; and while you're about it, a warehouse coat that can be washed.'

'I could wash that on a Monday when I do mine,' said Liz.

Bill was no fool; he did not reply for a minute and then said, 'Richard, I think you're going a long way round to tell me that Bert may have brought trouble here.'

'Bill, I cannot discuss another of my client's veterinary affairs with you, but of course you can draw your own conclusions. What I am saying is this, that with you not having taken sufficient precautions against the introduction of infection, it could be a possible route by which infection got into your herd this spring.'

Bill looked at Liz and said, 'So that's it, why didn't I think of it before? I know he had a cow calve in spring, so it could have come that way. Liz, we'll have to do what we thought of doing a bit since and that's sack him.'

'I told you you should do it, he's always off ill or he says he is and he's so unreliable as well; we've thought about him and his family too long.'

'Aye, I'll tell him he's sacked this weekend. I know Ted Robert's youngest lad at Sykes is looking for a job and he could live in and I know Ted's herd is clean.'

When Richard drove away, he was relieved that he had got that off his chest, but what he never knew was the indescribably filthy language Bert used to describe him when Bill sacked him that weekend.

Richard never went to No 2 Grange Cottages again, nor did he ever see Bert because he died four years later. Two years before that he had written off Bert's account as a bad debt.

On Friday at Halhead's he examined the cow's foot. The infected area was much cleaner and there was little smell, but Richard could see two holes in the swollen area between the claw and the fetlock from which pus oozed.

'I don't like it, Brian; the joint above the claw is now infected and it will take weeks of dressing and even then may not heal up.'

'What are you goin ter do?'

'Carry on dressing it about every four days for a bit and see how she goes on. Is she eating better?'

'Aye, an er's a drop more milk about her.'

'Then if you agree I'll carry on and bandage it up.'

'You do, Mr Holden.'

That evening Richard, smoking a cigarette, was sitting by the fire in the lounge opposite Flora who was knitting. He had been reading the *Veterinary Record* for a short while when the phone rang.

'I'll get it,' said Flora, picking up the receiver.

'Holden, veterinary surgeon – hello, mum, how are you?' After the reply, Flora said, 'That's worrying, so you've never heard anything since then.'

Richard, listening to the conversation, said to himself, I hope she is not coming over here, and at once began to question himself. Why don't you want her here? It would be nice for Flora if Jean came and stayed for a day or two and she never comes empty-handed. Well, I suppose it's because I am tired and things get on top of me.

Flora came back. 'That was Mum.'

'Yes, I realised it was; what did she want this time?'

'Nothing, don't be so edgy, Richard, you know, you're getting like you were a bit back. Mum's worried because she has not heard from our Mary for almost a month.'

'What does she expect, a letter twice a week?'

'Richard, don't be rude, she wanted to know if we'd heard from Mary; our Bill is fine and so are the Lawsons in spite of everything, except for Maggie who fell in the blackout the other night.'

'I'm not surprised, it's a damned nuisance. That reminds me, I'll have to clean my headlamp cowls and get the gateposts and steps whitewashed again before somebody walks into them.' He lit another cigarette.

'Richard, that's your third fag since we came upstairs.'

'Is it? Well I can please myself, can't I?'

'Dear me, you are bad-tempered side out tonight, aren't you?'

'No I'm not, I'm just tired, that's all.'

'So am I a bit, but I do wish you would smoke less.'

'How can I? Now even bloody sweets are rationed. Wilf thought I had a slate loose this morning when I asked for half a pound of Mintoes.'

'Of course he would, don't you pay any attention to the news and the notices in the paper?'

'Of course I do, I just damn well forget, that's all.' Flora got up.

'Where are you going?'

'Into the dispensary for a bit of nice company – my own.'

Flora walked out and banged the door shut. Both the cats and the dog were showing signs of fear at the unusually loud voices and the door being slammed to. Now they relaxed and dozed while Richard began to read. Much later Flora found him fast asleep with Ming on his knee and the paper was on the floor. She felt a twinge of remorse at being unpleasant earlier and was surprised to find his forehead wet with perspiration when she gently pushed back his thinning hair.

Richard awoke, blinked and yawned.

'I must have just dropped off.'

'Yes, you must have; I'll go and make a drink before we go to bed.'

Richard looked at his watch, but said nothing when he saw it was almost ten o'clock.

The appointment with Professor Bernstein in Liverpool was arranged for 10.30 a.m. on Wednesday 21st October.

'We will have to catch the train at eight fifteen from here, to be in time to get the 8.40 to Liverpool in Droughton. Flora, will you ask Marjorie to come early and I'll ask Tommy Knowles to do any emergencies; everything else I'll put off. I won't need anything, but Bill did say you had to take your night clothes so I'll get your case down for you.'

It was a bright cold morning when they walked out of Exchange Station, Liverpool and down Moorfields to catch the tram in Dale Street. Richard was amazed at the extent of the bomb damage in the city, but relieved to see that the Royal Infirmary in Pembroke Place was undamaged. As it was only ten o'clock, Richard showed Flora the Veterinary Hospital and then they walked up Brownlow Street and saw the bomb-damaged buildings and some more in the Quadrangle. When they walked into the Royal, Richard could hardly believe how quickly time had flown – it was ten years ago when he was here last. The professor and his staff welcomed them and quickly made them feel at ease. After all their personal details and medical histories had been checked, their physical examinations were identical with those which Mr Graham had done fifteen months earlier.

Later, when they had dressed and were back together in the professor's office, he came in and sat down.

'It is remarkable how close the results of my examinations today are to those of Mr Graham last year. Mrs Holden, to make certain that the bacteria present in your uterus and vagina are normal I have taken swabs so that cultures can be made and examined. Another D & C is not indicated, but I think an insufflation is, so that we can be certain that ova are reaching the uterus. To make sure it is in the correct state to receive a fertilised ovum, I recommend a course of injections.'

'Thank you very much, Professor,' said Richard. 'What do you want us to do now?'

'Oh, you can go home, Mr Holden, but your wife will have to stay here until tomorrow, because this afternoon under a light anaesthetic I will perform the insufflation. Do you agree to that, both of you?'

'Yes,' they replied. A man entered the room.

'Then in that case I will leave you in the hands of my deputy, Dr Ford here. Will you go with him, Mrs Holden. Goodbye, Mr Holden, Mr Graham will contact you next week.'

Richard picked up Flora's case and followed her out of the room. When they stopped at the entrance to a ward, they kissed and parted, Flora following Dr Ford and Richard making his way out of the hospital. Flora rang the next morning and said the train would arrive just after eleven o'clock. Richard met her at the barrier, gave her a kiss and took her case.

'I am glad to see you, Flora. How do you feel, and did you sleep well?'

'Let's get home and I'll tell you; right now I am dying for a cup of tea.'

Later, sitting in the lounge, she said.

'After I left you, I had to undress, put on a white gown and get into bed. Nurse gave me a tablet and soon I felt really drowsy. I was only half awake when I was taken down to the theatre and apart from a stabbing pain which only lasted a few seconds, I felt nothing. The professor and the other doctors talked together and someone said that it was quite normal and that was it. I was put back to bed, given a cup of tea and slept until the nurse wakened me and I had dinner. Dr Ford came to see me after breakfast and said he hoped the treatment would prove effective and, darling, I do so hope it does this time.'

'So do I, Flora,' said Richard, feeling that this was definitely their last chance to start a family. A message for Richard to go to Tom Collinson, Park Hall, to see a cow with very bad mastitis terminated their talk.

Tom was grumbling. 'Hello, Mr Holden. This is one of my show cows, she only calved last night and was a bit wrong on a quarter at six o'clock this morning, so I dosed her with two mastitis powders, but when I came to give her the next one just now, she's really ill.'

'Yes, she looks bad, Tom; has she had both injections of that mixed bacterin for mastitis?'

'Yes she has, but it's no damned good; this is three cows wi' mastitis this month and they'd all bin injected.'

The cow's temperature was over 106°F and she was breathing quickly. From the hot coloured quarter Richard squirted some pale yellow fluid into a sterile MacCartney bottle.

'What's tha' takin that for?'

'Because your cows have got a germ which is different from what you have had before. It makes them very ill in a few hours and Soluseptasine injections and mastitis powders don't stop it.'

'They damn well don't.'

'So I'm sending this sample to the laboratory as soon as I get home, because I want to know what the germ is and how to treat it. Now I'm going to wash out that quarter with this Proflavine solution and inject her with mastitis serum, and you must dose her every four hours with this fever medicine. She has a water bowl in front of her so she's all right for water.'

When Richard visited the cow at five o'clock, he was relieved to find that her condition had not worsened and next day he repeated the treatment. By Saturday the cow was eating and her temperature was down. He went from examining her to examine one at High Moor, Greyhurst, and Bob Barker said, 'I'm pleased to see thee, Mr Holden, because this cow's got a bad bag since six o'clock this morning.' The case was identical with that at Tom Collinson's but on Monday morning Bob's cow died.

It was a busy week for Richard, as he said to Flora later.

'It all started with Mavis not coming on Monday morning because her little boy had measles and on Wednesday Marjorie did not turn in because her dad was ill.'

'Don't I know it. If John hadn't helped and brought his sister Margaret I couldn't have coped – she did the shopping and helped in the house. You know, I never had a minute with the practice being so busy. I was getting proper depressed until Monty cheered me up with his bashing round like hell.'

During that week strangles broke out among the horses on the docks, in Richard's opinion brought in by new horses which had come from Scotland.

He visited the horses early each morning and then in the evening. On Tuesday he calved a cow at Greyhurst Hall and with Tom Crompton helping the calf was alive. When Tom sent for him again on Wednesday the cow was very feverish and had a bloody diarrhoea. Richard gave Tom a large bottle of fever medicine and another of anti-diarrhoea medicine and told him to dose the cow at two-hourly intervals using the medicine alternately. When he arrived at Jackson's, Shepherds Farm, Goswick, to treat a cow with milk fever just after 6.a.m. on Thursday morning it had already died. He went from there to Brookhouse Farm, Markhey to another milk fever and though in a bad way, it quickly responded to treatment, much to Harold Brigg's relief.

As he walked back into the shippon Tom Crompton shouted to Richard that the cow had just died and wanted to know what had killed it so quickly. Richard explained that it was a form of dysentery caused by a germ often present in the soil which did affect new calved cows mainly and that they sometimes died before they had time to scour. As he drove home to get some breakfast he was depressed; three cows had died in four days, which was not a good advertisement for his practice, but gave his bad temper a boost. He could scarcely conceal his vexation when his breakfast was interrupted by Eric Sugden from Lodge Farm. Blackhead had broken out among his turkeys, so he wanted a bottle of Nigosyl and a syringe so that he could inject them himself. When he got back to the kitchen table the phone rang again and Flora ran to answer it.

'It's Bob Dawson for you.'

'Well, I hope it's not more swine fever.'

Bob had something different this time. He asked Richard to do the veterinary inspection at the cattle market, Droughton next morning, Friday, because Mr Wilson was ill and one member of Bob's staff was absent. Owing to the summertime regulations it was only coming daylight when he left for Droughton and it developed into a wet cold day. He had a quick word with the RSPCA inspector and then went into the shippons to inspect the cattle. Some were in pens outside and he got very wet slowly walking along looking at them all.

He was glad to get into his car, where from his Thermos flask he poured a cup of hot tea which he drank quickly and it did help him to get warm. At Turner's coal-yard he bought a bag of slack coal and talked to the head horseman, who said that his name was Will and that he was the boss's son. He wanted a tin of electuary, a packet of alterative powders and some colic drinks. After he had carried these into the tack-room, he helped Richard get the bag of coal into the car. The next stop was on the main Mereside road at Old Hall Farm at Markhey. Tom Lee was ill, but still working, wearing a cap, an overcoat and a muffler round his neck.

'What's the matter, aren't you so well, Tom?'

'I don't know proper like; mebbe I've getten a bit of flu, there's a lot of it about.'

'There is that. Where's the cow?'

'Down theer at bottom end.'

Richard examined the cow which had diarrhoea and then gave Tom a large bottle of medicine to give to her, which contained Tinct opii and 5pts Aether nit.

'If she is not right in two days let me know.'

'Aye, I will that, Mr Holden.'

'And you look after yourself, Tom.'

It was a heifer with wooden tongue at Moss Edge Farm in Carden, so George Arrowsmith was given a medicine containing iodine and Pot. iodide for it. At Brian Halhead's, the lame cow was much improved in bodily condition, but she was still lame with a discharge coming from the outer claw.

'It looks as what tha said at start is reet, Mr Holden, it's not goin' to do.'

'Yes, that sums it up, Brian; you know, you now have two choices, either to send her for slaughter, or else I'll have to operate and take that claw off.'

'Would it do any good?'

'Some heal up and fatten well though they've only one claw, but of course some don't.'

'And how long afore it will be reet?'

'At least a month.'

'That will be two month tha's bin fettling it; hell, thy bill all be more than oo's worth; I'll cash her straight away 'cos she's getten a bit of meat on her now.'

'Yes, she has, you're probably right, Brian.'

Driving home, Richard thought, I'll be glad when this week is over, precious little has gone right and now I feel cold and shivery. He lit a cigarette but it made him cough so much he put it out. Flora said, 'You don't look well; go and sit by the lounge fire and I'll bring you some tea.'

He felt a lot better after he had drunk the tea which Flora had laced with rum and was halfway through his lunch when Arthur Gardner rang from Dunthwaite to say he had a mare in a bad way with something stuck in her throat. Leaving the rest of his lunch, which Flora put into the oven, Richard was on his way in minutes. As he got out of the car he began to cough and Arthur came out of a loose box.

'I'm glad tha's not bin so long, because mare's in a queer way.'

'Have you had another vet to this mare?'

'Nay, I haven't because I want thee to do mi work. Tha sees Major Townsend has bin 'ome, and theer's bin a bust up; Knowles has gone an a chap called Macrae is theer.'

'That's fine; let's have a look at her,' and Richard had another spasm of coughing.

'What happened?'

'Tom took two horses t' ut trough, goes back t' ut stable to put out chop and comes out to find mare in t' feeding passage in t' shippon gulping down rolled oats.'

Food was stuck to the skin around the mare's nostrils and she gulped and retched when Richard pressed on her neck just behind her jaw and saliva dribbled from her mouth.

'She's choked with dry food, Arthur; will you bring a bucket of cold water.' When he went out to the car to get his stomach tube and pump, the cold air brought on another fit of coughing.

'Now, Arthur, the danger in this condition is that if she has breathed food and fluid into her lungs she'll die from septic pneumonia and there's nothing can be done for that. The same risk is present in treating her; do you want me to carry on?'

'Aye, ger on wi' it, she's a gradely mare.'

Richard pushed the tube up the mare's nostril until it reached the obstruction.

'Now will you put the end of the tube onto the side tube of the pump and press the plunger down slowly about four inches. That's it, now pull it off.' Some food and water came back down the tube; the mare retched and snorted and more of the fluid mixture came down the other nostril. She struck out with a fore-foot, but missed Richard, who at once put a twitch on her nose and he began to repeat the treatment. Each time he pushed the tube a little further in, until after about six attempts suddenly there was no resistance, then he passed the tube down to the stomach and withdrew it.

'That's it, give her some water.'

The mare drank greedily and he watched the swelling travelling down the oesophageal groove each time she swallowed.

'We've been lucky, Arthur, but if she becomes off colour at all in the next day or two let me know at once.'

'Aye, I'll do that, an afore tha' goes will ta open a cow's big knee?'

'Yes, but I don't usually open them, I'll put a Seton through it.'

The front of the left knee of the cow was the size of half a football and when she was well secured he injected local anaesthetic into the skin at the top and bottom of the swelling. While this was taking effect, he pulled out of a jar some broad tape which had been soaked in carbolised oil. He threaded this through the eye of the twelve-inch long steel Seton needle, which was blunt at the end. With a scalpel he now made small holes at the top and bottom of the swelling and some yellowish liquid ran out. He now pushed the threaded needle through the holes from above to below, removed the needle from the tape and tied the piece of tape which projected from the top hole to the end projecting from the bottom one. He gave Arthur a large bottle of Iodoform dressing.

'Now, Arthur, all I want you to do is once a day pull the knot down, pour the dressing on the tape and then pull the knot up and the tape takes the dressing inside the swelling. It should steadily discharge and go down, so put plenty of bedding in front of her. I'll call in a fortnight to see how it's doing.'

'Aye, I'd like to see 'ow it does. Knowles lanced one, an it bled like hell then it got septic and she went for killing.'

At Wyresham Post office there was a message to go to Intack Farm, Middleton. Richard guessed it would be a cow with mastitis and realised that Jack Booth was getting too many cases, as were many other farmers like Tom and George Collinson, Crompton at Greyhurst Hall and Roberts at Sykes.

Jack was grumbling. 'I thought this 'ere new mastitis vaccine tha's given 'em would stop it, but 'ere's another wi' a bad bag. At Friesian sale t' other day we were talking an a lot of us is plagued with this. Why can't tha' stop it?'

'I'll tell you, Jack,' said Richard, loudly coughing and feeling bad tempered. 'For two reasons; you've got a germ in your cows that the new drugs don't kill and it's aggravated by machine milking.'

'So that's what ta' thinks, eh?'

'Oh, damn this cough. Yes, it is; they're the main causes but there are others, yet Harry Allen and Huddlestone hand milk and get no trouble.'

The cow had a very high temperature, so she was injected with mastitis serum, the quarter emptied and irrigated with Proflavine and Jack given the job of dosing her with the fever medicine and sulphanilaimide every four hours.

'I'm off now, I'll see her tomorrow, Jack.'

Richard with a cough, sore throat and chest, and a headache was soon home, and Flora, realising that he was ill, at once took charge. He had to sit by the fire and she made him drink a dose of Veno's cough cure and then a measure of Fenning's fever medicine. He lay back in the chair and dozed until Flora brought him a cup of tea at half past five.

As soon as evening surgery was finished, he felt so ill he didn't want dinner, so Flora made him go to bed and sent for Dr McConnell. Bill at once told Richard that he had an acute tracheo-bronchitis and gave him two tablets of a new sulpha drug with a drink of water and left some to be taken every two hours until midnight, then every six hours.

'Look, Bill, I have some repeat visits to do in the morning and whatever else comes in.'

'Richard, you will stay in bed until I come in the morning – you will have to ring somebody if you have an emergency – you are not to go.'

The cough kept him awake, but finally he went to sleep for some hours, until Flora had to awaken him to take the tablets, after which he had a very restless night. Ming sat near his pillow on the bed and rarely left him. In the middle of the night her continuous purring was strangely comforting. Flora brought Richard his breakfast and also the wireless set, to which he listened while he was eating sitting up in bed. His chest was less sore, and he felt somewhat better, especially on hearing the news that the Eighth Army was slowly moving forward fighting fiercely. Near the coast of Tripoli the Navy had sunk German supply ships, helped by the RAF.

Bill came after nine o'clock and, finding Richard's temperature down, allowed him to get up and gave him more tablets to take over the weekend.

'Listen, Richard, your condition has improved but you are not better, so do only the absolute minimum of work for the next two days. If you don't, you could have a relapse and remember you were near to broncho-pneumonia yesterday. Don't try to smoke, and take the tablets and medicine regularly. Also, when you go out put a scarf over your mouth and nostrils, and I'll see you in the surgery on Monday afternoon.'

'I will do that, Bill, thank you very much.'

That weekend he saw the cows at Tom Collinson's and Jack Booth's; at Higher Syke, Catley a milk fever case; and on the docks a horse with colic and one with strangles.

He spent Sunday afternoon fast asleep in bed until Flora brought him tea at five o'clock.

'You have had a good sleep. How do you feel now?' she asked.

'Really quite well, in spite of everything this week. How about you, love, you must be worn out?'

'I am a bit weary with all the rushing about, with Mavis and Marjorie not coming and then you ill. What I'd have done without John I don't know.'

'Neither do I. Nothing has gone right and things were beginning to get me down.'

'They were that and your temper showed you weren't well on Thursday and Friday.'

'You're right, I really felt lousy on Friday. You know, I think you should give John ten shillings extra for all the work he's done for us this week.'

'Yes, so do I; I'll give it him when he comes at six o'clock.'

On Monday Jean rang Flora to tell her that at last she had heard from Mary, who was well and that her unit was in camp in Scotland. The letter had been posted three weeks before and it was heavily censored. Jean made provisional arrangements for Christmas and told Flora all the rest of the news about the family. At his surgery Bill declared Richard almost better, but told him to take the tablets until he had used them up.

A day or so later when he read the laboratory report on the two milk samples Richard quietly cursed because the germs were virulent and difficult to kill with the new drugs. He visited both farms and explained the position to Tom Collinson and Jack Booth, advising them that the use of an autogenous vaccine might prevent more mastitis cases occurring. They both agreed to him taking a pooled sample from ten cows and sending this to the laboratory. Richard also insisted that all cows showing any sign of infection and any recovered cases be put into one shippon, thus isolated from the healthy cows. One milker and one bucket and cluster dealt with this shippon. For the Panel Scheme members he had got Marjorie to type out a list of conditions regarding their milking machines' maintenance that had to be checked every week. When he gave a copy to each farmer, he emphasised the importance of doing checks and also the infectiousness of mastitis. By the adoption of these measures he expected that there would be a reduction in the number of cases of mastitis, of quarters lost and of cows dying, but above all he hoped they would reduce the amount of grumbling, and even rudeness he received from some farmers whose herds were plagued by the disease.

Later that week at Whyngate he took a blood sample from the jugular vein of every animal in the herd. It all went very smoothly because Bill nosed the animals, young David Roberts held the rope, and Elizabeth entered each animal's particulars in Richard's loose-leaf book. When Richard stopped at the garage for petrol Gordon Hindle came out and asked if he could bring Blackie to the surgery that morning. When he arrived Richard immediately noticed that the dog was thin.

'How long has he been losing weight, Gordon?'

'I don't rightly know, because as he's the guard dog for the garage I don't handle him much.'

'Is he eating?'

'No, he's eaten very little this last day or two, but he's drinking a hell of a lot of water and sometimes brings it all back.'

'Lift him on the table.'

The dog's stinking breath confirmed Richard's suspicions.

'I'm sorry to tell you, Gordon, he's got Stuttgart Disease.'

'And what's that?'

'It's a condition which starts in the kidneys and then spreads throughout the body. There's only a palliative treatment, it doesn't cure them and they always die. He is slowly dying now.'

'In that case, I'd rather you put him to sleep; I don't want him suffering.'

'Very well, Gordon, just go in the other room, and I'll do it and then you can see him after.'

When Gordon stroked his dead dog, he gulped and in a choked voice said, 'Thanks Richard,' and then hurried out of the surgery, as John came rushing in.

'It's on t' wireless there's bin a big victory at El Alamein, an t' King's sent congratulations to th' Eighth Army.' They all cheered and were excited by the news. 'It's the best we've had for years,' said Flora. It must have acted like a tonic, because that night their married life became very passionate and loving and Flora sleepily said, 'It would be a lovely wonderful night to conceive.' Richard most sincerely hoped that she would do so.

The six o'clock phone call from Tom Jackson at Goswick amused Richard.

Tom said, 'Wilta cum as quick as tha can? I've a cow goin balmy, it's trying to run up wall, I've never sin owt like it afore.'

'Yes, Tom, I'll be along inside half an hour. Just leave her alone and quiet for now.'

Richard drove rapidly to Shepherds Farm and his clinical examination of the cow revealed that she had advanced acetonaemia.

'What the hell's wrong wi' 'er, Mr 'olden?'

'She's got an advanced severe form of slow fever, can't you smell it?'

'Aye I con, but I've had cows wi slow fever afore, but ne'er one like 'er.'

'When did she calve?'

'Near on four week ago.'

'Well now, this is what you must do; she gets no proven until she is getting better, and only milk her once a day for three days. Will you nose her for me, Tom?'

Richard gave the cow an intravenous injection of glucose solution and told Tom to give her the pink powder in a quart of water in two hours' time.

This had to be followed three times a day with a slow fever powder which was composed of 1 oz of Sodii bicarb and ¼ oz of Pulv anisi shaken up in a pint of cold water.

'Have you any black treacle, Tom?'

'Aye, I've some in a drum in t' barn.'

'Good; give her eight tablespoonsful in some bran mash twice a day. If she's not right by Tuesday next week, let me know.'

'Aye, I will that.' Richard drove home quickly; he really wanted his breakfast, being cold and hungry.

Later in the day a cow was found dead at Moss End Ryton; Richard with Tommy Birtwell drove along a green lane to a field on the moss and there took a blood sample from the cow's ear. It was negative for anthrax.

'What's killed her, Mr Holden?'

'By all the froth round her head, it is fog fever; who collects your dead animals?'

'Bob Whiteside fray Southall.'

'Then I'll ask him to confirm it and I'll let you know. For now, all you can do is take them out of this field, there is too much clover in it.'

He went to the Home Farm to arrange their private herd test for tuberculosis. On walking into the office he found Bill Griffin with his spaniel at his feet and old Heather stretched out in front of the fire.

'Hello, Richard, I know what you've come for.'

'What, Bill?'

'To arrange our tuberculin test – look, I've marked it on the calendar.'

'You're right. Will next Monday be convenient to start at half past eight?'

'Yes, I'll have everything ready for you.'

'Thanks, Bill, I'll see you then.'

That evening he ordered a book of TT Certificates from H.R. Grubb Ltd. of Croydon, because after the test, the Colonel often sold animals. They had to have a certificate giving the date the test had been carried out, the number and full description of the animal, and that it had passed the test.

The second Sunday in November was Remembrance Sunday, so Richard set out to do his farm visits at half past seven. He planned to be back in time to go with Flora to the service and this he managed to do. In St. Luke's more than half the congregation were in uniform and though he felt that somehow he was not actively fighting to defeat Hitler, he did not feel guilty when on looking round he saw Dick Hayes, Jim Lord and Dick Harrison in the congregation. He enjoyed the inspired singing and the vicar's sermon on faith in the future. He used Churchill's words 'that it was the end of the beginning', saying that surely this was true when after more than three years of losses and defeats, the tide appeared to have turned in both Egypt and Russia. After the service they talked to the Reverend Evans and Edna and exchanged family news. Edna told Flora that two members of their WVS Unit had died, and she invited Flora to start again to attend on a Monday afternoon and help in their many activities. That evening on the wireless it was announced that a large invasion force of Americans had landed in North Africa and that the Germans were still retreating as the Eighth Army steadily advanced. 'And that calls for a drink,' said Richard. After he had poured them out, they drank cheerfully to success to all the forces of the Crown.

On the Monday, Richard first injected all the animals which were tied up, while Bill wrote down the measurements and two men helped to hold them. He then put on his overcoat and went outside where in the yard were the dry cows and the in-calf heifers. Three feet from the shippon wall there was an iron railing about ten yards long which made a passage, closed at one end by a door. The animals were driven one at a time behind the railing, secured, tested and then marked with a blue paint stick. When all had been done, they were driven out into another yard and the big calves, heifers and some bullocks took their place. These were more difficult to test, because being smaller they tried to escape by turning round or lying down, so one of the men went inside to hold them.

Each animal was injected with 0.1.c.c. of tuberculin into the thickness of the skin, which made a small nodule form. This was achieved by setting the adjustment screw on the piston rod of the syringe to deliver the requisite amount for each animal. It was a finicky procedure to have to perform especially if one's hands were very cold and there was also an element of risk when injecting an animal. Richard discovered this when trying to inject a particularly fractious heifer, when he injected the tuberculin into the end of the thumb of his left hand. It was only like a pin prick and he sucked his thumb hoping to extract any tuberculin along with the little blood which oozed out.

He then cleansed his thumb with surgical spirit and carried on working. Later he was injecting another heifer when there was a shout, 'Look out!' from one of the men, but at that very moment he received a powerful blow on his bottom, which lifted him off his feet and sent him sprawling on the concrete; the syringe was smashed when it was knocked from his hand.

Two men rushed forward wielding brushes, shouting 'Ger off, you young devil!' and drove the young bull down the yard. Bill helped Richard to his feet. 'You're not hurt, are you, Richard?'

'No I'm not, but for a second I wondered what was happening. That little bull is terribly strong, it was as bad as being kicked by a horse.'

'I'm sorry, Richard, he's only eleven months old, I should have tied him up, but Les the cowman thought one of those big heifers was riding this morning, so we let him out to see which one it was, I never thought he would attack us.'

'Bill, I never appreciated until now just how powerful even a young bull is; he just tossed me like a bale of hay. I'm glad I was wearing my overcoat, and his horns are still short.'

'Yes, we are lucky; no harm's done except to the syringe, I'll pay for that. Bring that bull back and drive him in, we'll do him next, so you can get a bit of your own back.' Richard got another syringe from the car, and then finished injecting all the animals as well as the bull.

By Tuesday afternoon his thumb was swollen and painful.

'That looks sore, Richard.'

'It is, Flora, and very uncomfortable. I've failed the test all right, having got a local reaction and a general one – I've got a mild headache. I'm not surprised I've reacted because all the time I am dealing with infected cattle. I'll wear an old glove tomorrow – I don't want to prick it again.' The next day his thumb was more painful, so he was careful to avoid knocking it. The young bull and the big heifers were tied up, which made it easier to inject them again. On Thursday, as he picked up folds of skin to measure them, his thumb ached all the time, but he worked on and completed the test. Two animals which had been purchased some weeks before failed the test, which annoyed the Colonel as they had been accompanied by a test certificate stating that they were free from tuberculosis. Richard advised him to isolate them at once, and to contact the farmer from whom they had been bought. The Colonel said he would, but in future he would not buy any animals, he would keep a closed herd.

Having found another tuberculosis cow while doing a herd examination, Richard had to go to Southall to make a post mortem examination of it. It was an advanced case and Bob Whiteside said,

'I can't understand them keeping a cow till it gets as bad as this. You took one from there last year.'

'I know I did and both times I've had a row with Harry Allen over the value I put on his cow. He seems to think I can give him any price he wants. Really, £10 is too much for this.'

'Aye, it is; it's only a screw.'

'You know I told him to go TT last year when he restocked after the outbreak of foot and mouth disease he had. It was a golden opportunity to get rid of the damned disease, but he wouldn't listen to me. He said TT cows were too dear.'

'They'd hev bin cheaper than losing an £80 cow every twelve months.'

'They would, Bob. By the way, was Tommy Birtwell's cow fog fever?'

'Aye, it were; when I cut lungs open, froth ran out everywhere.'

'I was certain it was, I'll let him know now. Thanks, Bob.'

The laboratory report on the blood test of Bill Meadow's herd revealed two doubtful reactors, and that one sample had haemolysed while in the post. The result pleased Richard, and when he told Bill he said that it was the best news he'd had all year, and asked when the retest would be. Richard told him January, when his TT was due. Because the end of his left thumb had burst open and was raw, he went to Jim Lord's and bought a leather finger stall, which he wore after bandaging the raw flesh. The next day he cut out the Seton from the cow's knee at Dunthwaite, and told Arthur to dress the wounds in the very much smaller knee until they had stopped discharging, when he could let them heal.

Mary, having got a weekend pass from her battery, told Flora that she would arrive on Friday evening about nine o'clock. Flora was thrilled by the news and phoned Jean, telling her to come and stay for the weekend. She came bringing some braising steak, but would not divulge how or where she had obtained it. That didn't worry Flora, who at once made it into a dish with onions, carrots, mushrooms and seasoning arranged in layers in a big earthenware cooking pot. After adding an Oxo cube and water it was closed by a lid and put into the oven to simmer for hours.

Having received the autogenous vaccine, Richard delivered one package to Tom Collinson, and the other to Jack Booth. He showed both men how to inject their animals, warning them not to inject any which showed signs of mastitis and to continue to practise the preventative measures he had given them earlier. He gave syringes, needles and disinfectant to them, and then went on to Cross Road farm at Wyresham, and Old Hall at Markhey; there was a cow to cleanse on each farm. During the last three months he had manually removed an afterbirth from a cow at least two or three times a week. Many could not be removed completely at the first visit, so he had to go a couple of days later to try and extract the rest of it. Within a few weeks the cow sometimes developed a low grade metritis, which he had to treat. As a result of this continuous exposure to infected material, his arms were often sore, and retained the foul odour of putrefaction, even though he used Dettol liberally, and also his obstetric cream.

After the evening surgery, he changed his suit and then joined Flora and Jean upstairs. He poured drinks for the three of them, and they all began to feel hungry as the delicious aroma of cooking steak pervaded the house. Richard found that week's *Veterinary Record* and saw on the front cover an advertisement for Isovacuil – a hormone product for the easy removal of the placenta in cows and mares. At once he went into the office, and wrote out an order for this product, thinking that he had found a way of preventing his arms becoming sore.

It was nine thirty, half an hour after Mary's arrival, when they sat down round the dining table. After the vegetable soup, they all enjoyed the delicious braised steak served with potatoes and brussel sprouts. Richard noticed that the fibres in his steak were coarse and thick, and the suspicion soon became a conviction in his mind that it was horsemeat, but he kept his thoughts to himself and joined in the talk which followed: Mary's description of masses of ships which had assembled in the Clyde during the previous five weeks and which had disappeared one night. On Sunday 15th November the church bells were rung for half an hour for the first time in years to celebrate the victory at El Alamein. They were all in good spirits and before lunch drank a toast to the success of the Eighth Army which was still forcing Rommel to retreat. Richard recalled his childhood, when he used to lie in bed at midnight, listening to the church bells ringing in Christmas Day, trying to stay awake long enough to be able to discover what presents his parents had brought. For a fleeting moment he felt very sad that those happy days with his family were gone for ever. As it was barely six weeks to Christmas they asked Mary to come and stay with them then, but she could not promise to do so, though Jean said that she would come definitely.

The next morning Richard looked in the walnut chest which they used as a wine cupboard and was surprised to find how little alcoholic drink they had left. Before lunch he went to Jim Lord's shop, where he had often seen Wincarnis, Stone's Ginger Wine, and small bottles of whisky and brandy on sale. Jim came in. 'Hello, Richard, come on through and see Isabel and our James Edward' was his welcome. They were very well, and Jim was obviously very proud of his baby son. Richard felt very jealous of his good fortune, and turned the conversation round to supplies of drinks for Christmas. Jim promised to get some, adding that the price of all alcoholic drinks was rising steadily.

For Richard time passed quickly, being taken up by work for the Ministry of Agriculture & Food, and under the Panel scheme. The troubles among horses, cattle, calves and pigs made him very busy, added to by an outbreak of distemper in dogs. He gave John Lamb the job of whitewashing the kerb stones of the pavement in front of the house, the lamp post, and the gate posts leading up to the front door. The walls each side of the entrance into the yard and the doorposts of the garage were also whitened. Another major job was the removal of the soot-encrusted privet hedge from all round the garden. The bushes were piled in the back garden, with all the other rubbish, and when dry made a great bonfire one Saturday afternoon.

To the list of rationed materials were now added towels and tea cloths, so one evening Flora with Richard's help checked all the linen and bedding they had brought from Auntie Winnie's house a year ago. The blankets were shaken and refolded with many moth balls put between the folds. The linen and cotton sheets were refolded and Flora counted fourteen Irish linen tea towels, some new and most little used. But Richard made the major discovery – towels of every size from guest to bath sheet which he pulled out of an old steamer trunk. Flora was delighted and said she would use a few as Christmas presents, or swap them for clothes with Jean or her friends. For the surgery Richard had twice bought a big roll of surgical gauze, which was used for other things than routine surgery; it was cut up into lengths for use as dusters and washing up cloths.

It was pitch black and raining very hard at 5.30 a.m. when George Dobson at East View at Catley rang and Richard was soon on his way to a cow down with milk fever. Between Wyresham and Goswick the road was flooded in places and he had to slow down and drive with caution.

'Tha's bin a long time Mr 'olden.'

'I know, but the road was a foot deep in water the other side of Goswick. Where's the cow?'

He followed George across the yard and into the box.

'Hell fire, she's gitten her calf bed out.' The uterus already was bigger than a large bucket.

'Quick, George, get two men and a sheet, some buckets of hot water, a bale of straw and a plough line.'

Richard secured the cow's head by tying a calving rope round her horns and fastening it to a ring in the wall. He began to inject the milk fever solution intravenously very slowly, and the cow was beginning to respond when George and two men came rushing into the box.

'Ow's 'er doin' Mr 'olden?'

'She's coming round, George. Now bring a pulley block and hang it on a chain on that beam.'

'I evn't one.'

'Then get mine out of the back of the car, hurry up.'

The injection finished, Richard let the cow loose, and with a push she sat upright.

'Torch 'as gone out, but we've gitten block.'

Once everything was in position, the cow's hindquarters were quickly raised and rested on the bale. Richard rapidly replaced the uterus, put pessaries into it and put on the strappings. While they were carrying all the equipment out of the box the cow suddenly got to her feet.

'Well, that's super, Mr 'olden, come and have some tea wil'ta?'

'I will that, George, it's a raw cold morning.'

When they were in the warm kitchen George said, 'Mr Holden dusta ever git a strong dog brought to thee to be killed 'cos folk who own it can't manage it?'

'Yes, I do now and again. Why do you ask?'

'Well, tha's sees, it's like this: wi' so many airmen and workmen round 'ere now, I'm losing too many birds and eggs from mi cabins, so I want two real bad devils, tha' knows, each side of gate inta yon field. They should fricken any poachers away.'

'George, I'll remember that and try and find you a couple soon.'

Later that morning at Smithy Farm in Greyhurst, Tom Jackson explained,

'I only got 'er 'a Friday in Droughton Auction but she's given nowt this morning and 'oo ne'er touched 'er proven.'

The cow's temperature was 106.8°F, and her heart beat was 100 per minute. Her eyes were very dull, and her horns hot, and though the cow was very ill, Richard could not make a diagnosis.

'Will you bring me a bucket of hot water and some soap, Tom?'

'Aye, I won't be a minute.' Richard now had a big towel in his car, which was drier and cleaner than the towel from the dairy which most farmers produced. After pouring disinfectant into the water, he examined the cow's vagina and uterus and found both were normal. After he had withdrawn his arm, the cow suddenly passed a lot of very dark reddish-brown coloured urine.

He turned to Tom. 'There's the answer, she's got redwater, and she is very ill.'

'I thought 'oo were, but what is it, I've niver ad one afore?'

'She's an Irish cow?'

'Aye, there were some come o'er last week.'

'I thought so, it's a germ gets into the blood, and it's spread by ticks. She's very feverish, so you must dose her with this medicine every four hours, and give her a powder in a pint of milk twice today. I'll be back in the morning to see her again.' Next morning Tom sent a message to say the cow had died.

He had almost finished the herd examination at Fred Noblett's Highgate Farm, when he heard a cow cough and, quickly looking round, saw that it was a big roan shorthorn in moderate condition.

'I don't like the sound of that cough, Fred, so I'll examine her chest.'

Using his stethoscope he could hear abnormal sounds as she was breathing, and when she coughed again, he noticed a blob of yellow mucus appear on the wall in front of her.

'Her lungs sound rough, so I'll make a slide of that phlegm, and examine it tonight.'

'As 'er got TB?'

'It's suspicious.'

'But 'er's milked well, an' 'er's still on two a day.'

'That does not matter; by law I've got to give you this Form "A", and you read the instructions on it.'

That evening, using his microscope, he found the little red rods of TB bacilli in the stained preparation.

'I didn't expect to see thee, Mr 'olden.'

'Maybe you didn't, but I'm back, Fred, because she has TB and will have to go. Next thing is we have to value her.'

'Then I want fifty quid for her.'

'I'll give you £38.'

'Nay, that 'ull not do. I want fifty quid.'

Richard went to £40 and then to £42, but Fred would not budge and began to get mad.

'Yer a 'ard devil, Mr 'olden, tha' knows I only got £5 for that 'un last year.'

'I know you did because she was rotten.'

'Well, I still want £50.'

'Look Fred, I don't want to fall out with you and argue all day. The best thing you can do is pick an arbitrator from this list and his value is final.'

Fred looked at the list and said,

'Oh, I'll 'ev John Tunstall frae Droughton Cattle Market, I knows 'im.'

'Right, I'll arrange for him to come.'

Later that day, the auctioneer who sold hundreds of cattle a month, took a long look at the cow, ran his hands along her back and said, '£45 is all she is worth.'

'Nay, she's worth more than that, John.'

'She's not, put £45 on that valuation form, and then Fred can sign it.' This he did reluctantly. Tom Noblett the manager of the Droughton abattoir said the cow could go in for slaughter the next morning, and Richard arrived as she was being unloaded from Robson's truck. She was led into a bay in the abattoir which was well apart from the area where the healthy cattle were slaughtered. She was pole-axed, bled and then dressed; Richard took notes of the findings made by Charlie White, the meat inspector. TB was found in the mesenteric glands so the intestines were condemned, as also was the head. The liver was healthy and put on a hook, and then the butcher opened the chest and cut out the lungs. Charlie ran his hands over them and, finding some lumps, cut into them. They were round hard abscesses about an inch in diameter, and they had a TB soft cheese-like centre; the lungs were condemned.

On the chest walls were red velvety areas, so the butcher sawed the carcase into two sides, and Charlie tore off the lining membranes. Walter, using the same cloth and bucket of water, washed the two sides, then Charlie examined them carefully, and as no TB lesions were found they were passed. When Richard completed the post mortem form stating the case was not an advanced one, it meant that Fred would receive £34 for his cow which would cause him to have another grievance. That did not worry Richard as much as the poor hygiene practised by the butcher; if the water in his bucket or his cloth had picked up any tuberculosis material, he had wiped it all over the carcase – that made it fit for human consumption? – like hell it did.

On his way back to Sandhaven he called at Cross Roads Farm, Wyresham and Bill Harrison met him in the yard.

'It's another to cleanse, Mr 'olden, and I want thee to wash out that 'un you injected last time, because she held onto it for a week; yon stuff didn't work.'

'But it's the latest treatment, Bill.'

'Maybe, but I'd rather tha' cleansed 'em properly.'

As luck would have it the cleansing came away easily, and then he irrigated the uterus of the second cow. On leaving the farm he decided to keep a record of the cows he injected to see if the Isovacuil helped them to cleanse or not.

Later that week it was early morning when Droughton police rang and asked Richard to go at once to the egg packing station on Shipton Road where a horse had been injured in an accident. He put the humane killer into the car and then drove very fast to the place where he found the horse lying on its side having suffered a compound comminuted fracture of the right humerus, and a fracture of the fetlock of the right hind leg.

'It's hopeless, isn't it, Mr Holden?' asked Eric Vickers.

'Yes, it is; I'm going to shoot it now on humane grounds,' and a few seconds later he put the horse out of its suffering. By this time PC Hibbert had arrived on his bicycle and both he and Richard wanted to know how the accident had happened. Eric didn't know, because he had just taken some milk into the packing station when he heard a crash. He had run out and found the horse down; the shafts and milk float were smashed and milk was running away. The lorry had stopped down the road, and some American soldiers had come back.

'Have you rung Whiteside, Eric?'

'No, but I'll go inta t' station and do it now.'

'That's it, then; I'll be on my way.'

He had just finished breakfast when George Duke arrived with the half year's accounts, which he described as satisfactory, though the turnover had not increased very much. Richard said that as he had been ill on and off he realised that he had not done as much work as earlier in the year, and that the distemper outbreak had reduced the number of his canine clients.

At the weekend when he went to Higher Syke at Catley, Bill Wallbank said that he had bought the big Friesian cow a week before, and that she had been uneasy since early that morning, but had started to calve about nine o'clock.

'I've had a feel in 'er, Mr 'olden, and I've niver felt owt like it afore, there's nowt but legs; it must be twins.'

Forewarned, Richard examined the cow carefully and found there were six legs – a sterno-abdominal presentation, so it was a monster made up of two calves fused together. He explained this to Bill, and asked for plenty of hot water, and the help of two more men. While he was waiting for them to come he gave the cow an epidural anaesthetic, and decided to try and cut off each part of the monster as it came within his reach. He threaded a rough cutting wire through one tube of his embryotome and tied a calving rope onto it. When the men arrived one held the embryotome while he pushed the calving rope into the cow's passage and along the nearest leg right to the top, and over a large lump of the monster which he could feel there. He cursed under his breath because his left thumb was still tender though covered by the finger-stall. After a struggle he grasped the loop on the underside of the swelling, and pulled it towards him, but it came out without the wire which had become detached.

'That's a devil, Bill, it's come off; I'll have to start again. Will you hold the tubes and feed the wire through when I pull on the rope.'

'You want me to hold tubes an t' wire.'

'Yes, like that; that's right, push it in.'

This time the rope remained attached to the wire, so Richard untied it, and threaded the wire through the parallel tube, and attached a handle to it. He now cut the wire about two feet from the other tube from off the roll, and attached a handle to the end.

'Now the wire is right round the leg, you keep that rope which is holding the leg tight. Now I'll hold the tubes, and you and Bill pull the wire to and fro like you were sawing with a double handled saw; have you got that?'

'Aye, course I hev.'

'Then Bill, start pulling, towards you; that's it, you pull; let it go back, Bill, keep it going nice and steady – don't pull too hard or it will jam.' After about a dozen times the lump was sawn through, and the leg drawn out after the embryotome.

''ow many more are there?'

'I think five.'

'At this rate we'll be 'ere all t' day.'

As he spoke the cow lay down.

'Damn it, that's going to make it a lot harder; make her get up, Bill.'

But in spite of being hit with a leather strap, and then a stick she would not rise. Down on his knees, Richard struggled to repeat the procedure threading the wire round the top of the next leg. It was some time later before the leg with a lot of bone and skin at the top to which a tail was attached was pulled out of the cow.

'Bill, that should have made it a bit less, because we have cut the back end off one calf.' Richard got to his feet. 'Try again and make her get up.'

The cow would not, so he lay down on his stomach and, pushing his arm into the cow right up to his armpit, felt round the mass. There were two more legs as big as the ones which had been cut off, and two smaller ones. He attached rope to the latter and told the men to pull on them while he pushed the other two backwards. The mass moved round enough to allow the small legs to enter the vagina.

'Hold it there, don't pull.' At the top of the legs he felt along a neck and to the poll of a head. 'It's two calves definitely grown together, Bill, and we've got half of the back end out. I must cut these two small legs off, and then swing it round and get the others off – it should come then.'

It took an hour to cut off the small legs, which brought with them some ribs, and then to turn the mass round and rope the other legs. After securely fixing into the mass two sharp hooks which had ropes attached to them, he cut off the legs which were pulled out.

'Thee hev a rest and I'll go for some baggin, get some more 'ot watter, you two.'

Richard wearily got to his feet and was grateful for the hot sweet tea and bread and cheese sandwich. After they had eaten Richard put handfuls of Lux flakes into the cow's uterus and rubbed them all over the mass.

'Now for the last lap. Pull gently – that's enough, stop.'

He felt round as much of the cylindrical shape as he could reach and, finding nothing sharp, told them to pull. He guided the mass into the passage, and after he had withdrawn his arm, they pulled hard, and it came out of the cow.

'What a bloody freak,' said Bill.

'It is that, but it's not what I thought it was. I thought they were joined together back to back from nose to tail, but they're not, you can see the back end of one has fused to half of the front end of the other, partly pushed into its chest.'

'I don't care what the 'ell it is, it's out and that's all that matters.'

'True, I'll just feel that she is not torn at all.'

'Is oo?'

'Yes, there is one about the length of my hand, but it's not bleeding.'

He removed some calf intestines and liver-like material and put pessaries and sulphanilamide into the uterus.

When he had washed and dressed he told Bill to get her up, and after a few hefty clouts with a stick and all their assistance she got to her feet.

'Dusta know it's one o'clock?'

'It is, damn it, that's half the day gone.'

'Aye, it is, stop an 'ev a bit of dinner.'

'That's nice of you, Bill, but I must get going.'

'All reet then, Mr 'olden, tha's done a good job gerrin that bugger.' Richard laughed, got into his car and drove back to Sandhaven feeling very pleased with himself, but very hungry.

'Where on earth have you been?' said Flora.

'At Wallbank's at Catley getting a freak calf; well, really, two fused together. It's taken all the morning.'

'Oh, that's where you've been, because Bob Dawson has rung twice and wants you to ring him back.'

'Let's have some lunch first, I'm starving. He can wait half an hour.'

Bob asked if it would be convenient if the superintending inspector and he called about eleven o'clock on the next morning. Richard assured him it would be.

'What did Bob want, Richard?'

'To know if it would be convenient for him and the superintending inspector to come and see me tomorrow. I wonder what I've done wrong.'

'Why should you have done anything wrong?'

'I don't know that I have; I'm just guessing at the reason for the two of them wanting to see me.'

'Why? Are you really worried?' asked Flora.

'A bit; you know that the Ministry cheque is a good slice of our income most months, and I do not want to lose it.'

'You won't; you've always done all they ask you to do; don't look on the black side. Eat up while I get the apple pie out of the oven.'

Next morning Richard was back in the surgery before eleven o'clock, when Flora answered the door bell and then led Bob Dawson and the superintending inspector into the room. He was wondering if he should ask the two men to go upstairs and have a coffee in the lounge, when Bob said, 'Richard, let me introduce Mr Campbell Morrison.' They shook hands, and Bob continued, 'We can't stop long because Mr Morrison has two other appointments to keep before lunch.'

'Very well, come with me and we can sit in the waiting room.'

Mr Morrison looked round and then said, 'I am very pleased with your surgery and waiting room; it must make a very favourable impression on the general public – it is a credit to you.'

'Thank you very much, I do try to run it as though it were an outpatients' department and a pharmacy; that's why everything is painted white as in a hospital which is what the public expects.'

Flora knocked on the door, and came in carrying a tray on which were tea cups, saucers, a plate full of slices of cake, a jug of milk and the tea pot.

'Help yourselves, gentlemen,' she said as she withdrew and closed the door.

'I am pleased to hear your ideas, Mr Holden, because I want the public to get a better grasp of our profession's aims and objects, and eradication of TB in cattle, and clean and hygienic premises, will help no end.'

The cake and tea were being consumed rapidly and he continued, 'Bob has been telling me about the good number of diseased animals you find while doing herd examinations. It is sterling work, but I must ask you to keep your valuations as low as possible.'

'I do try, but you must know how difficult some farmers are to deal with.'

'Oh I do, but £18 is too much to pay for a screw cow.'

'But sir, you can't always decide on a physical examination that the animal will be an advanced case.'

'I grant you that; don't get the idea that I am finding fault, because I'm not; it is just a general recommendation I am giving to all inspectors. By the way, two practices in this area are behind in doing herd examinations; can you do more if Mr Dawson sends more to you?'

'Yes, I'll try and do any you send me as soon as I can.'

'That will be a great help, because we're short of inspectors even though we are trying to recruit more from members who have been in practice for a few years. Now, Bob, have you any questions?'

'Yes. Richard, are you getting enough petrol coupons?'

'On the whole, yes, but some months I have to apply for some supplementary ones.'

'And what about car tyres?'

'I've stopped putting gaiters inside because I was getting too many blow outs. I apply before they get down to the canvas, with a certificate from my garage to say that they are very worn.'

'Good, but if you are having difficulties, let me know.'

'Thank you, I will.'

'Then we will be on our way,' said Campbell. 'You will thank your wife, Richard, for the tea and cake, won't you? I am pleased we have met and that you will be able to keep up the good work,' and with that Campbell and Bob left.

'Well, what was it all about?' asked Flora, picking up the tray.

'Really a chance to meet one of his LVIs; a polite ticking off for paying too much for TB cows, and an indirect invitation to join the M of A & F.'

'But you wouldn't want to, would you?'

'No thanks, I like running my own show too much; anyway I'll go and get two visits done and see you at one o'clock.'

That evening Ted Croft the Estate Agent came into the surgery with his Airedale which was muzzled and on a lead.

'Hello, Mr Croft, has Reeth come for his distemper injection?'

'No, Mr Holden. I am sorry to say I want him put down because he's got too vicious. I daren't let him out into the garden alone or he attacks everybody who comes to the house and even my wife is getting afraid of him.'

'That seems a shame, seeing he is not five years old.'

'Yes, it does, but what can I do with him, nobody wants a dog that bites.'

'He could go to a farm as a guard dog,' and Richard told Ted what George Dobson wanted at Catley.

'Oh, it would be great if he would have him. I don't really want to have him destroyed, he's such a loyal pal.'

'Then go and sit in the waiting room, while I try and get hold of him. Being next to the airfield, he has got a phone.'

As a result of the phone call, Ted handed Reeth over to George in the surgery next morning.

'Be careful he doesn't bite you.'

'Eh, I will that, Mr Croft, but tha knows, I con manage mi bull on t' farm so I'll manage him all reet, and thanks. Now come on thee, as long as tha' knows I'm boss we'll get on gradely,' and George led Reeth out of the surgery to begin a very different life.

It was the Saturday morning before Christmas about six o'clock when George Meadows from Boundary Farm rang to say he had found a cow dead, and he thought she had hanged herself. George had begun to build up a milking herd in 1939, and was now producing a lot of milk, most of which was retailed in Sandhaven. The dead cow was in a stall in the twenty shippon right opposite the central door.

'It's a bad do, she were one o' mi best milkers. Conta manage, Richard, I'm short-handed this morning. One of mi men 'asn't turned in; it were t' fur and feather in Middleton last neet.'

'Oh, I'll manage. Can I take my microscope into the kitchen?'

'Aye tha do, Winnie's theer.' Richard as usual made a smear of the cow's blood on a glass slide, let it dry, went across the yard, and then stepped into the warm kitchen.

'Come along in, Mr Holden. Did she hang herself?'

'I don't know yet, Mrs Meadows, but I will know when I've prepared and examined this slide.'

When he did black anthrax bacilli came into view.

'Dear me, I didn't expect to find that.'

'Why, what is it, Mr Holden?'

'It's anthrax, Mrs Meadows, I must go and tell George.'

'Where the hell's that come from?' he said.

'I don't know, are you feeding any cake?'

'No, at the moment they are eating vetch silage and home-grown cereals.'

'It's a mystery. Then I'll just take a swab of blood, and I'll let the police and the Ministry know. For now I'll block her passages with tow so no fluid runs out, and tie the cows from each side of her somewhere else. You'd better block up that drain; the Ministry chaps will be here soon and will deal with her. I'm sorry you've lost her, George; but all the best for Christmas to you all. Cheerio.'

When he arrived back at Cross Street, Flora was busy checking the Christmas decorations.

'So that's the next job, is it? I'm hungry.'

'Of course it is, there's only six days to Christmas so we must get on. After breakfast you must go to Lord's and get the drinks. You did order them, didn't you?'

'Yes, I did. I'll get them this morning because I want some bandages and things.'

'And call at Eric Sugden's and see if he has a turkey for us.'

'I don't know if he will have, he lost a lot with blackhead, and I've been told a fox got in and killed some.'

'Anyway, call and if he hasn't got one order a capon, a big one from Frank Wood, and some meat pies and get some sausages if he has any, or else black puddings.' He arrived home at lunch-time with bottles of drink, two small meat pies and two black puddings, after being told to call next week to see if a bird for Christmas would be available.

'Bob Dawson's sent you a Christmas present.'

'Oh yes, what is it?'

'Two suspect swine fevers, one at George Whiteside's at Seedhill and the other at Rigby, Greenacres, Causeway Lane.'

'What a damned job for a cold wet Saturday afternoon.'

'It is; come and have your lunch now and you can go straight after.'

At George Whiteside's the ill pigs were eight to twelve weeks old, stores, and two had died. Richard examined the movement book and then said, 'Will you bring me some water in an old bucket, not one you use for feeding?'

'Aye, I won't be a minit.'

When George brought it, Richard poured in some Toxenol disinfectant, soaked his hands, and then cut open the chest of the dead pig. He took out the lungs, but found nothing diagnostic.

'Nowt wrong wi them,' said George.

'No, there isn't, I'll just open the belly.' When he did, pink fluid ran out; the stomach and bowels were very inflamed; and when he cut the latter open they contained many cream-coloured roundworms.

'What made you think they had swine fever, George?'

'Wi mi pigs deeing. Tha sees, I bought some in th' auction two week back, and they started to scour, and one of 'em deed, and I thought it had spread to these.'

'Well, I don't see any signs of swine fever here; it's just acute scour aggravated by roundworms. They could even be causing it; how old was this one?'

'Near on nine week, it's out o' this lot here.'

The pigs were bright and alert, though there was some scour on the floor, and the trough was empty.

'They look well, so I'll give you a bottle of worm medicine. Now, dose them as it says on the label. When you've dosed them they will pass worms. Sweep the worms and droppings up, and burn them. From now on you'll have to dose every litter when they are six weeks old. Here are some anti-scour powders to mix in the feed of this lot twice a day. Where are the other pigs?'

'Out back, follow me.'

Some of the windows in the dilapidated building were missing; inside it was cold and damp, and puddles of water were on the floor.

'George, before we go any further, this is a bad building, you must not keep pigs in here.'

'I knows that, Mr 'olden, but they're only here temp'ry like, till two pens of fat 'uns go. They were to go yester morn, but Tom Latham didn't turn up, he's comin' Monday.'

'Where's he from?'

'T'other side o' Burton; he allus shifts mi pigs, he's my wife's cousin's husband, we're all related like.'

There was some scour in this pen too, and the pigs looked ill. George dragged the dead twelve-week-old pig out of the pen into the passage. Richard found the intestines very thickened and there was inflammation through much of their lengths, and in places they were almost blocked by a yellow material like blood-soaked cheese.

'I've not sin owt like that afore.'

'No, it's not common; it's what is called necrotic enteritis. The inside of the bowel dies and becomes this yellow stuff.' The kidneys, bladder, lungs and heart were all fairly normal. 'I don't think there is swine fever here, but I can't be certain with all these pigs being ill, so I must take some samples'. A piece of lung, a length of bowel, the larynx and the kidneys were put into grease-proof paper and put in a cardboard box.

'Now, here are the powders to put in their feed three times a day; give them small feeds and don't move them into the big piggery or the germ will spread in there as well. What are we going to do in this shop? First, George, no more swilling water everywhere; use your sawdust for sweeping out and then burn it. Next, nail sacking over those broken windows; put two paraffin heaters on at full, one at each end of the building, and give the pigs plenty of bedding and sawdust. Here's your licence to move those two lots on Monday.'

'Reet, I'll do that, and I'll let thee know how they fare.'

'Good, but you must report it, if any more die.' After disinfecting himself, Richard left quickly.

It was almost dusk when he got to Causeway Lane, and the car lurched and bounced from pot-hole to pot-hole until he reached Green Acres. Tom Rigby was a big fair-haired young man with a red face and a happy disposition.

'Hello, Mr Holden, I were thinking tha wouldn't get 'ere before tomorrer.'

'I decided to come because I knew you had electric light along with Alan Williams and Hall so we can carry on, though it's going dark quickly. You've reported that you think your pigs have got swine fever.'

'That's reet, they've bin going back for more than a week coughin' and scourin' like, two hev deed.'

'Then I want to check your movement book; have any pigs gone off the place since you bought those?'

'No.'

'That's a help; now I want to examine the ill ones, and do a post mortem on those two dead ones.'

'They're in th' old stable down t' yard.'

Two horses were in the first two stalls, but the last one had been made into a pen. Though the stable was warm and dry, the pigs were huddled together partly hidden in the straw bedding and were very quiet. The two dead pigs were lying in diarrhoeic liquid; their ears were blue and their bellies and legs were a reddish brown colour.

'These are in a bad way, Tom. Did you breed them?'

'No, I bought 'em in Droughton o'er a fortneet gone, they were grand then. I allus put any I buy in 'ere for a bit in case 'owt goes wrong, like tha' told me a good bit sin.'

'I'm glad you did with this lot; bring me some clean water in an old bucket.'

At the post mortem all the diagnostic signs of acute swine fever were present and so another cardboard box was filled with specimens.

'You know, I am fairly certain that these have swine fever.'

'Aye, I were comin round to that way o' thinkin' misel.'

'Have you any others ill?'

'No, they've all bin tut' trough this arternoon, and they're goin in a Monday morn for t' Christmas trade, most are fat.'

Richard looked them over in the big clean piggery, and then gave Tom a movement licence for them.

'Now, don't bring any more on until the Ministry lets you know the result. Will you bring me some more water, so I can disinfect myself, and don't you go to any other farm where there are pigs. If you have to go, you must thoroughly disinfect your boots and anything you take with you and wear a clean suit, and leave your car on the road outside the premises.'

'Aye, I'll do that.'

At the surgery Richard wrapped up his malodorous boxes, then sealed and labelled them. He took them to the railway station, realising that he had a headache and was cold and tired. As he drove down Victoria Street he saw a big van outside the Market Hotel, and wondered what was going on there. It was pleasant to get back home and into the kitchen, but it was not really warm. He moved Tommy and the cats out of the way, and was putting the coal and coke mixture into the stove when Flora came into the room.

'Stop it, Richard, don't put any more in.'

'Why not? I'm cold and it's not very warm in here.'

'I know it's not, because I live here, and it's not warm because I'm trying to save some coal for next week – it's Christmas and we are practically out of coal; you've not brought any coal or slack home lately. What am I to do? Burn the bloody furniture to keep warm?'

'I'm sorry, love, don't get mad. I didn't know it was as bad as that.'

'Well, it is, there's not much left, and coal is getting really scarce. Some children are down at the sidings gates picking up any lumps of coal which fall off the lorries as they come out. It's getting now that if I keep the stove going in here, there will be no fire in the lounge.'

'Oh no; then I'll damn well do something about it next week.'

'You do; now come on and have your tea, and before you start grumbling about it, it is the best I can do.'

It was corned beef stew with dumplings made from soya bean flour and homegrown potatoes and carrots, with a thick slice of the off-white coloured national loaf with which to mop up the gravy. In the autumn Flora had boiled and sweetened blackberries with saccharine and sugar and bottled them. They were the sweet, served with custard. They were washing up when a wave of nausea swept over Richard; he felt dizzy and hot, but said nothing though inwardly he was cursing, thinking that this was the beginning of another cold. The phone rang – it was Ted Wearing from Smithy Farm, Greyhurst with a cow not well.

'Who's that?' asked Flora; Richard told her that it was only in Greyhurst, not too far away.

'I'm glad it is, because you don't look too well tonight, Richard.'

'Oh, I don't know, I've probably a bit of a cold. I won't be long.'

He drove away into the very dark night and took longer than usual to arrive at the farm. The cow had not eaten her hay at midday, so Ted had dosed her with fever medicine, but since the afternoon milking she had begun to breathe quickly. It was a case of pneumonia; the cow's temperature was high and her pulse and breathing rapid.

'Will you bring me a quart of water in a jug, Ted?'

When he returned, he held the cow's horns while Richard passed the stomach tube. When he had mixed a double dose of M & B 693 powder in the water, he pushed a funnel into the end of the tube and poured the fluid into it, following this with a pint of fever medicine.

'That's it for tonight, Ted. As it is airy in here, she'll get enough fresh air. I wouldn't wrap her up because her temperature is high.'

'Dusta think ool git o'er it?'

'I don't know, Ted, I'll be able to have a better idea in the morning when I see how she responds to that medicine. I'll say good night now.'

He was nearly in Wyresham when a back tyre went flat, so he had to change the wheel and was pleased to find that the spare was fully inflated.

Feeling weary, he got back into the car. 'It's bed for you, my lad,' he said to himself, and drove fast to Sandhaven. He stopped at the garage, and put the wheel with the flat tyre against the garage's side door. It was an arrangement he had with Gordon, who always repaired them as soon as possible, giving Richard and also Dr McConnell priority.

When he opened the door and walked into the kitchen at Cross Street he found Flora fast asleep in a chair near the stove, so he very quietly withdrew the key, closed the door, and stood looking at her. She was so lovely, his heart was strangely moved, and he realised just how strongly he loved her. She stirred and opened her eyes.

'You've been a long time, love.'

'Yes, I know, but I had to change a wheel; the tyre went flat.'

'What a nuisance for you. Anyway, now we can have our bedtime drink.'

Richard passed a restless night, awakening twice to find he was wet through with perspiration, and his legs were painful. Nevertheless he could not stay in bed on Sunday morning because Tom Atherton had a horse with a thick leg at the Marsh Gate steelworks. So after a breakfast of porridge followed by reconstituted scrambled egg on toast, he drove to the garage and collected his wheel, Gordon having done the repair to the tyre. The drive to the works on this pleasant mild morning was not appreciated by Richard who still had a headache and felt weary, but he cheered up at Tom Atherton's hearty greeting. 'Now, mi lad, it's great to see thee.' Soon the horse had the stomach tube passed and gallons of saline laxative medicine were pumped into him. At Wearing's farm he repeated the treatment he had given the night before, and then told Ted he would be back in the afternoon. From Sandhaven he went to Bob Hall's at Long Dyke, Pelham, to a case he could have done without. It was a farrowing, and though his knees were painful he delivered the sow of one dead and eight live piglets. After lunch he went into the office and cashed up, and filled in the paying-in book ready to be taken to the bank on Monday morning.

Flora came into the office.

'Have you finished, Richard?'

'Yes, I have, do you want to use the desk?'

'No, I've come to ask you; don't you think we should ring Mum, and ask her over for Christmas?'

'By jove, yes; give her a ring now.'

'And while we are about it don't you think we could have our friends in one night?'

'Oh I do, but what can we give them?'

'Just a drink and a sandwich, I thought.'

'But which night?'

'I thought this Wednesday, because there are only two days to Christmas.'

'Good Lord, it does seem to have come quickly this year.'

'I know, so let's get the decorations out, they will probably do for this year, though I found they were shabby and dropping to bits when I looked at them the other day.'

'Yes, they are; I'll try and get some holly and mistletoe on my travels – they will help out.'

'Oh, they will; you do that.'

Richard dosed Ted Wearing's cow again, it was getting better.

Jean said that she would come on Tuesday and bring whatever she could lay her hands on. 'Thank God for Mum,' said Flora to herself, because rations for two would not go very far in giving their friends a buffet supper. Not all their friends could come; both Tom and Edna Duke were ill with flu. Flora was disappointed, because now and then on a Saturday night they had been to the Dukes' for the evening. If because of this they had missed going to the pictures, Richard and Flora always tried to go on the following Wednesday night, mainly to see the newsreel – the Pathé Gazette.

On Monday, a pleasant mild day, anthrax was confirmed at George Meadow's farm, but the source of the outbreak had not been found. Richard on his way back from the steel works went to Turner's Coal Yard. Young Will sold him two bags of coal called 'bright nuts', and two of slack, which they shoved into the car, regardless of the black dust being scattered on the upholstery. He gave Will some diuretic powders for a horse which was passing 'thick water', and some greasy leg dressing. When he arrived home Flora was overjoyed to see four bags of fuel. Richard emptied the coal into the bunker and then went to the gas works and got the bags filled with coke, which he stored with the slack in the disused outside lavatory next to the garage. Flora remarked that now they would be warm for Christmas, so she had better go and find some food. She was disappointed when Eric Sugden from the Lodge Farm left a note with Marjorie to say that he could not supply a turkey because he had lost too many from blackhead and to a fox. Flora went to Melling's shop and bought a small chicken which she put into the oven to roast as soon as she got home. She calculated that this would feed the three of them, and probably there would be some left over with which she could make sandwiches the next day. To get a bird for Christmas Day, she went post-haste to Wood the butcher where she bought a large capon which Frank with his back towards her wrapped in newspaper. She thought it was dear, but when she unwrapped the bird at home, she was delighted to find that there was a big piece of beef suet with a kidney in the parcel – no wonder it was dear – but even so she told Richard that Frank was an angel! In the afternoon Jean arrived and brought half a leg of mutton, and an ox tongue.

'Mum, however did you manage to get that mutton, there's more than half a month's ration there?'

'Never you mind how I got it. Ruth from the Sitting Goose asked me if I wanted some, do you think I'd be daft enough to say no?'

'Well, Mum, you are a pet; we are having a few friends in for a drink tomorrow night, so now I can make some sandwiches, and as Frank Wood has let me have a big piece of beef suet I want to make some mincemeat straight away. Make a pot of tea while I go and get some apples out of the coach house loft.'

Mother and daughter worked happily together in the kitchen; Jean cut up the suet and then put it through the mincer, and after peeling the apples made the mincemeat. Flora, while keeping an eye on the chicken, cleaned the ox tongue, cut away the fat, then washed it well and put it on to boil. When the chicken was well roasted it was taken out and the mutton was put into the oven. During the evening surgery, the aroma of roast mutton drifted into the hall, making Richard so hungry he could hardly wait for his dinner. The last person in the waiting room was a man from Bishop's bakery, who gave a sealed envelope and a square box to Richard, who thanked him and, after showing him out of the house, locked the door and hurried into the kitchen feeling ravenous.

'What have you got there?'

'I don't know, it's just come from Tommy Bishop.'

He opened the envelope and found a note saying Tom and Joan were very sorry but they would not be able to come on Wednesday evening because their baby Thomas had developed a very bad cold. Meanwhile Flora had opened the box which contained a small iced Christmas cake from Tom and Joan, and six mince pies of the Misses Bishop at the Market Café.

'Isn't that kind of them, Mum,' said Flora, 'I'll just go and phone them to ask how the baby is. Richard, empty the water out of the pan into a basin, take the tongue out and skin it. I'll be back in a minute.'

'I'll believe that when I see it,' said Richard to the departing Flora. Jean laughed and said, 'I agree with you, she's a great talker when she gets on the phone.'

'I hope she's back soon, I'm dying of hunger and yet I am surrounded by more food than I've seen in weeks.'

He dutifully cut all the skin off the steaming tongue. Jean dissolved the isinglass in the hot gravy and when Flora came back they rolled up the tongue and pushed it into a round casserole; it was covered with the gravy solution, a plate was put on top and on the plate a heavy flat iron. The casserole was put in the larder until it went cold.

The long awaited dinner of roast mutton with home grown potatoes, carrots and sprouts was excellent. This was followed by a steamed blackberry pudding. After washing up the pots, they went upstairs to the lounge where Flora had made a good fire. Richard soon dozed off and slept soundly until he was awakened at ten o'clock to have his bedtime drink. He felt better.

On Wednesday morning Jean and Flora only managed to decorate part of the house, because some of the four-year-old coloured paper chains dropped to bits when they were opened. Flora went and bought some holly and mistletoe from Betty Heyes and as this was not enough, she stripped some ivy off the wall of Number 4 Cross Street. Soon it was all put in place and the house looked very festive.

When Richard arrived home for lunch, he found both Jean and Flora upset.

'What on earth has happened, love?'

'Jimmy Lawson has been wounded – you know, Uncle Jerry's eldest lad. Margaret rang from Holme and asked for Jean who took the message. She was rather white and trembling when she came back from the phone to tell me, because it's given Uncle Jack another bad angina attack and he is in bed.'

'And where's Jean now?'

'She's gone to lie down; it's so sad just at Christmas again.' Tears ran down Flora's face as Richard drew her to him and said,

'Don't cry, darling; tell me what exactly has happened to Jim.'

'They were bombing the Ruhr on Monday night when their Lancaster was hit, Jimmy and the rear gunner were wounded, and the pilot managed to get the plane back to England – that's all we know. It's such a blow for Jerry and Gladys.'

'Come on and sit down and I'll make a pot of tea, or would you like a drink?'

'No, make some tea, Richard, and I'll take a cup to Jean and then we will have some lunch.'

They were very subdued while they were having the meal, but decided to have their friends in that evening but not to mention what had happened. Richard thought it was the best course of action because it would take the women's minds off the news about Jim. Flora later made biscuits with Quaker Oats and Jean got out the cutlery and small plates ready for the buffet. After he had finished his afternoon visits Richard went across the road to the Market Hotel when it opened and was pleasantly surprised to see Ben Belcher behind the bar. He was the new landlord, having come from the Wheatsheaf in Wilsdon. They chatted for a few minutes, and Richard bought half a dozen bottles of beer. When he arrived back in the surgery Flora told him that Bob Dawson had sent a message to say that swine fever had been confirmed at Tom Rigby's.

There were only a few animals brought that evening for treatment, but even so Richard was still making the punch at a quarter to eight when the Heyes, Kings and Meadows arrived. They began to tease him, saying that he was a poor barman not having drinks ready when guests arrived; and should they go to the Market pub for half an hour? But it was ready when the Reverend Evans and Edna arrived at the same time as the Lords who had brought their baby son, who ran in when Flora opened the door. She took their top clothes and put them on the table in the waiting room, while they followed little Jimmy up the stairs and into the lounge. Later Dick Harrison the bank manager and Mary his wife came in with Dr McConnell whose partner was a stunning looking blonde: Peggy Pape, the only child of the wealthy soap manufacturer Will Pape of Droughton. It pleased Richard and Flora when in a short time all their friends were obviously enjoying themselves, and the sound of laughter and conversation became much louder. As they moved among their guests they noticed that the daily worries of rationing, fuel shortage and the war were temporarily forgotten except by the Reverend Tom who was complaining bitterly about the low level of heating for the church and the vicarage. Richard stopped this diatribe by promising to ask the Colonel at the Hall to apply for more fuel, especially as he was the senior church warden.

For Flora and Jean the evening was made perfect when Richard opened the front door to find Bill Dickenson standing there. After closing the door Richard turned on the light and saw that Bill was now a sergeant wearing the black beret of the Tank Corps and looking very big and tough. When Richard called upstairs that Bill had come Flora and Jean came running down to greet him, Flora saying it made the evening perfect.

He had surreptitiously given Richard a bottle of whisky, much to the latter's relief; he diluted half of it with twice the amount of water and added it to the punch, which ensured that it would now last the night. The buffet of cut-up meat pies, mutton and chicken sandwiches, followed by oat biscuits and mince pies, quickly disappeared. At half past ten they formed a circle and sang Auld Lang Syne, which awakened Jimmy Lord who had been asleep in a bedroom. Isabel brought him into the lounge, and Flora gave him a bar of chocolate, after which they led the exodus amid much merriment as Christmas greetings were exchanged, and kisses were given under the mistletoe.

Flora brewed tea, and the four of them agreed that the evening had gone off well – it had been a good party. Bill said he thought the victories in Egypt, North Africa and Russia had raised morale generally, and people were more cheerful as the tide of war appeared to be turning in the Allies' favour. Flora said maybe he was right even though shortages were getting worse, and the blackout was a confounded nuisance.

On Christmas Eve Richard received a letter from Norman Robinson in which he sent seasonal greetings, and the information that he was now a Pilot Officer flying on offensive missions and actually enjoying his life in the RAF. After reading it, Richard reflected that Norman was the only close friend he had, that none of his many acquaintances came into this category, and he vaguely wondered why this was so. He slowly realised that professional work consumed all his time and energy, because he wanted to get rid of the mortgage – he still owed many hundreds of pounds. This dedication meant that he was giving his life to veterinary practice, never refusing a call whatever time it was of day or night, and disregarding how he felt mentally or physically. He told himself that he was improving veterinary services in the area, and that he hoped this would make his practice grow. His reverie was ended by the phone ringing – it was Mary who said that as she had not got Christmas leave, she could come on Tuesday night to spend New Year with them. Richard called Flora and Jean to talk to her and wished her a Happy Christmas.

At twelve o'clock on the 25th the four did justice to the roasted capon, which was accompanied by home grown vegetables – even the sage and onion used for the stuffing were home grown. The three of them drank a bumper toast to Mrs Greenfingers – 'to our Flora, the blushing head gardener.' With a glass of whisky and water in her hand, she stood up and thanked them for the toast, and said that in 1943 a lot more digging and gardening would have to be done.

Lunch over, the presents were distributed by Richard who gave to Flora a bottle of perfume which Jim Lord had procured. She also got two books – one on antiques, the other on gardening. They gave to Jean two towels, and one to Bill who also got a tin of Ogden's pipe tobacco. Richard thanked Flora for his present which was a pair of brown shoes. They were made to war time utility standards, and Richard considered them to be a bit shoddy when compared with the lovely brown shoes he used to buy in J.H. Lees Store in Liverpool before the war. At three o'clock they listened to the King's speech on the wireless, after which they decided to stay round the lovely fire in the lounge, rather than go for a walk on this raw chilly day.

Bill left on Sunday because he had only a seventy-two hour pass, and had to be back before 'Lights Out' that night. On Monday Richard drove Jean to the station after lunch to catch the ten past one train which would enable her to arrive home before dark. 'It's back to work with a vengeance,' said Flora that night as she carried all the sheets and pillow cases downstairs. While she put them to soak in a dolly tub, Richard dismantled the folding bed in the lounge and put it away behind the wardrobe in the small bedroom. Being almost year end he had spent the afternoon in the office planning work for the future, paying accounts he owed, and then cashing up.

Next morning at six o'clock George Meadows rang to say that he had found another cow dead. Richard's examination of a stained blood film showed that it was anthrax again.

'Where the hell is it coming frae? The Ministry men worked hard to get shut of it and all t' place has bin scrubbed wi' disinfectant.'

'I know, George, but they did not find out how the germ was getting here.'

'Did ta find out at Crooks at th' Oaks?'

'Yes, it was from cattle bones dug up when they made the trench to take the pipeline to the new factory.'

'Well, how many more cows will dee of it?'

'I don't know.'

'Ye don't – hell fire, 'ow did yer stop it at Crooks?'

'By injecting every cow with anti-anthrax serum.'

'Reet, when con ta do 'em?'

'As soon as I can get some serum sent from London.'

'Blast it, how long ull that tek?'

'It could be here tomorrow on a fast train.'

'Thee get some.'

'I will, George, but don't forget it's dear.'

'What dusta mean by dear? I've lost near on two hundred pounds worth of cattle in a fortneet.'

'Probably forty or fifty pounds, depending on how many cattle you have.'

'That's nowt, thee order it straight away.'

'How many cows and heifers have you got?'

'I'll go and git mi book and tha con count how many doses tha'll need.'

On his way home he stopped at Sandhaven Police Station and reported this second case of anthrax; later in the surgery he informed the Ministry of Agriculture and Food.

He had just finished breakfast when Mr Walmsley rang from Seaton, and asked Richard to go as soon as possible to treat his dog which was acting very strangely. The Walmsleys who owned two very large ladies' fashion shops – one in Seaton and the other in Sandhaven – lived in some style at Meols Hall on St. Anne's Lane. Richard put the dog catcher in his car, and checked that he had some morphine hydrochloride hypodermic tablets in his bag.

He was soon stopping at the top of the drive in front of the Hall. Mr Walmsley came down the steps and explained that Jane their Dalmatian bitch had been rather quiet for some days, and had taken one of his slippers to her bed, and growled when he tried to take it off her. This morning she had run into the dining room and, standing under the table, was snarling and snapping at anyone who went near.

'Very well, Mr Walmsley, this is what I will do. We will go into the room together, and while you distract her attention I will push this loop of my dog catcher over her head and drag her out.'

So it happened and Richard dragged the very aggressive dog roughly into the hall, where she struggled and snarled.

'Don't hurt her, please,' called Mrs Walmsley from the safety of the stairs.

'I'm not hurting her, I'm controlling her – she will soon calm down when I have given her an injection. Mr Walmsley, hold this handle, keep the dog away from you, and keep the rope pulled tight.'

The injection of morphia soon took effect, the bitch vomited, and then slavering copiously lay down; Richard removed the dog catcher and examined her. Her mammary glands were very swollen.

'Has she had pups?'

'No.'

'Then she is suffering from phantom pregnancy, a condition related to her sexual cycle, which can be treated.'

'Mr Holden, my wife and I are now afraid of Jane, and the children won't go near her. Will you please take her away and put her to sleep.'

'How old is she?'

'Two and a half.'

'I don't like destroying a healthy dog when it could have a good life elsewhere. Would you let her go to a farm where she will be well looked after and will be a guard dog?'

'What do you say, Violet?'

'I think it's a great idea, Mr Holden. Would you do that, please,' said a more composed Mrs Walmsley.

'Very well, Mr Holden, she is all yours.'

'Then I'll take her to Mr George Dobson at East View Farm, Catley.'

George came for the bitch later in the day and said, 'Thanks, Mr 'olden, 'er ull mek a good pal for t' other devil.'

'How do you manage him, George?'

'All reet, he knows who's boss when I've gitten mi stick, and he's a damned good guard dog. This 'un will soon larn I'm t' boss, and I were thinkin I might hev some black and white Airedale terriers afore long. Esta iver sin one?' It kept Richard amused for hours thinking what they would look like.

At lunchtime Flora was happy; she was singing in the kitchen when Richard walked in, and she told him that from Jean she had learned that Jim was much better, but would be in hospital some weeks until his badly broken leg healed. Uncle Jack had recovered and was going back to his office in the Town Hall in Holme; and Mary was coming alone at four o'clock, because her friend Rosemary was going home to her family for the New Year.

On Wednesday morning Richard was at the station to meet the 10.50 train, and got the box from the International Serum Company from the guard after signing for it. He then went to the Railway 'A' stable and treated a horse which had a septic wound on its near hind leg. He at once went home for an early lunch, and that afternoon injected every beast at Boundary Farm. He fervently hoped that it would end the anthrax cases; time proved that it did.

It was pitch dark when he had finished there, but he went on to Whitehouse Farm at Carden. Tom Greaves met Richard with, 'I thowt tha'd forgotten mi, Mr 'olden.'

'No, Tom, I've been delayed, that's all, by having to inject nearly a hundred animals this afternoon, and it's taken longer than I expected. Where's your cow?'

'In t' back, thee follow me.' The oil lamp which he took off a hook gave very little light as he walked up the passageway between the line of cows. Richard, feeling rather tired, followed the dim outline of Tom. As he said, 'She's along 'ere,' the light almost disappeared, and at that moment Richard, unable to see the two steps down, stumbled forwards and crashed his head against the stone lintel of the doorway.

'Blast it,' he shouted as he fell on his back. Tom and the light reappeared in a second.

'As ta' hurt th'sell? I should ev said mind step.'

'By God, you should, I damn well saw stars.'

'Let's hev a look; by gum, it's a fair lump all reet.'

'Is it? Then I'm glad the neb of my cap cushioned it a bit.' Tom helped Richard to his feet.

'Ow dusta feel?'

'A bit dizzy and my head hurts.'

'Then thee cum an hev a sit down.'

'No I won't; let's get on.'

Richard soon treated the case of slow fever and was glad to be setting off home.

'Damn it, whatever have you done this time?' said Flora. 'Look, I'm getting fed up with you coming home kicked and battered for me to look after. Do you think your so-called farmer friends appreciate what you do for them?'

'Oh they do, I'm certain.'

'Then they've a damned funny way of showing it when you are treating their animals. You're the one that always gets hurt, not them. I don't think it would matter to some of them if you dropped dead.'

'Flora, you are not being fair; you know the Royal College says you've got to be available twenty-four hours a day, and that's why I get so bloody weary that I walked into a door lintel at Tom Greaves. I missed the steps down because I couldn't see because he had the lamp inside his coat because of the bloody black-out.'

'Come on and sit down, that's going to be bathed straight away.' After she had finished he took two aspirin compound tablets and ate his tea. There were only two for surgery which pleased Richard whose head was aching continuously, so he took two more tablets and went to bed at half past seven.

Next morning the lump on his forehead was bluish red in colour and so sore that he could not wear his cap. He searched his wardrobe until he found an old woolly tam-o'-shanter which was more comfortable. He went to Sands House Farm at Ryton to see Leslie Howarth who would not tell Richard on the telephone what was wrong. Leslie, over six feet tall, was an impressive figure, well respected in the community, being a local preacher for the Methodist Church and chairman of the Parish Council. Driving an old Bean car he and his sons delivered milk to most of the three hundred or so inhabitants of the village.

He came straight to the point. 'Mr Holden, my Henry was stopped the other day and the milk sampled, and I've got a summons saying I've added water to my milk. I've never done such a thing, so I want you to help me, and find out how it's happened.'

Richard thought for a few seconds.

'There are five ways I can think of – a leaking cooler; old cows giving milk low in fat; a can not having been drained properly after it had been cleaned; or water getting in on a very wet day; or you or somebody with a spite against you did it.'

'I've never done anything like that in my life; don't you start accusing me.'

'Calm down, Leslie, I'm not accusing you; you asked me how does water get there, and I've answered your question, so now what do you want me to do?'

'Well then, as you're on my side, try and find out how the water got into the milk.'

'This summons, are you going to plead "guilty" or "not guilty"?'

'"Not guilty"; I've done nowt wrong.'

'I believe you; I only asked because you'll want your solicitor to defend you, and vouch for whatever I do.'

'Oh, I'll soon get him, he lives near, in that big house at the Cross Road on Wyresham Road.'

'Then you go and get him to come and bring some labels and sealing wax with you.'

At that moment, there was the sound of a car coming into the yard, 'Eee, that's lucky,' said Leslie, rushing outside. 'Ernie!' he shouted, 'thee tak me up to Oakfield this minit.'

'Wora about customers?'

'Let them wait, come on, git goin.'

Richard now went into the dairy; it was spotlessly clean. The milk cooler had been scoured for so long over the years that most of the nickel plating had disappeared, exposing a gleaming copper surface and white soldered seams. He examined it carefully and the hose which carried the cold water. He could not see any cracks or holes, and two empty ten gallon churns had been left upside down after scalding – so no water could have got in from them.

Soon Ernest and Leslie with Mr Ward the solicitor arrived, and after being introduced to him Richard explained that he wanted him to witness the collection of the milk samples, and the testing of the cooler. They all walked into the thirty shippon, which was very clean and the walls had been recently white washed. All the cattle were Friesians, and Richard noticed that most were old and had pendulous udders.

'Do you always buy old cows, Leslie?'

'Yes. I do that, 'cos they're cheaper, and they give a lot of milk, and now Will Turner at the Grange has got a Friesian bull, it serves them and I've had some good calves.'

'I appreciate your reasons, but the longer old cows milk the poorer their milk becomes, with less fat and it's almost water.'

'I don't believe you.'

'It's right, Leslie. Now, which are the oldest in this lot? Let's have a look.'

By looking at their horn rings they chose sixteen cows, and Richard said, 'Ernie, will you get a bucket and milk a few squirts out of each quarter of these sixteen cows. Leslie, has your bulk milk gone yet?'

'No, it's on the stand.'

They went into the yard and after Leslie had stirred the milk round, Richard poured milk from the dipper into two large sterile bottles, then tightly corked them, and using a lighted match sealed them with red wax on which he pressed his signet ring. When he had labelled them he gave one to Leslie. As soon as Ernest had finished milking, Richard sampled that milk also, again giving one bottle to Leslie.

'Now, Leslie, I'll send my two bottles to the laboratory for analysis and you can either keep yours, or send them to another laboratory.'

'Right, I understand, Mr Holden.'

'Then next we will test the cooler.'

After Leslie had blocked the bottom pipe he brought a jug and Richard mixed methylene blue with the water. This was then poured into the cooler at the top, and they waited to see what would happen. From the third corrugation a slight dribble of blue water began to run down.

'Well I never,' said Leslie, 'who'd believe that?'

'I hope the magistrates will,' said Mr Ward, 'and use it as a mitigating circumstance when they reach their verdict.'

'So they should, I haven't added water deliberately.'

'That's not the point, Mr Howarth, water unknown to you was added to your milk.'

'And as Mr Ward will notice, the hole has been made by your attention to cleanliness, and you've scrubbed the solder away at that spot.'

Leslie looking rather crestfallen said, 'Well, Mr Ward, you can tell them the truth, can't you; that being so clean has caused that hole, and I didn't know.'

'Yes. I'm taking in all these points.'

'Very well, gentlemen, I'll leave you to discuss what you will say,' and Richard left.

Some weeks later in the courtroom, one of the magistrates was a farmer. It made no difference; they found the charge– proved, after taking into account that the milk from the old cows contained only 2.9% fat. So Leslie was fined, and the reporter from the *Farmer's Times* was the first person to leave the court room, which resulted in a long report in the next edition. The notoriety did not last long, nor do Leslie any harm – his sales of milk increased!

Richard visited another farm and two stables that morning before driving back to Sandhaven and round to the garage. Gordon Hindle came out.

'How many do you want, Richard?'

'Four gallons, that should fill her up.'

'Have you heard that private motoring is going to be banned from tomorrow?'

'No I didn't; does that mean less petrol?'

'I don't know, Richard, but it looks like rationing is going to be even stricter.'

'And yet people are selling petrol coupons on the black market.'

'Yes, I know they do, but that's because they can't run their cars. I don't think that racket will last long.'

'What about me, Gordon, should I apply for more coupons straight away?'

'I would, Richard; I've only coupons for fourteen gallons left for you.'

'I'll do that, then. Happy New Year to you and Pat when it comes!'

'Same to you, and keep sober.'

Arriving at the surgery he was just in time to wish Mavis and Marjorie all the best. Flora remarked that he sounded a lot more cheerful.

'Oh I am, my headache has stopped, though this lump is still very tender.'

'I bet it is, but what do you expect? I was telling Joan Bishop and she said you should get danger money. By the way, Baby Tom is better; they are so relieved after spending Christmas nursing him. Anyway, lunch is ready, so come on in.'

He had hoped to spend the afternoon in the office and the surgery, but he had to go to Birchnott Farm at Ridgeton. A heifer was unable to calve because one of the legs of the calf was turned back. Richard soon corrected this malpresentation, and helped by Harold Fowler and his man he delivered a live heifer calf. Harold was pleased.

'It's a good 'un is that; it ull suit mi dad, yer see he bought it a month sin – full pedigree heifer, and 'e wanted a heifer calf out of 'er, and he's getten one. 'e's trying to upgrade our 'erd and get it in t' 'erd book.'

'Then it's a good sign for the New Year, and all the best to you and your wife.'

'Same to you Mr 'olden.'

Richard drove the nineteen miles home in a buoyant mood; he was feeling better than he had for some weeks. After surgery he and Flora passed the evening warm and cosy in front of a large fire in the lounge. After supper they switched on the wireless, and listened to the service. Richard poured out a whisky for Flora, and a brandy for himself, and as Big Ben rang out the last strokes of 1942, they clinked glasses, and drank to a Happy New Year. Putting down his glass, Richard kissed Flora passionately.

1943

Richard found that what Gordon had said about the ban on private motoring was true; when on his way to Mereside he saw only one other private car in two miles, but a lot of the Air Force's vehicles. He liked John Tomlinson at School Farm, – a very pleasant young man who came quickly to the point.

''Ello, Mr 'olden, yon injection didn't work,' so Richard had manually to remove the retained cleansing from his cow. He then examined two calves with pneumonia, injected them with pneumonia serum, and went out to the car to get some powders for them. Looking across the yard he was alarmed to see that little Alan Tomlinson who was about four years old had got into a pen and was walking about among some yearlings. He ran back into the calf house shouting, 'John, quick, your little lad has got into a pen across the yard.'

''as'e? I'm not surprised; 'e's done it for six month; they won't 'arm 'im. Mi wife's father sez e's a stockman already.'

'He jolly well must be; now those are the powders for the calves, mix them up one at a time in a dessertspoonful of custard or rice pudding and scrape it onto the back of the tongue – don't drench them.'

'Reet, an' I want some mastitis powders.'

When Richard gave them to him he asked, 'And how are they at Shepherd's Farm? I haven't seen them for some time.'

'They're all reet; they've nowt wrong; and tha' knows Tom being a butcher and all, knocks owt int' head that looks a bit dicky.' And Richard thought, I bet he will have a good market for it as well. The rest of the morning was spent doing semi-urgent work. He opened the blocked teat of a newly calved cow, saw a young horse with 'a bad cold' which proved to be strangles and scouring calves and cows. For the calves he gave medicine and for the cows Phenothiazine powders to be followed by astringent powders. When later that day he checked his notes on Isovacuil, he decided to stop using it, and to cleanse mares and cows manually again. He now changed the composition of his cream for use in all obstetrical work, using Dettol in place of AC. Carbolic glyc. He applied regularly now for a permit, so that he could get the very mild soft soap from Field's before he used up all his cream. When he went into the kitchen after evening surgery, Flora told him that the news was that the German Army at Stalingrad had been surrounded by the Russians.

'My word, that is a good start to the New Year.'
'It is,' said Flora, 'and I hope it goes on getting better.'

The week after, when a supply of tuberculin had come from the Royal Veterinary College he did Bill Meadow's herd test at Whyngate, and took the three blood samples. Richard noticed what a willing intelligent young man David Roberts was; no infection would be brought onto the farm by him. Yet two cows were doubtful reactors to the tuberculin test, so would have to retested in sixty days time; the best news was that the three blood samples were negative for contagious abortion. At lunchtime Flora said she was going from two until four o'clock to the WVS to help, and Marjorie would now come every Monday afternoon.

The next day he went to Pirton Hall Farm and met the two Hodge brothers. They told him that Tom Lee at Marhey had recommended him to be their vet, because they had sacked Mr McCrea from Wiiton. They showed him a big Ayrshire cow, six weeks calved and in very good condition, which was not eating well and its milk yield was going down. It was a case of slow fever, which he treated with glucose intravenously, and left them the usual powders. A second cow was thin though eating well, but had a history of scouring twice in the last month. Richard took a dung sample from the cow and gave them tonic powders for her. That night a microscopical examination of the sample revealed that she had Johne's disease. He idly wondered why the first animals treated for a new client invariably died or had to be slaughtered. He rang the Hodges and told them to get the cow killed. Very politely he was thanked for the speed with which a definite diagnosis had been made; this cheered him up, as did the news on the radio that the German Army at Stalingrad was being liquidated by shell fire, starvation and the bitter Russian winter – it could not break out of the ring of steel which encircled it.

On one or two fine days Flora worked in the garden nearest the house – she called it her kitchen garden. She raked together all the dead leaves, bits of twigs, and rubbish and burned them, then she overhauled and oiled all the gardening tools and rang up Liz Meadows and ordered some manure to be delivered at the end of February. By now she had read the Christmas present gardening book twice, and had planned her garden work for the coming season.

On an early morning visit to Smithy Farm at Greyhurst, Richard soon discovered what was wrong with the six calves.

'Ted, these calves have ringworm, what have you been putting on them?'

'Train oil and creosote.'

'Fat lot of good that will do – you've nearly poisoned them.'

'Gerr away, it's cured 'em afore.'

'Maybe, but their tongues are nearly raw. Don't use it again. I'll give you some M&T mouth wash; dab it on their tongues with a piece of clean cloth. You know, you can catch ringworm, so put some old gloves on, and clip away all these scabs and matted hair and burn them. Then gently rub in this dressing once a day for five days. If it's a mild day let them out to graze for a bit – Johnny Green helps a lot.'

'Reet, I'll ger it done.'

'And burn the gloves afterwards and scrub all the muck off these pens with hot soda water.'

Ted had a circular saw in the yard and a man, having attached the driving belt to the wheel on the milking machine engine, started it up, and began to saw up tree trunks, of which there were plenty.

'You don't mean to be cold, Ted.'

'By gum, I don't; there'll be six months firing there when they're all cut up. Dusta want some?'

'I would like some very much. We get very little coal, so they would help a lot.' Soon Richard had stacked as many short logs as he could into the car. On the way back, he called to see a cow at Sykes on Beech Hill. He had seen her the night before, and she had a bad mastitis. He opened the gate, drove into the yard, and then closed the gate. A voice shouted 'Help, Help.' Richard looked down the yard and saw a few cows drinking from the trough or wandering about, and among them was a young Ayrshire bull.

'Where are you?'

'In the midden, come and 'elp me!'

Richard ran across, and as he looked over the wall, the voice said, 'Watch yon bloody bull.' A man was lying on his back with one leg lying at an acute angle – obviously broken.

'Mr 'olden, wil ta go and git boss, es in t' house.'

Richard ran out of the yard, closed the gate behind him, and crossed the road to the house, where his knocking brought Ted Roberts to the door.

'What's up, Mr 'olden?'

'Your bull has tossed your man into the midden and I think he's got a broken leg.'

'Hell, has ee? Misses, phone doctor quick, while us goes and helps him.'

The leg was broken, but Richard would not let Ted move the man until the doctor arrived, hurrying down the yard with Mrs Roberts. Now the bull and cows had been driven into the shippon. Harry was given a drink of tea, and then under the doctor's directions carefully lifted out of the muck, and lowered onto a door, where the leg was immobilised and Harry was given an injection of morphia. Ted had the young bull slaughtered that day because his father had died after being gored by one. What had happened was that the bull and the cows had been let out to drink; Harry was wheeling a barrow full of muck across the yard and had almost reached the midden when the bull had charged and tossed him over the wall, where though injured he was safe. He was back at work six weeks later: as he said, thankful to be alive.

The cow with mastitis recovered but the quarter was lost. Richard began to question his treatment of mastitis cases; he was getting more and more on some farms in spite of everything from injecting every cow with autogenous vaccine, to having the milk machine serviced regularly. What more could he do? He decided to take a milk sample from every mastitis case, and to examine the sediment when stained microscopically. The next case was at Dobson's at East View, Catley. As he drove up the drive to the farm gate, he could see the two guard dogs beyond it watching his approach.

'I'm not getting out to open the gate,' he said aloud. 'Come on, George.' He blew the car horn, and the dogs frantically jumped up and barked. George appeared, stick in hand, and shouted at them. They at once dashed into their respective barrels, one each side of the gate, which George opened. Richard drove well up the yard, stopped the car and got out.

'You've got two good sentries there, George.'

'Aye I hev that; they're worth their keep. So far I've gitten 'arf a blue trouser leg and a bit of a khaki one.'

'And I bet not lost one bird.'

'Yer reet theer, I 'aven't.'

'Good, let's have a look at the cow.' It was an acute mastitis. Richard took a sample of the milk, injected the cow with a big dose of Soluseptasine, and gave George mastitis powders with which to start dosing her at once.

By microscopical examination he found streptococci, yet he had to treat the cow three times before she recovered and was left very light on that quarter. He decided that every case would be injected with mastitis serum and Soluseptasine, be given suphanilamide powders, and if possible the infected quarter would have Euflavine aseptically pumped into it. As the clusters were passed from cow to cow, he used to emphasise that they must be disinfected and then dipped in clean water between each cow and not used on infected cows. Over the next few weeks he did his best to convince Tom Collinson, Jack Booth, Tom Priestley and others.

At the end of the month Bumble started calling, so he took her to Tom Billsborough's in Droughton. When he rang the door bell, the door was opened by a young man – a Flight Lieutenant in the RAF who was Tom's son and on leave. After the cat had been put in a cage Richard asked him how difficult it was bombing Germany and told him about Jimmy's injury. Young Tom said that it was getting more dangerous, and that Jim had been lucky in that they had got back to England. He had been in a squadron which kept attacking Berlin and had had many losses, but now the Americans were helping, he was certain the opposition from the ground was slightly weaker. That evening it was announced that Berlin had been attacked the night before, and that three of our aircraft were missing. Richard wondered if the Germans in Russia knew of the damage that was being done in their homeland – I bet they don't, he said to himself.

When the laboratory report stated that both blood samples were negative, Richard was pleased and Bill Meadows at Whyndyle was delighted that his herd was free at last from the abortion disease.

February saw another tightening of the people's rations – milk now was only a pint a day per person. George Meadows told Richard to collect some at the farm if ever he was short. The herd inspections produced two more TB cows, and Fred Noblett at Highgate had two cows abort at seven months. The blood samples were positive from these two which were going dry. They had been tied up along with six others in a small shippon. Fred sold the lot at the next Friday auction, 'because owt is better than gerrin it through my 'erd.' Pity the fellow who brought them, went through Richard's mind. The week after Richard brought Bumble home, George Street was closed for repairs to be made to a sewer, but it did not cause much inconvenience because there was so little traffic.

The first morning of the Tuberculin test at George Arrowsmith's went smoothly and quickly because all the adult cattle and the heifers were tied up. Only the calves had to be caught and held while they were dealt with. So at ten o'clock they stopped work and went into the kitchen in the farmhouse. Richard ate the cheese sandwiches and drank his tea with relish. Looking at the north through the kitchen widow he could see men working on a tall chimney.

'Are they taking the isolation hospital chimney down?'

'Nay, they're meken it 'igher, worse luck. It spoils view for t' missus 'evin to look at it every day.'

'So they are making the hospital bigger, are they?'

'Well, they've built a bit on the back, but its not really th' isolation 'ospital now, because TB cases are 'ere now. Tha sees they won't 'ave em in t' new American 'ospital at Wilsdon; that's for pilots that's bin hurt. So our lads and theirs that's gitten TB are 'ere now. If tha goes up to th 'ospital, tha con see 'em in all weathers on t' balconies in bed wrapped up in red blankets. Rather them than me. Now we'd better ger on.'

When Richard arrived home at lunch time, Flora met him at the door.

'Have you seen our Bumble?

'No, why?'

'Well, she's missing; she went out about seven o'clock last night and that's the last I've seen of her.'

'That's strange, I wonder if she's in the coach house.'

'She isn't. Mavis and I have looked everywhere, but there is no sign of her. I do hope nothing has happened to her, she's so much my cat.'

In the late afternoon, Richard walked along Cross Street, up George Street where the sewer men were finishing work, then along Manor Road, and finally down Victoria Road to the surgery. As there was no sign of her, he walked across the road to the Police Station and reported her missing.

'A Siamese cat wearing a blue collar, with a disc with her name and address on it; it should be easy to spot. I'll tell the lads to look out for her, Mr Holden,' said the Station Sergeant, 'because the weather has turned bitter today, she will be feeling cold.'

'She will that, she likes being near the fire; I hope you find her soon.'

'We'll do our best.' But after a week of night frost and very cold winds she was still missing, and Flora was very depressed and tearful. This was forgotten amidst all the distress of the death of Uncle Jack, who collapsed the next morning as he was walking to the Town Hall and died immediately. Again Jean rang Flora with the news, and when Richard called in the surgery at half past ten he found her distraught.

'Oh Richard, poor Auntie Margaret, it's dreadful for her now after Ben and Mark; Uncle Jack has gone, and they were such a great family,' and she sobbed and sobbed.

'Flora, come on, listen to me, you mustn't get so upset. I'll get you a drink and then tell me what you want to do.' Sipping her drink she became calmer, and decided to go to Holme the next day. Richard took her to the station to catch an early train. 'You will tell her, Flora, how sorry I am and that she has my sincere sympathy.'

'Yes. I'll do that, I'll come back on the five to five train.'

'You do, I'll meet you love, take care.'

As he drove away to do his farm visits, he thought that this appeared to be one of those weeks when the unexpected happens. First Bumble disappears, and now Uncle Jack has died – I wonder what will be next. The day quickly passed dealing with the winter ills of livestock, most of the morning being spent at Blacklands farm at Ryton where four cows were suffering from proven poisoning. Tom Bolton was happy-go-lucky in his attitude to his stock – doors tied shut with string; cow ties made of old binder twine; pigs' pens constructed of old corrugated iron sheets; and gaps in the hedge blocked up with old bedsteads. No wonder his sheep grazed all over the parish!

Richard arrived at the farm to find one cow down and obviously dying and three others swollen up and ill owing to the food fermenting in their stomachs.

'Aye, they git loose in t' neet, and pushed proven house door open.'

'And how much have they eaten?'

'I don't know like; tha sees I mix mi proven up in an old bath, an it were pretty full last neet, so they've had a fair do.'

'Then, Tom, they have a frothy sticky mass of food inside them; it's fermenting and poisoning them, and it will kill them before they can pass it.'

'What dusta think I should do?'

'Send them for killing at once before they die on you.' At that moment the cow which was down died, and as they watched it Richard said, 'You see what I mean, Tom.'

'Aye I do, and worra about 'er now?'

'I'll take a blood sample and then tell Bob Whiteside to collect her.'

'Reet, I'll get them to Droughton as fast as I con.'

'Then I'll ring Tom Noblett, and tell him that they are coming.' The blood sample was negative; and two cows were passed fit for human consumption, one condemned.

A very sad Flora said that Jack and Brenda were with Auntie Margaret, and Mary who was in the Wrens was on her way from Plymouth. The funeral would be on Monday at St. John's Church in Holme.

It was a bitterly cold morning when Richard went to Arrowsmith's to read the results of the test, and was glad to get into the warm shippons where the cows were tied up. They quickly worked their way through them and all passed the test. They had a drink of tea and then crossed the road to the big wooden building, half of which was the heifer shippon for twenty and the other half part workshop and part implement shed. With his callipers dangling at the end of a piece of string round his neck, he squeezed between the first two heifers to measure the skin fold. One was doubtful and the other was a reactor – it had failed the test.

'Thee measure it again, Mr 'olden, it can't be right,' said George, but it was, and out of the nineteen heifers only two passed, six were doubtful, and eleven failed the test. Consternation reigned; voices were raised.

'But where the hell has it come frae? They're all home bred and never bin off shop.'

'You are sure nobody's cattle got among them last year?'

''Course I am, nowt con git in this heifer field – it's a good hedge an' a fence.'

'And what about water?'

'There's piped water frae this building to trough in t' middle, sethee there in t' field.'

'And they can't get to the brook?'

'Nay, it's t'other side o' t' hedge.'

'Have you had any casual workers helping you last year?'

'Nay, we're all t' same as we 'ave bin for four year.'

'It's a mystery now, but there must be some explanation.'

'I wish tha' could bloody well think what it is, Mr 'olden – it's a mystery to me.'

'I know, but it's such a strange result that I'll have a word with Mr Dawson of the Ministry in Droughton. Until we have found out where it's come from, you will have to keep them in quarantine here; don't let them out, keep one set of shovels and brushes for them, and only one man looks after them; and don't forget he disinfects his boots and hands every time he has been among them. Now, let's have a bucket of water and we can disinfect ourselves before we go to the calves.'

All the calves passed the test, and Richard was annoyed with himself because he could not think of a reason why the heifers failed. Arriving home, he talked to Bob Dawson on the phone, who was at once very interested in and puzzled by these results, and arranged to meet Richard at the farm even though it was a private test. He examined the animals himself, and then they went into the house, and he questioned George about the heifers more thoroughly than Richard had done. Robert, George's son, gave the first hint of a solution, but none of them appreciated the fact.

'Dad; dusta' think someat were left on t' grass when t' brook flooded bottom 'alf of field last year?'

'What dusta say, Mr Dawson?'

'It could have come down the brook, I suppose, but it must have been a lot of infection; who is your neighbour at the next farm up the lane?'

'Billy Gregson at Corner Farm.'

'Mr Holden, did you take any TB cow from there last year?'

'No, he's a healthy small herd; I don't go there often.'

'And what's the next farm?'

'That's Ralph Crompton at the Mill in Pickhill,' said George.

'And you've had no trouble there?'

'No,' replied Richard.

'Does your land border the isolation hospitals?'

'Nay, it's nowhere near it.'

'But Mr Dawson, the other day Mr Arrowsmith told me the hospital is now taking TB patients.'

'Hum, maybe they are, but they are always very careful that no infection escapes; there are traps and filters everywhere, and they incinerate everything they can. But I think it might be worth making inquiries. However, for the present, Mr Arrowsmith, I would advise you to keep these animals isolated here; and let Mr Holden retest them before you turn out in a couple of months.'

'If this sort of weather keeps on, there'll be nowt to turn out to any road.'

'Yes, it is bitter today and last night's frost was severe. Thank you very much for the tea and cake, Mrs Arrowsmith, it was very kind of you; now I must be off. Good day to you all.'

'Good day,' said George, 'and thanks, Mr 'olden, for gerrin him 'ere, becos he must have sin a lot of failures, but he hasn't condemned them heifers. I'll do as he ses, and wait for t' spring.'

'I think that's the best thing you can do, and I hope he can find out why they failed.'

On that cold afternoon, Richard and Flora arrived at Cross Street at the same time, and while she was making an evening meal she recounted the events of the day.

'It was such a big funeral, he must have been very well liked by everybody. The Mayor and Mayoress were there with members of the Corporation, and of course all the staff from his office. Among the family wreaths on the coffin I could see ours when he was carried into church. It was wrapped in the Union Jack, and the British Legion carrying their standard were there, because he had been in the East County regiment in the Great War.'

'I never knew that, Flora – he never talked about it.'

'No, he didn't, I know; we were in the pew behind Auntie Margaret and all her family, with Uncle Terry and Gladys, and cousin Jim had come limping along on his crutches. He was with poor Mark as usual; they have been great friends since they were children. After the service I saw Bob Mattinson and Bill Bond, and they told me that Charlie Dean had died just after Christmas. They asked how you were.'

'Dear me, Charlie dead, that is sad; he couldn't have been more than fifty. Where did you have lunch?'

'In the Assembly Rooms, and then I went back with all of them to Auntie Margaret's with Uncle Jerry; being a solicitor he is dealing with everything for her.'

'Yes, it's lucky she has him to help her. By the way, what is Mark doing?'

'You wouldn't believe it but he runs the kiosk in the station entrance – it sells tobacco and newspapers. I was talking to his sister Jean and she says he has enough sight in one eye to let him get about. Of course he carries a white stick, but he is obviously doing quite well.'

'That's great; but let's have tea, and you can tell me more when I've done surgery.'

Next morning Mavis was so excited that she could hardly get her words out as she rushed in through the front door.

'Mrs 'olden, yer must come quick, I think our Bumble is under the grid at the end o' t' street. I 'eard her crying and when I called her name she answered me.'

Breakfast was forgotten in the rush. Flora and Mavis ran all the way, Richard bringing up the rear carrying a basket. People stopped to see what was happening as Flora on her knees was shouting, 'Bumble, Bumble,' through the manhole cover.

'It's her, Richard, come on, get her out quick. Oh, do something, for God's sake.'

Richard ran to the workmen in George Street and told them what he wanted. They grabbed some handles and came running, then they lifted off the heavy metal cover.

'Aye, poor little devil's 'ere all reet.'

Sitting on the top of the broad stone steps which led down into the sewer was a dirty, pathetically thin, Bumble, her head flopping on the step. She was mewing plaintively. As Richard knelt down and picked her up, she began to twitch, so he put her quickly into the basket. Flora thanked the two men, who said that she must have got into the sewer when they had it open in George Street the week before. Mavis ran ahead to the surgery to get a hot water bottle ready, and Richard went into the consulting room and put the basket on top of the warm radiator. When he raised the lid the cat was having clonic spasms.

Flora begged, 'Richard, can't you do something? Don't let her die.'

'She's not dying, she's thawing out; put the bottle in and then the blanket when I lift her. That's it, now we'll leave her for a bit and then I'll give her some normal saline.'

An hour after this Bumble was sitting up in the basket and feebly lapping milk from a saucer held by a jubilant Flora – so happy to have got her cat back.

The next day the weather turned milder so when the half load of manure was delivered during the next week John began digging it in on the Saturday. That night at the pictures Richard and Flora saw the Sword of Honour which the King had presented to the citizens of Stalingrad for its heroic, unyielding resistance to the Germans.

Those last days in February, and the first few in March were very wet and windy, poor weather for the lambing which had just started on the farms near to Sandhaven. Early one morning Bill Gregson from Corner Farm brought into the surgery a semi-conscious ewe with her lamb which was still wet – she had never licked it.

'I found 'er doin nowt though both legs were showing, so I pulled lamb out, but oo couldna ger up.'

'Yes, she can't because she has got something like milk fever in a cow.'

As Richard injected 50 c.c. of solution intravenously the ewe began to revive so he completed the treatment by injecting 50 c.c. under the skin on both sides of the neck.

'I think that will be enough for now, and get that lamb to suck as soon as you can. Here, rub him dry with this old towel.'

'Could I 'ev some of that stuff, Mr 'olden, for when I sees one staggering about? I 'ev a syringe, tha' knows.'

'Yes, Bill, but you must be clean. Keep your syringe in weak Dettol and water, then all you have to do is wash it in clean water and put it together. You must also rub that rubber bung with pretty strong Dettol and also both sides of the ewe's neck, then you should be all right.'

'Thanks, Mr 'olden, oos comin round fast.'

Not all did even when Richard treated them. Later in the flooding which followed the heavy rain some lambs were drowned, and many wet cold ones were revived by the warmth of the bread oven on the farm, and a feed of diluted cows' milk. It was not only lambs which were affected; Richard considered it a factor in outbreaks of scouring among calves and young pigs kept in damp, cold buildings, and many died. Many a post mortem showed very severe inflammation of the bowels, they were red raw inside, and the laboratory report almost always said that the germ causing it was the bacillus Coli.

He used polyvalent vaccine for pigs to try and prevent it; and medicine, vaccines and serum in calves – often to no avail – it was dispiriting and frustrating for both the farmer and his vet.

When the handle fell off his leather bag, Richard took it to Bob Wilson, the saddler, who was grumbling because he had so much work to do.

'Wi more 'orses about, folk are bringing in a lot of old collars an girths and such, an they want 'em repaired quick, an I can't do it. Seetha, Mr 'olden, I've even to mek mi own tacking ends.'

Richard watched as with practised skill he rubbed three yellow threads along his thigh with his hand until they made one long thick thread. He then rubbed it along its length with beeswax.

'I'll 'ev thi bag ready i' two days' time.'

Richard said nothing because Bob was an ill-mannered, bad tempered man. This delay in getting his bag repaired brought home to him the fact that as he was treating more horses, the increase in numbers was helping other people. He said to himself, I bet Bob and Albert are busy in the smithy. More horses was the consequence of fewer private cars being used, but their absence was made up for by American Army cars being used, but Dr Bill McConnell was furious when one ran into the back of his Vauxhall Six saloon. He was not hurt, but it was weeks before he could get it repaired. The RAF were now continuously bombing Germany, and the Germans responded by bombing towns on the south coast and sometimes London, inflicting damage and causing casualties. It was no wonder that families moved from the south and east, to the north and west, some arriving in Sandhaven which was crowded, the shortage of houses now very marked. Frank Wood the butcher always blamed the population increase when the meat ration was on the small side, much to Flora' vexation – and even more so when the skin on his sausages was so tough after they had been cooked that you could not cut them with a knife, let alone chew them!

Tom Whittaker at Brick House, Mereside died after a long illness, and afterwards his widow had a sale of live and dead stock. One morning she phoned Richard and asked him to go and destroy the farm cats. When he asked her how many there were, she did not know. Having four cat baskets, he took them with him, and at the farm asked her where the cats were.

'In the loft over the long barn. When you get to the top of the steps, do be careful because they are a bit wild.'

'Thank you for telling me, Mrs Whittaker,' and to his surprise she closed the kitchen door. He went to the car and got his twitch with which to defend himself, but even so he was not prepared for the sight which met him when he opened the door and walked in, because cats seemed to dash everywhere, and there was an overpowering stench of cat urine and faeces. As he tried to approach a cat it would run to the top of some old bales of straw and turn and hiss and spit at him. He closed the door, and went back to the farmhouse and knocked on the door.

'Mrs Whittaker, it is obvious that those cats can't be caught without traps. I'll let the inspector of the RSPCA know and I'll arrange for us to come back together soon.'

'Oh, I see, yes, will you do that because I can't leave them to starve when I go soon, it may be the end of next week.'

The inspector did not sound very enthusiastic. 'One of them jobs is it, they'll tek a bit of catching, because I've only got two tunnel cat traps at this branch.'

'In that case it will take a long time, because my guess is that there are at least thirty up there.'

'Thirty! Good Lord, it could take days. Couldn't we gas them or something?'

'I don't think so; but you have given me an idea which will solve the problem, so when can we do it?'

'I think some afternoon when t' light's good. Warra 'bout Tuesday?'

'Yes, I can meet you there at two o'clock.'

'Reet, I'll be there, Mr 'olden.'

As it was a sunny day, Richard could see quite well in the loft when he and the inspector set the traps baited with pieces of rabbit. They withdrew and stood on the landing outside the door for a while. When they reopened the door they were disappointed to see that they had caught only one small cat. Richard filled a 5 c.c. syringe with Scheele's prussic acid and squirted a little on the cat's face; it died quickly.

'By gum, that's quick.'

'Yes, and a bit dangerous, but you gave me the idea when you talked about gassing them. Now I want to walk slowly towards the ones we can see and squirt it on them.'

With the inspector standing besides him holding the twitch, Richard killed seven in half an hour. The more wary cats disappeared into the holes among the bales, and when you moved a bale they had gone.

'At this rate we'll be 'ere tomorrer, Mr Holden.'

'I agree; don't you think it would be a good idea to bait both traps again, and go and ask Mrs Whittaker what's further along the loft beyond the bales?'

'Aye, let's do that, and gerout of this stink.'

She told them that there was a room at the far end of the loft where the Irish men slept in summer. The plan was made to take the dogs up and drive the cats into it, and try and destroy them there. Two days later the inspector had caught three cats in the traps, so with a relative of Mrs Whittaker's helping with the two farm dogs, the cats were driven into the room. Moving the rotten old bales was a dirty stinking job, but eventually more and more cats were sprayed with the cyanide and died, or were killed by the twitch or the dogs as they attempted to dash between them.

When it was all over the bodies were put into two sacks which the inspector took to the destructor. As they left Mrs Whittaker watched them from the kitchen window, but did not come out. It was a long time before she paid Richard's account, and he never went to the farm again, because the new tenant employed the vet from Runfold.

'I've one 'ere can't lamb, Mr 'olden,' said Tom Lee from Old Hall at Marhey, 'Conta 'ear, mi line's bad?'

'Yes, I can hear you, Tom; bring her here as soon as you can.'

'Aye, I wain't be long.'

When Richard examined the ewe in the trailer, he found that she had ringwomb – the neck of the uterus would not dilate.

'What's wrong wi' 'er?'

'The womb won't open. You don't often get this happening; last time it was in two heifers at Tom Nuttall's at Higher Conden eighteen months ago.'

'I 'eard about that, yer ad to kill em. Will I ev to kill this 'un? I don't want to 'cos she's a pure bred 'un.'

'Yes, I didn't know you had Suffolks, Tom. Now you've two choices: either you have her killed or I do a caesarian operation on her.'

'Warra 'er chances if tha does that?'

'A lot better than evens, I should say.'

'I'll ev it done then.'

'Then get her out of the trailer and take her into the room at the far end of the yard.' Richard brought the sterilizer which was ready for use.

'Now, Tom, we must quieten her. I don't want her struggling all the time so will you drench her with this.'

It was half a drachm of chloral hydrate dissolved in water.

'That will soon take effect and until it does you clip the wool off here on her left side. My clippers might not be so sharp as you'd like.'

Tom began to clip. 'I'll manage wi' these.'

When he had finished they lifted her up and laid her on the right side on the table and then tied her securely. Richard was feeling that tingle of excitement he always got when he was operating, and quickly disinfected the skin and injected local anaesthetic.

'Tha meks a big cut.'

'I must, otherwise I couldn't do the job properly.'

When he pulled the lamb out of the womb backwards it was a ram and alive, so he gave it to Tom.

'Rub it dry, quick, then it won't get cold.'

'Aye, I will; cut were only just big enough.'

'It's a good lamb.'

'Aye, 'tis that, one more for t' flock. Tha' sees, I'm meking a pedigree one o' Suffolks.'

'I like them, they are a good breed. You don't see many up here, but you do in the south, being lowland sheep.'

By this time the wounds had been stitched up, and she was released; when they pushed her upright, she looked around and began to bleat for her lamb.

'It's all reet, sher up,' and Tom steered her back into the trailer and then put the lamb in a sack.

'Owt I ev to do?'

'No, Tom, she should be all right; I've put pessaries in her womb, so I think she'll pass that cleansing soon, and I dusted everything with sulphanilamide powder. When I'm passing in a week I'll come and take those stitches out. Now off you go and put her by herself with her lamb for an hour or so.'

'I'll do that, thanks, Mr 'olden.'

Breakfast never tasted better. John arrived on his bike.

'Morning, John, what are you going to do?'

'As it's a nice day, Mr 'olden, I'm going to dig in more muck, in t' big garden 'cos it ull be April i' ten days.'

'So it will, come in for your baggin at quarter past ten.'

For Richard the endless rounds of visits to calves with scour and pneumonia, sows with mastitis, and cows not well went relentlessly on, and he began to feel weary again after three months being so well. He was so busy he had no time to read the *Veterinary Record* which was getting thinner and thinner, and had only five pages of papers and articles.

Bob Dawson, having made an appointment, arrived after lunch one day.

'Hello, Richard, nice to see you again. I've come because I want to tell you about the Arrowsmith results; I daren't say on the phone what I've found out.'

'Really, do sit down, and Flora will bring us some tea.'

'Fine, now the story is this. I've been making inquiries and apparently building work was going on at the hospital last back end.'

'That's right, George told me about it.'

'He did, so that's true; now it became very wet, and operations had to be suspended. It appears that mortar and cement got into the drains either having been thrown there by the workmen, or washed into them and blocked them, and this was not noticed. So the flood water brought down a lot of tuberculosis material which the heifers ate. Apparently there was hell to pay when this was found out, but it didn't get into the papers.'

Flora came with the tea.

'Good afternoon, Mrs Holden, it is good of you to do this.'

'Would you like some cake?'

'No, thank you. I've just come from a late lunch.'

'Very well, I'll leave you to it.'

'Now, where was I? The drains overflowed because the filters were blocked so it was all human infection.'

'So what am I going to tell Mr Arrowsmith without letting the secret out?'

'Good question, but what I said was that it was human infection which was in the flood water. What we may have got in those heifers is one of three or all three.'

'I hadn't thought of that with all the others passing.'

'Does he employ any labour apart from his family?'

'Yes, he has a man working for him.'

'So he could have brought bovine infection, the poultry running around avian and the flood water human – it's a real teaser.'

'What should I do, then?'

Bob didn't reply for a few seconds and then said, 'I would test all the heifers and any with a doubtful or positive reaction, tell him to get rid of them. If he's any left with no mammalian, but a big avian reaction, I'd let him keep them, but do a complete herd test in six months' time.'

'I'll do that, Bob, and thanks for your advice. I hadn't thought that bovine infection could be there as well.'

'Always suspect it. I needn't remind you of the number of TB cows there are around, with infected markets and cattle trucks, and people bringing the organism on their boots.'

'I will, and I'll find out where his man lives, and let you know the results of the heifer test.'

'Yes, do that; I'd like to know the result. I must go. You will thank your wife for the tea, won't you?'

'I will; thank you for coming.'

When Flora removed the tea tray she asked what Bob had come for. Richard told her the secret but said she had not to pass the information on to anybody. 'It was nice of you to bring him a cup of tea.'

'Well, it is vital for us to keep in his good books, because he is our best customer, but

I can't go on providing tea unless they increase the ration. Tea's very short this week.'

'So it's going to be a week of weak tea.'

'Get out or I'll throw the pot at you.'

Richard left, grinning all over his face, but stopped in the garden to admire the golden yellow forsythia in full bloom brought on by one or two lovely sunny days.

When he arrived at Seedhill he said to George Whiteside, 'That's the worst foul I've seen for a year, George, why didn't you send for me before?'

'Becos when oo started it wasn't bad and I put bran poultices on it, and she were gerrin better, but this last few days she's got a lot worse.'

'That often happens; will you wash all that bran off, please. Now, hold the nose for me.'

Richard passed a sterile probe into one of the bigger holes above the hoof which were discharging pus. About two inches in, it encountered resistance and he could feel it rubbing against something rough. He withdrew the probe. 'Let her go, George. It's a real mess is this foot, the foul's got right into the joint.'

'What can you do? I've only ed 'er a few week, and I don't want to be shut of 'er 'cos she's a grand milker.'

'As I see it you've got two choices; either you kill her before she loses any more flesh or else I've got to cut that claw off.'

'Ee dear, I didn't know it were as bad as that, I'll go and an' ask missus.'

She came back with George and was very business like, wanting to know if the cow would get over it, how long it would take to get better, and the cost. They agreed to have the operation.

'Very well, she gets nothing to eat until I get here in the morning.'

'Con oo drink?'

'Yes, and bed those two empty stalls thickly with straw because I'll put her down there. So I'll see you about nine o'clock in the morning and I'll want two of you to help.'

'Then I'll ask Jack Booth to let their Richard come, he's a useful lad.'

'That will be fine, and give her this medicine in a pint of water at half past eight in the morning.'

When Richard arrived the cow was a bit unsteady on her legs owing to the effect of the sedative medicine, so she was easily pulled over and laid on her left side. Her head was kept down by George, while the left leg was pulled out of the way and secured; then the right was tied securely across a bale. The leg was then washed, shaved and disinfected, and Richard injected plenty of local anaesthetic over the plantar nerves. A loop of thin rubber tubing was put above the hock and tightened with a piece of stick to make a tourniquet.

'George, you keep her head down in case she vomits, and Richard help me. Take the lid off the sterilizer; now wash your hands and arms in that Dettol water and don't faint.'

'I waint do that, I've helped Tom Hardman a few times at 'ome when es killed a pig for us.'

'Good, now tighten that tourniquet, and hold these forceps.'

They held a big gauze swab. Richard quickly rasped away the horn below the coronet all round, and then starting at the top cut through the skin over the swollen claw and right down through the coronary band. He cut two flaps of skin loose starting below the band and turned them back. He told Richard to tighten the tourniquet, and then swabbed the blood away. He sawed through the os corona, and cut away the claw and some rotten flesh and dropped it on the floor.

'Let the tourniquet slacken, Richard,' and as the blood squirted out he seized the arteries with forceps, and then tied them off firmly with catgut. When the stump had been dusted thickly with sulphanilamide powder he folded the flaps of skin over it, and stitched them in position.

'Now, Richard, put the forceps down, and release the tourniquet. Hold the leg up.'

He covered the skin wound with boric and iodoform powder, and bandaged a large gauze pad over it, and then covered the whole with Elastoplast.

'That's it, let it go, and move the bale then untie the other leg. Now move this blood and straw and let's have some clean in its place.' It was soon done; the cow's head was pulled round, and the three of them pushed her into a sitting position, when she immediately began to eat the straw.

'Bring her a bucket of water, George, and Richard, bring some hay.'

'It's bin a lot quicker than I thought it ud be,' said George. 'When wilta come and see her?'

'In three days time to change that bandage. Leave her here on dry bedding because I don't want it to get wet through.'

'Aye, I'll see she's kept dry.'

There was a lot of talking in the Cock Inn in Middleton that night about a cow with only one claw on her hind leg, many doubted it would be successful.

To save petrol Richard sold bottles of dextro-calcium and a syringe to farmers who were far from Sandhaven, so they could treat staggers cases in new lambed ewes. They were on Icken Fell, but the news soon spread in Droughton auction, and Harold Fowler at Birchnott, and Stan Earnshaw at Ashfield asked to be supplied. Apart from saving petrol it gave Richard more time to get his herd examinations done; to put setons in big knees in cows; and to try to find the reason for adult cattle scouring. He treated them with Phenothiazine and astringent powders, but some still died; others he found had Johne's disease and were slaughtered. George Waring at Beacon Farm on Icken Fell began to lose lambs of two to four weeks of age, so brought two dead ones to the surgery. Richard sent samples of the bowel with its contents and of the kidneys to the laboratory. They confirmed what he had suspected, that they were dying from pulpy kidney disease. As he could not find a specific serum in the veterinary price lists, he gave George the lamb dysentery serum to use, and told him to treat all lambs when they were a week or two old. He doubted whether it would be effective in stopping the outbreak, but to his relief it was.

When he called at Tom Lees at Old Hall, the ewe and lamb were doing well, so he took the stitches out. Later that day he changed the dressing on the cow's foot at Seedhill; and was going home down Beech Hill when Bill Meadows with David Roberts beside him came round the corner near Boundary Farm at high speed and made Richard swerve to avoid him. What the hell's got into him, he said to himself.

Later that evening Bill rang up to apologise and told Richard the sad news that Ted Roberts at Sykes had just started milking when he collapsed in the shippon. Mrs Roberts had rung the doctor and then Bill asking for David to come home. He was in time to go with his mother in the ambulance to the Memorial Hospital in Sandhaven, where his father died at six o'clock.

'Thanks for letting me know, Bill – it's a tragedy for Mrs Roberts, though she will have David to help her, but she's still the younger children to bring up.'

'Aye, it's very sad, and I'll have to get another man to replace David, but I'll be hard put to find another as good as him.'

'You will; he is a good lad, Good night, Bill.'

Next day Richard called at Bob Wilson's for the second time to see if his bag had been repaired.

'Aye it's here among this lot. It's teken a bit of fettlin I con tell thee.'

'How much, Bob?'

'Seven and six.'

'Here you are, and thanks very much.' Bob grunted in reply and went back to his bench. Richard realised that the repairs had been ridiculously cheap. Bob had made a new leather handle, sewed up two side seams, and then rubbed dressing all over the bag.

Later, when Richard drove into the yard at Sykes he found more cars there than he had expected, and wondered whether he would be intruding. Before he could knock on the kitchen door, it was opened by Tom Lee,

'Good morning, Tom, this is a sad do.'

'Aye, it is that; that's why I cum over as soon as I'd finished milkin to help out, seeing oos mi sister. Anyway, cum in.'

'Well, I never knew that.'

'No, tha couldn't know, sit down.'

Mrs Roberts and Mrs Dobson came into the room, and it was obvious that they were sisters. Richard got to his feet.

'Mrs Roberts, I must say how sorry my wife and I are over your tragedy; so I've come to tell you that you have all our sympathy, and if there is anything I can do to help you, I will be only too ready to oblige.'

'That's very nice of you, but Tom and my sister are here, so really I've all the help I need. David did say there's a cow to cleanse if you'd attend to that.'

'I'll come and help thee, Mr 'olden,' said Tom.

As Richard was working he said, 'She's taken this blow very well, Tom. I didn't expect to see her in such control of herself.'

'Aye she's 'ard, both lasses are if it comes to that; but we've all 'ad to be ter git through this last twenty year.'

'Yes, I remember my Uncle Ezra saying that when I was on the farm, when I worked there. That's it; I'll put some pessaries in her now, and then she will be OK.'

David came in, 'I see mother told thee, tha's done, 'asta, Mr 'olden?'

'Yes, I have, David, I really came to say how sorry I am about your dad, and I told your mother if you want any help you've only to ask.'

'Thanks, Mr 'olden, I'll remember that.'

'When is the funeral?'

'We don't know like. Tom Long the bobby from Middleton told us there'll be an inquest, tha' sees mi dad had never bin ill.'

'Yes, I understand. I'll be off now. Good morning to both of you.'

That evening the newsreader on the wireless announced another RAF and American raid on Germany. They were obviously following up the first raid they had done on Essen the month before, and were bent on destroying the great industrial area of the Ruhr. When he got up to switch off the set, his knees ached, and he felt a bit dizzy, so he held onto the table. Flora looked at him anxiously.

'What's the matter?'

'Nothing, I just felt a bit unsteady when I got up.'

'You're not starting again like you were before Christmas, are you?'

'No, I don't think so; I suppose I'm just a bit tired, it is bedtime.'

'Then I'll make a drink.'

Really he was not being truthful; it was the same condition and as the days went by it got worse, but he said nothing and just got on with an increasing amount of work. Yet as the weeks and months went by the warning signs of lassitude and discomfort became more pronounced, but he still worked on.

'Is that Mr Holden the vet?' the soft Irish voice asked,

'Yes, speaking.'

'Well now, this is Mary Doyle the housekeeper for Father O'Meara. Would you come and look at his cat, it is scratching itself bald.'

'Yes, I'll come, where is it?'

'At the Presbytery next to St. Peter's on East Street.'

The young cat was black with four white paws, and reminded him nostalgically of Sooty, his favourite at Ezra's farm all those years ago.

'He is a nice cat; how old is he?'

'About four months; the kittens were born at Christmas at Bishop's bakery across the road and they gave the Father one because he does like cats.'

'Well first, he has got ear trouble due to ear mites.' Richard then combed him with a nit comb, and though he didn't see any fleas, the shining black grains of their excrement betrayed their presence. 'Also, he has got fleas.'

'Oh dear me, whatever shall I do?'

'I'll show you how to treat him, Mrs Doyle. Hold his front legs, with his head to me.'

He dripped a little Otoryl into each ear.

'That will soften that brown wax, while I deal with the fleas. Will you bring a newspaper to stand him on. He lightly sprinkled Derris powder on the cat's fur and rubbed it in. When the cat struggled a flea dropped onto the newspaper, and was quickly killed by Mary.

'Now, hold him firmly, while I clean his ears.'

With a wisp of cotton wool wrapped round the points of a pair of fine sinus forceps, he extracted a lot of wax, though the cat struggled.

'Keep still, Noel,' said Mary.

'Why did you call him Noel?'

'Because he was born at Christmas,' said Father Patrick O'Meara who had come into the room.

'Good morning, Father.'

'Good morning, Mr Holden, I am pleased to meet you. Can you cure his trouble?'

'Yes, put a couple of drops into his ears and massage them gently once a day for five days like this, and use the flea powder once a week as I've shown you, Mrs Doyle, and don't forget the blanket he sleeps on.'

'I'll see that's done, and at what age will he have to be operated on?'

'At about six months, Father.'

'You will arrange that for me, Mary; now will you please excuse me?'

Mary paid, and wanted a receipt. The Father kept a tight ship.

Early on Tuesday morning Marjorie sent a message by the milkman that she could not come to the surgery because her father had become ill the night before, and was now in the Memorial Hospital.

'That means I can't go and represent you at Ted Roberts' funeral at eleven o'clock.'

'No you can't, that's awkward,'

'No it isn't; you'll have to go, so take your dark overcoat, and don't forget to take your wellingtons off.'

'As though I would.'

'Knowing you, you could, running in at the last minute.'

'Flora, you've made your point, now let's have breakfast.'

It was windy but pleasant as he walked up to the porch of St. Nicholas' Church in Middleton. There were very few people about in the village, and the muffled bell of the church was being slowly tolled. Inside, the church was packed with farmers and their wives come from near and far to pay their respects. The vicar gave an address worthy of the occasion, and then the coffin was carried to the graveyard by David, Tom Lee, George Dobson and Smith Priestley, followed by the family and a long procession of mourners. After he had seen Ted Roberts laid to rest, Richard chatted to many of his clients, but he had to refuse David's invitation to go to lunch which was being held in the upper room of the Cock Inn in the village. One thing he learned was that he would have to buy a bowler hat before the next funeral – a battered trilby or a cap would not do.

When he rang Flora from the phone box outside the pub, she told him to go to Churchlands at Underley to see a cow which was down. He drove fast to get there, expecting it to be a case of milk fever but it wasn't, the cow would just not get up. He examined her carefully and then per rectum but could find no reason. Stan Rainford helped and then asked,

'Is oo all reet inside?'

'Yes, there's no creaking of her bones when you move that leg about, so I'll give you this drench; give it as one dose straight away, and then the medicine once a day for a week. Now, don't forget to turn her regularly.'

'It's funny, sometimes ul turn ersell, and t'others we ev to shove her over.'

'Yes; she's not paralysed, she can move her legs well enough but she's not enough strength in them to support her. I'll look in towards the end of the week and see how she's getting on, but if she does get up let me know.'

'Aye, I will that.'

Flora had spent more of the morning sowing the seeds of sprouts, cabbage, carrots, beet, lettuce and summer spinach. She was determined to get as many vegetables out of the garden this year as she possibly could.

John had planted early seed potatoes she had got from Dick Hogarth, and upstairs in the coach house she had planted scarlet runner beans in pots, and onion and leek seed in trays. She did not think it was worth while trying to grow tomatoes when Richard could get them all summer from the growers who had glasshouses in Newton and Pelham.

George Whiteside was pleased that his cow was doing well, when the dressing was changed; and said that she was giving almost four gallons a day again, and putting a bit of meat on her back. Richard went on to Reedly Lodge in Wyresham, and found Harry Helm's Shire gelding had fistulous withers developing which were more swollen on the near side.

'It is fistulous withers, isn't it?'

'Yes it is, Harry.'

'Where's it come frae, saddles's not bin rubbing and collar don't touch it.'

'And nothing's been dropped on his back?'

'Nay, nowt I knows of.'

'There is another reason I've read about.'

'Oh what's that?'

'The germ that causes pick in cows. Have you had any this last six months?'

'Aye, there were one last summer and then one at back end; I soon got shut of 'em I can tell thee.'

'He could have got the germ from them; the only way to tell will be to blood test him and if it's a positive result to treat him.'

'I'll ev him tested then.'

It was soon done, and later sent to the laboratory.

At Fell Top Tom Walker was annoyed.

'I bought er i' February in t' Auction, an' I were told she were due for fost week of April. Well, tha con see oos not mekin a bag, though she's a big belly, an I can't bump a calf in 'er.'

'Yes, it is a bit maddening; Bring me a bucket of warm water, will you?'

After thickly smearing his arm with antiseptic cream, he examined the cow.

'Owt there?'

'No, Tom, she's empty, so I'll give a certificate to that effect.' A thumping noise in the yard made Tom tell his son John,

'Go and open the field gate afore yon two smash door down, an let 'em out.'

Richard, having washed and dried his arms, put on his jacket, and walked out of the shippon as John reached the box door and opened it quickly, stepping back as two big Shire colts plunged out of the box and galloped across the yard and into the field in which about thirty yards from the gate there was a rocky outcrop.

'They're a lively pair, Tom.'

'Aye, tha'll ev to cut 'em next month.' As he spoke the leading horse tripped over the outcrop, did a complete cartwheel and fell heavily with his head under him, his legs shooting out stiffly.

'Good God, he's killed hi sell.' All three men ran to the horse, as his legs fell limply to the earth, while the other colt was coming round in a circle back to where Richard, touching the eye of the fallen horse, could get no reflex, nor hear his heartbeat through his stethoscope.

'He's dead, Tom.'

'Blast it; I thow't he war way he fell down.'

'Was he insured?'

'Nay, only mi mares are for foaling.'

'That's a pity, he's a lovely animal, and worth quite a bit at today's prices, I'd say.'

'Aye, he'd a full pedigree; he'd a fetched more than a 'undred pounds at sale.'

'I am sorry. I'll just give you that certificate. Get off, will you.' He had to drive the other colt away because it was trying to chew his newly repaired bag. Driving down the Elmsham road he noticed prisoners of war working the fields on two farms, guarded by soldiers, and at once he decided to tell Bill Meadows at Whyngate; he could do with some extra help at the moment. When he spoke to him later, he said that he had been on to Tom Priestley seeing he was on the War Ag. Committee, and that he had promised to try and get some POWs to help him.

As Marjorie had not come to work for three days Richard went to the Elms to see how her father was getting on. Mrs Parsons asked him in, and then told him that her husband had got kidney trouble and would be in the hospital for some time, so Marjorie could not now come back to work.

'But Mrs Parsons, I must have somebody to do the books and run the office soon. Do you mean that she is never coming back to work?'

'Yes, Richard, I'm afraid it does. Marjorie is needed here all the time to help me in this big house and of course as I can't see very well she has to do the shopping.'

'Then in that case, I will have to get another secretary.'

'Yes, you will. I'll tell Charles you called, he will be pleased.'

The conversation had taken place in the hall; Marjorie had not appeared and so Mrs Parsons opened the front door and said goodbye to Richard who walked away feeling dumbfounded at Mrs Parsons' casual attitude.

Flora was annoyed when he told her.

'The bloody cheek. She might have let us know before this that if they became ill Marjorie would leave; it's damned inconsiderate. Anyway, you're not going begging for her to come back. You can get down to the *Evening Post* office and put an advert in for a good shorthand typist today.'

'I will, you write out an advert while I put some stuff in the car; shall we have a box number?'

'No, we won't; they'll see we don't need their daughter's help.'

Richard went straight to the office with the advertisement, sorry in a way that the feeling of permanency had been shattered.

When he got back to Cross Roads Farm he found Bill Harrison's cow had slow fever, so he treated her, and then gave Bill a packet of powders.

'Dusta think it ull ev tainted mi milk? I'm asking 'cos 'es 'ad one or two o' t' women grumbling this week.'

'Of course it will.'

'Reet, I won't put it in then; an another thing I want to ask thee: What's mekkin mi milk blue? They say it is.'

'Let's have a look at your cows, Bill, seeing they produce it.' Many were old. 'And is that silage you're feeding?'

'Aye, it is, it's mi fost attempt and it weren't so good, but it fills their bellies.'

'And you're feeding cereals?'

'Aye.'

'Then there are two things you can do at once. One is dry off those old ones, and start feeding something with oil in it – linseed meal, and a bit of good cod liver oil will help. Those two are in good condition; I'd fatten them off, they won't need much finishing, and buy two young new calved Guernseys to take their place. As the weather is mild I'd turn them out days, that will help your milk as well.'

His son drove into the yard. 'Are they still at it wi' their grousing?'

''Course they are.'

'Well, don't let it git yer down. Mr 'olden's just told me what I ev ter do to stop it.'

Richard learned later that it had worked.

The cow at Harry Carter's at Squires Farm which he had treated the day before for milk fever was still down, and they could not make her get up, though Richard could find nothing wrong with her.

'Do you know, Harry, this is the second one this week like this, and they're both Friesians. Now, give her this drench first, and then the medicine once a day. If she's not up soon, let me know.'

At George Whiteside's, the cow's foot had healed.

'That's it, George, she doesn't need any more dressing. I see you are letting them out days; I'd let her go out last until she gets used to using that leg, you don't want a rough one knocking her over.'

'I don't that, believe me, Mr 'olden, but I want you to look at a good lamb, I think its leg's bust.' It was a well grown seven-week old lamb with the leg broken at the elbow. 'You're right, it's broken; get it killed because I couldn't set it being all round the joint.'

'Wilta do it for us?'

'You mean dress it?'

'Aye, wilta?'

'Yes, but I'll want a table to put it on, and then somewhere to hang it.'

Richard shot it and bled it and then, using his PM knife, skinned it.

'Tha's mekkin a good job o' that, Mr 'olden; it looks as though tha's done it afore.'

'I have, George, in an emergency.'

'I thought tha' had. Wilta split it and cut t'hind legs off while I go to t' house?'

He came back with a sheet of brown paper, wrapped one of the legs in it, and gave it to Richard, saying,

'Ere yar, gi it tut wife, tha deserves it for t' way tha's fettled yon cow.'

'Well, that's very good of you, George. Thank you very much, my wife will be pleased.'

She was; her comment was, 'Why don't you do this more often?' She had been working at the front of the house, digging away the turf to make a border on each side of the path up to the front door.

'What are you making, love?'

'I'm making this border; it will look more attractive when people come to the surgery, and then I'll get some bedding plants from Dick later.'

'It will look nice, then, but I haven't time to help you now.'

'You never have; you've never done a hand's turn in this garden since you rooted the old hedge out years ago, and it will be less to cut; I'm sick of pushing that old lawn mower about.'

'You tell me next time it wants cutting, then I can do it.'

'The saints be praised, I'll keep you to that.'

The blood sample from Helm's horse was positive for infection with the abortion germ, so he decided to go and vaccinate it that morning. First he had to go to the lodge where Sugdens wanted a bottle of white liniment and a packet of mastitis powders. As he drove up to the gate he could see Father O'Meara blessing the twenty shippon, shaking the water on the door, which he then opened and walked inside. Richard got out of the car and ran across the yard because he knew the fifth cow in was 'a mucky bugger'. She watched you walk behind her and at that very moment she would cough, which caused her to shoot out a stream of faeces. Before Richard reached the door Father Patrick came out, the green liquid running down his jacket and trousers.

'Oh dear, I am just too late to warn you.'

'Yes, you are; I did not think this would happen.'

'Stand still while I get a towel from the car.'

As he was wiping off the Father's clothes, Mrs Sugden came running in. 'Oh, Father Patrick, I am sorry this has happened, come along into the house now. Mr Holden, will you put the powders in the dairy, please.' Richard did, and gave his towel a good wash under the tap, lest Flora should have some pointed comment to make on wash day.

'Yes, Harry, those two cows left the germ over your pasture all right and it's infected this gelding. Bring him out, will you, and I'll inject him, and I'll come again in a fortnight and give him another one.'

'What ull 'appen?'

'It might burst and run, or just start to get less, we'll just have to wait and see.' This one was a 'gentle giant'; he never moved when Richard pushed the needle into his neck.

When he arrived home Flora told him that Stanley Rainford had rung to say the cow was up, but he wanted the horns taking off another cow the next morning; also three girls were coming for an interview that evening after seven o'clock in response to the advertisement in the *Post*.

Flora and Richard together interviewed each girl separately, and rejected the first out of hand because she had no testimonials, and appeared lacking in intelligence. The second was very smartly dressed in a blue and white two-piece, and was immaculate. She was a receptionist and assistant secretary in a London hotel. Her testimonials were very good. The third was older, wore glasses and was very polite. She had worked in a large store in Manchester until it was bombed, since when she had been working part time at the Droughton Royal Infirmary. They chose the second girl, and dismissed the other two after thanking them for coming. Flora now took over, and went with the young lady into the office, where she gave her a letter to type, and then tested her shorthand; she did both excellently. Flora left her, and went upstairs to tell Richard that she would be just what they wanted.

'Right, bring her up here where it is warmer, and we can give her a cup of tea and find out more about her.'

Flora brought her upstairs.

'Come in, Miss Collinson, and sit down, would you like a cup of tea?'

'Yes please.' The phone rang.

'Will you excuse me while I answer that?'

'Of course.' It was George Arrowsmith wanting to know when Richard would test the heifers.

'I want to turn 'em out soon, afore grass gets ahead of 'em.'

'Of course you will. Now, next Monday about ten o'clock, it won't take that long. Is that OK?'

'Aye that ull do grand. Good neet.'

Flora and Miss Collinson were chatting away, each with a cup of tea, when Richard went into the lounge.

'Guess what I've found out, Richard?'

'What? You tell me.'

'Miss Collinson is the younger daughter of Tom at Park Hall, and George at Church Farm is her big brother.'

'Well, I'll be blessed. I thought he had only one daughter who was a nurse at Droughton Royal.'

'That's right, that is my elder sister Doris, she is a Sister now,' said Miss Collinson.

'She is doing very well then.'

'Yes, Father is very proud of her, Mr Holden.'

'So how long have you been in London?' asked Flora.

'Nearly four years.'

'What, through all the blitz; I would have been terrified.'

'Yes, I was there the whole time. Mother wanted me to come home, but I had a good job and stayed because they looked after us very well, and we had a deep shelter to go to if an air raid started.'

'So why do you want this job?'

'Because I want to be near home now.'

'Well, you couldn't be nearer than this, because my wife Flora and I would like you to accept the position.'

'I've got it! Oh, that's great, wait till I tell Dad and Mum; they will be pleased.'

'That's good, now there are certain things we will tell you. You will have to sign an employees' agreement in which you promise to keep secret all professional matters. Your hours will be 8.30 to 12.30 and 1.30 to 5.30 during the week and then 8.30 to 12.00 on Saturday. We will provide you with a white coat and a locker, and we all have a break for tea in the morning and afternoon. One thing I do want to stress is that you have to try and not make mistakes. Now, when would you be able to start?'

'In two weeks' time. I've already served one week of my notice, though it is my holiday – it was due to me. So I've got to go back on Sunday and work another fortnight.'

'Is there anything else, Flora?'

'I don't think so, except you may sometimes have to assist in the surgery. You do like animals?'

'Of course I do.'

'And you don't faint at the sight of blood?'

'No, I don't, Mrs Holden.'

'I think then you had better go home and think about it, and let me know your decision in the morning,' said Richard.

'I will, thank you both very much, and by the way, my name is Joan.'

'Good night, Joan.' Flora took her downstairs and saw her out of the house.

Richard stood in front of the fire annoyed with himself, because his conscience had suddenly said, 'So you have not forgotten her, have you? Joan Winifred Matthews from Weston.' He couldn't.

The next morning Joan Collinson became the new secretary, to start work in a fortnight's time.

Helped by George Arrowsmith, and his man, who was called Dick, Richard quickly carried out the Tuberculin test on the heifers. He found out that Dick was one of the Warburtons from Fir Trees Farm, which was really a smallholding on the north side of the village. They were in every branch of agriculture: they kept poultry, pigs, goats, sheep and a few heifers. They grew vegetables: potatoes, tomatoes, cucumbers and marrows; sold flowers in season and jars of jam, pickled onions and red cabbage. There was nothing they couldn't turn their hands to, some were ploughmen, hedgers and ditchers, two travelled with a threshing team. It was a big family of seven men and two girls, who wrung the last drop of profit from their eighteen acres. Richard was curious about them; they must have a house cow for milk. He rang Bob Whiteside that night and asked if he could let him know in strict secrecy if he had removed a screw cow from Fir Trees some time last year.

There was a pause, then Bob said, 'That's that little shop wi' a few glass houses on t' 'igher Carden Road.'

'Yes, that's the place, Bob; he's called Tom Warburton.'

'Aye, now I come to think on I did; it were an Irish cow that ud gone a screw about last October time.'

'Thanks a lot, Bob; you won't let on I've been asking.'

'I won't, Mr 'olden; by the way tha's done a good job on our George's cow.'

'Yes, it's done very well, to say that it was going downhill so fast with that foot. How did you know?'

'I hevn't sin him, but they were talkin' about it in the XL t'other neet.'

'News travels fast. Good night, Bob, and thanks.'

The first staggers case of the spring was at Tommy Crompton's at Greyhurst Hall, and Richard drove up Brookwood Road at sixty miles an hour, making a cloud of dust as he drove into the yard. One of the men shouted,

'Go in t'at field; Tom's theer wi' 'er,' and the car bounced and rattled as it was driven over the hard-baked earth in the gateway. He grabbed his bag and hurried over to the cow which was on her side shaking all over. As he reached her it suddenly stopped.

'Blast it; oos a goner,' said Tommy. 'An oos just given o'er two gallons; tha' wouldn't believe it, would ta?'

'Yes, Tom, and it's always worse if they have just been milked. If one comes up for milking and she's nervy and jumpy, don't milk her. By the way are you feeding minerals?'

'Nay, I'm not.'

'Then get plenty and drench every one of them with a good handful in water today, and put some in a box in the field so they can help themselves.'

'That ull be a hell of a job, Mr 'olden.'

'I know, but it's the only preventative there is. They do say new leys make it worse, so don't put them on one.'

'But they're in one,'

'Than you will have to get them out or ration their grazing. I'll take a sample of blood or Whiteside won't move her.'

So he was late at Stan Rainford's, but the cow was tied up in the shippon when he came in.

'Bin held up, Mr 'olden?'

'Yes, the first staggers this spring and it died as I got there.'

'Thats a poor do for 'em then; is there 'owt I can do to stop it?'

Richard was telling him about minerals when his son Harry walked in wearing a bandage over one eye.

'Hello, Harry, what's happened to you?'

'This un clouted mi one in t' face wi' its 'orns last neet and bust mi glasses.'

'Has it hurt your eye?'

'No, it 'asn't. Doctor said I were lucky.'

'Ee were, Mr 'olden; she's a bad devil, so them 'orns hev got to come off.'

'Is she an Ayrshire?' asked Richard, looking at the strong curved jointed horns.

'Nay, oos 'alf Red Friesian an 'alf Ayrshire.'

'So that's why she is so big and strong. Stanley put these bulldogs in her nose and, Harry, go and put this iron in the kitchen fire.'

Richard injected plenty of local anaesthetic round the base of each horn, and then tied binder twice very tightly in a figure of eight in the same place. Harry came in.

'Ow 'ot dusta want iron, Mr 'olden?'

'Just glowing red, bring it in a bucket when I shout.' What with a cow tie, bulldogs, and a halter holding her the cow didn't struggle much as Richard sawed off each horn an inch above its base, and then seared the stump with the hot iron.

Mrs Rainford appeared at the shippon door. 'Mr 'olden, wilta go to Meatham 'all at once; there's bin an accident.'

'Yes, thank you, Mrs Rainford, we're just finished. I'll give you a bottle of antiseptic oil to pour on those stumps every day for a week, and cut that twine off tonight. If it bleeds, put it back on. Got that?'

'Aye, Mr 'olden.'

'Good. I'm off.'

As he turned onto the Brookwood Road Richard thought the quickest way would be straight down to Wyresham and onto the main Droughton-Mereside Road. He drove very fast and didn't slow down much as he entered Wyresham. But he did when the car which passed him waved him down. He wound down the window as the police inspector approached – the same one who had stopped him two years before.

'Good morning, Mr Holden. You were going far too fast as you came into Moor Street. Will you please curb your speed? This is the second time I've told you; next time you will be in Court, do you understand?'

'Yes, but there's been an accident at Meatham Hall.'

'Maybe, but do what I say or it will be worse for you. Good morning.'

Richard was fuming; how the hell can I get from one emergency to another if I don't drive fast, he said to himself, wait till they ring up for an emergency and I'll make them wait, I will that. Seething with anger, he really put his foot down going along Mereside Road.

Dick Smith was standing beside a cow down on the side of the road talking to a policeman.

'Good morning, Mr 'olden, wilta tell me if she's getten a broken leg?'

A quick examination revealed that the hind leg was broken above the stifle.

'Yes, it's broken; she must be killed.'

'I thowt so. Tommy and Leslie are bringing a gate out to shove 'er on, then we'll get 'er in t' wagon.'

'What happened?'

'Well, it were like this. Tommy and me 'ad four heifers and three dry cows in t' yard. I were going to turn 'em out in ta field across road. Six were out but this 'un ran back in, so Tom came back and we chased her out, and Ley's van from Droughton were comin like hell and hit 'er.'

'So there was nobody on the road when the van came round the corner?' asked the PC.

'No but there were six beasts there; silly bugger musta sin I were drivin 'em out o' t' yard.'

'He could he? They could ev git out for all he'd know.'

'Don't be so daft, tha don't leave beasts loose on t' road. He were comin' too bloody fast I tell yer,' shouted Dick getting red in the face. 'I'll sue him, I will that.'

'Then let's go in and I'll write you a certificate for the manager of the abattoir because it sounds as though the wagon's here.' It was, and three men rolled the cow onto the gate and secured her, and she was winched into the wagon. Richard had taken all her particulars, so that he could type a certificate in the office and then send a copy to Dick.

Months later he was furious when he lost the Court case. Richard was the only professional witness who gave details of the animal's injuries and Dick paid him reluctantly a long time afterwards.

Richard was still bitter and worked up by the events of the morning when he arrived at Harry Carter's whose cow was still down. He was grumbling in a light-hearted manner which Richard resented.

'You've no need to blame me, Harry, you are not helping her to get up, are you? This floor is so damned slippery, she'll never get up. Get some sand or ashes down, and bring some straw and somebody else to help us. Come on, hurry up, the damned day's going.'

'All reet, Mr 'olden, there's no need to be like that, keep thi shirt on.' He hurried out; and soon sand was scattered on the floor and covered with straw by his man.

'That will do, now grab that lump of skin in front of her stifle, are you ready?'

'Aye.' Richard grabbed her tail, hit her hard with his twitch and shouted, 'Lift!'

The startled cow scrambled to her feet.

'There, that's all she needed, Harry.'

'Aye tha's reet, any road I'm glad oos up; now gi' me a bottle of scour medicine, I've two calves on t' loose side.'

'Here you are; don't give them any milk for twenty-four hours, only warm water and medicine.'

'Aye, I will. Good day, Mr 'olden.'

The cold manner of his dismissal by Harry – a most pleasant man – made Richard cool down and act more sensibly. This was fortunate because next morning it was George Arrowsmith's turn to be annoyed.

'That means five av failed, seven are doubtful, and seven passed thi test. Blast it, three o' them that's failed are full pedigree.'

'Yes, that's a shame, but they will sell well. All five have to go, you know, and I wouldn't keep the doubtfuls.'

'Mebbe tha wouldn't but its me oos trying to mek a pedigree herd, not thee.'

'I know that, George. What I was thinking was that the money from selling the five and the doubtfuls would buy full pedigree stock. I expressed myself badly.'

'Aye, tha did, but I see the point. But Mr 'olden, I've gitten a closed 'erd; I've brought nowt on for three year, and I don't want to be buying pick and garget, dusta see?'

'Yes I do, but you must buy them with a veterinary certificate and a recent one at that, that they have passed the Tuberculin test and the abortion test, and bring them in your own trailer, not a dirty cattle wagon.'

'I'll think it o'er, but I still don't like idea o' bringing owt on. Wilta test em again soon?'

'I was thinking about this, and I'll tell you when I've had a word with Mr Dawson. Two heads are better than one even if they are sheep's heads.'

'Gerra way; yer daft!' They both laughed, and Richard left and went back to the surgery to see George Duke the accountant, who had been there working all the previous day.

'Yes, Richard, you are making steady progress, it's been a good year for you. See, there's your nett profit, and the turnover has grown, while debtors and bad debts are much less. The analysis shows more horse work and less small animal but the growth is in cattle. You have got nine new farm clients in less than four years.'

'That's very pleasant to hear, George. Now I haven't told you, but I've engaged a new secretary to start in a fortnight, and she will be working regular hours, not like Marjorie was. She's left because her father is ill, so she has to look after her mother. Now, how much will I have to pay the new woman?'

'First, how many hours a week is she going to work?'

'Forty-three and a half: I want to let Flora have a bit more free time.'

'So you should; now, the new girl is a shorthand typist?'

'Yes.'

'Is she going to have to do other work?'

'Of course, you know, help in the surgery and in the dispensary.'

'I think you should see Tommy and get an agreement as to hours of work; nature of the work; time off; holidays; wages and bonuses; sick pay etc. That will have to be her starting salary.'

'As much as that? It seems a lot.'

'No, it isn't, it's the rate for the job at the moment; and another thing I have here is my notes – you are not making any provision for a pension or for life assurance.'

'Must I, when really I want to get rid of that mortgage as soon as I can.'

'Yes, you must; if anything happened to you where would your wife be?'

'I hadn't given it a thought, George, so would you find a good one and work out how much I can afford.'

'Yes, I will, and you'll see Tommy about your new employee. By the way, what's her name?'

'Joan Collinson; Tom at Park Hall – his daughter.'

'I think you have done well getting her, both his girls are bright and jolly good looking; she should be an asset for the practice that will increase in value as she gets to know the clients better, though I expect she will know a lot of them already.'

'I expect she will. Thanks, George; I must go.'

The cow at Ryton Grange responded rapidly to the intravenous injection for milk fever and soon got to her feet. Richard got up more slowly.

'Is thi' leg troublin' thee, Mr 'olden?' asked Mr Turner.

'Not my leg, Will, it's my knee; it's a bit swollen and kneeling on rough floors doesn't help.'

'By gum, it don't; they con be the very devil.'

'Why are you limping, Richard?' asked Flora later that evening.

'Because my knee is swollen, like it was last year; all this kneeling down has set it off again.'

'It may have, but I think you're tired out. Do you know you've never stopped since

Christmas; and though the cows have gone out you are still busy. I think you're making yourself ill; can't you get someone to help you?'

'Well, not now; things will quieten down in a week or two; they always do, but it might be a good idea for the back end. I think we could afford it because George showed me the figures for last year and they are good. By the way, he says I should take out a life assurance policy, in case anything should happen to me, so I told him to get on with it. It must be a good thing to do.'

'I think it will be, too.'

Richard sat by the fire thinking what an increase in the size of the practice would mean. He now had a salaried secretary, then there was Flora's wage. The car would have to be kept if he got an assistant and where would he live? So he would have to buy another car, more equipment, warehouse coats, and wellingtons and ... but he had dozed off.

It was a lovely morning in the first week of May when very early he had to visit a cow with milk fever. By half past seven he was home enjoying breakfasting with Flora, who said, 'You do look a lot better this morning, love.'

'Thanks, I feel OK; it was great driving to Tom Priestley's and things are quieter, which helps.' To prove him wrong the phone rang. It was Joe Fowler who wanted a visit that morning to see a lame stallion.

'Good morning, Joe, let's have him outside.'

One of his men led the huge horse from his box.

'Walk him on; now turn him to your left and bring him back. Joe, I can't see he's lame.'

'No, he isn't; it don't show on t' yard. We'll tek him into t' other yard on t' cobbles. Tek horse round t' back; we'll go this road then we con see him come towards us.' And as he did, he was lame.

'He's lame off fore.'

'I knows that, but thee tell me where.'

Richard examined the horse's leg from its shoulder down to its hoof, but found nothing wrong.

'Will you walk him away again.' The man did, 'Bring him back. In my opinion he is definitely lame in the foot.'

'He can't be; yon farrier's searched it twice and found nowt.'

'Then I'll search it myself, it must be in that foot.'

Richard brought his farrier's bag from the car, and then hammered every clench; Joe watching him intently. He did the same to the sole, but the horse was only slightly sensitive when he hammered the frog.

'Joe, have you another man to hold this foot?'

'Aye, I'll find one.' Richard was glad of the rest for a few minutes. When they came back, the man picked up the foot.

'Hold it as still as you can.' Richard put a steel punch on the point of the frog and told Joe to hit it with the hammer; the horse showed no reaction. Richard carried out the search this way, moving backwards from the point of the frog toward the heel, and was about halfway there when the horse tried to snatch the foot away.

'You touched summat there.'

'I'll have to cut the frog away until I can find it.' He began to cut strip after strip away from the black frog, but found nothing.

'I don't think there's owt there, ta's gone far enough.'

'We'll soon see.' He continued to cut off thin strips, and was getting worried that he might draw blood if he went any deeper when his knife scratched something, 'What's that?' asked Joe. Richard didn't answer but very carefully cut away another strip when something a bit bright was revealed. He pushed it out with his knife and it was a short felt nail with only half a head, and that half was pressing into the foot. He gave it to Joe and straightened up. 'I told yon farrier there were summat there.' Richard watched the spot for a few seconds but there was no bleeding.

'It's lucky that nail was lying flat, Joe; if it had been pointing in it would have killed him. I wonder where he picked it up.'

Joe said nothing, so Richard told the man to put the foot down.

'Asta done wi' 'im?'

'Yes.'

'Put 'im back in his box.'

'Now, Joe, that frog is so thin anything can prick through it, so paint it with Stockholm tar, and get your farrier to nail a piece of tin sheet to protect it, and leave it on for a couple of weeks.'

'I'll do that, Mr 'olden, an' I'll tell him a few things too, believe me.'

Joe did not tell him that he himself had nailed new felt on the hen cabin which was in the paddock where the stallion grazed alone.

A message came from the house that there was a cow with milk fever at High Moor, Greyhurst, and as he was already only five miles away, he soon reached the farm. Bob Barber came out of the diary.

'Yer con drive to her, Mr 'olden, she's not far in t' field an our Tom's wi' 'er.'

Richard soon reached her, and with Tom's help was injecting her intravenously when Bob walked up.

'Oo's not bad, is oo?'

'No, she's coming round, Bob; I'll soon finish injecting this.' After a few minutes the cow sat up, belched and moved her legs. Bob gave her a kick, but she did not move.

'Come on, gerrup,' he said as he kicked her again; still the cow did not rise.

'I'd leave her for a bit until it works, Bob, but if she isn't up by milking time, let me know.'

'All reet, Mr 'olden. I'll see what 'appens.'

Nothing did, so at four o'clock Richard had to go back and inject her again, but still she didn't get up.

Late that evening the phone rang.

'This is Mr Holden? Then I want you to come and see my pekinese, Poppy. I live at White Gate, Wilton just before you get to the crossroads in the village. My name is Mrs Foster. Now, you will come, won't you?'

'Before I answer that, will you please tell me if another vet has been treating her.'

'No there hasn't, she's been very well since we got her last year. It was Mr Bainbridge from Duckworth Hall who told us to ring you.'

'And what is wrong with her?'

'Nothing, but I want her checked over, and her nails are long.'

'Very well, I will come to see her tomorrow.'

'What on earth was all that about at this time of night?' asked Flora.

'A woman in Wilton wanting me to go and see her peke tomorrow. She must have more money than sense.' Unknown to Richard his words were very near the mark, she was extremely wealthy; but she had a lot of sense though she acted as though she were silly.

He planned to go to the east end of the practice next morning, but he had to go west to a staggers case at Mill Farm, Nenton. The cow was down and twitching all over, so he injected a bottle of solution on each side of the neck.

'She's in a bad way, George, so leave her alone and be quiet while that takes effect because she could go into a fit at any moment.'

'So there's nowt for me to do.'

'Nothing; I'll be back later in the morning.'

As it was already half past nine he drove at top speed until he reached Wyresham, and then fairly crawled through the village.

'It looks like yon's a gonner like 'er we ed two year gone, 'er's still down,' said Bob Parker as he and Richard walked down the field to the cow.

'I hope not, Bob, that did get Robson worked up, though there were no hard feelings afterwards.' The cow was normal in every way, eagerly eating a heap of grass which had been cut for her.

'Why don't she gerrup; come on, you lazy bitch, come on wi yer,' shouted Bob giving her a real clout with his stick. To their surprise she did and walked a few paces away, then turned round and gazed at them.

'Well, I'll be damned,' said Bob. 'Any road, bugger's up; that's what counts.'

Richard silently agreed, and went on his way, after telling Bob to start feeding minerals to his cows.

Harry Helm led the horse out for Richard to examine.

'Aye, Mr 'olden, it burst day after tha were 'ere last time and ran a lot, but it's dried up since, and tha' con see it's gone down.' It obviously had.

'Yes it's working well so far, so I'll give him another injection. It may be enough, so

I won't come for a month.'

'Thanks, Mr 'olden, if owt different 'appens I'll let tha know.'

As he was approaching Wilton village he saw an old man slowly riding a bicycle coming towards him, so he stopped and asked him for White Gate House.

'It's 'alf a mile up road on the right. Tha means Frank Foster's; there's a long drive up to it.'

Richard thanked him, and admired the beautiful garden and immaculately cut box hedges as he drove up to the front door. He rang the bell, and after he had announced who he was he was asked inside. Mrs Foster came to meet him across the large hall.

'Good morning, Mr Holden, I am Doris Foster; it is nice to meet you,' and as he reciprocated the greeting they shook hands.

'Do come this way,' she said and led the way into the morning room where Poppy stood up in her silk lined basket to meet them. She picked her up, and placed her on the table. He thought the dark-haired woman must be about forty-five years old. She gave him the impression of doing things in a languid, often silly manner, but it was a cloak adopted by a single-minded very determined woman. She wore two large diamond rings on her right hand, and a very large square aquamarine above her wedding ring on her left. The diamond brooch on the lapel of her jacket flashed in the sunshine.

'As Frank my husband would say – he's an engineer – give her a good overhaul.'

Richard was still suspicious of the woman's motive in asking him to come all this way to examine an obviously healthy dog, so he meticulously went over the animal while Mrs Foster held her and talked to her in this manner:

'And who's my poppet Poppy then? Mummy's girl, aren't you? Go on, wag your tail; there you are, she knows every word I say.'

'She does, Mrs Foster, and I find her very well; nothing is wrong, but the dew claws on her hind legs were not removed when she was a puppy and need cutting.'

'Do it then, please.' Richard did. Poppy took no notice; she was watching a Siamese cat which walked into the room and looked round – in that supercilious manner characteristic of the breed – as though she owned the place.

'So you have a Siamese, Mrs Foster.'

'Yes, I got him from Mr Billsborough in Droughton; I think you know him.'

'Yes, I do, because I've got two Siamese.'

'How often should my animals be vaccinated?'

'Really, whenever there is an outbreak of disease in the area, but they have been done when they were young?'

'Oh yes, I think so, but I don't really know – it will be on file in the office.'

'If you are not certain I do advise them to be done at once.'

'Very well. Now, Mr Holden, will you call about once a month to keep your eye on them?'

'Yes, I'll do that with pleasure.'

'Then I'll say goodbye. I must go, my maid will show you out,' and putting Poppy under her arm she swept out of the room. As Richard was getting into his car, an Austin Six came at full speed round the house, and went down the drive, Doris at the wheel. She did not wave.

Flora was curious that evening. 'And what was the new client like in Wilton?'

Richard told her the story, and as he liked jewellery, he described the rings in detail.

'Strikes me you spent more time looking at her hands than at the dog.'

'Well, it's not every day I have a chance to look at a thousand quid's worth of diamonds, it's usually a cow's backside.'

'I'll ask in Bishop's who they are when I go shopping in the morning, but if they are wealthy as that it's got to be £2 a visit.'

'Yes I suppose it must, it is a long way.'

'And that takes a lot of time; think of all the visits you could have done around here in that time, and anything else she...'

'Be quiet, Flora, what's he say?' They both listened as the announcer said on the wireless that Tunis had been captured.

'That's good; sorry, what were you going to say?'

'Only this, that that is the minimum charge, and anything else will be extra.'

'Oh it must be, because she wants a visit every month.'

Flora found out that Mrs Foster, a wealthy woman in her own right, was a director of Frank Foster (Drop. Forgings) Ltd with factories in Droughton, Glasgow and Wolverhampton.

On Sunday morning, there was a case of staggers at Tom Collinson's, and though Richard was there in ten minutes it was dead when he arrived.

'That was quick, Tom, doesn't give one a chance.'

'No, it doesn't, an' t' worst of it is, she were one of mi show cows.'

'Just bad luck, it's the second one like this I've had already this spring.'

'I 'ope I don't have any more. Our Joan's home, she's looking forward to starting work for you tomorrow.'

'I hope she likes the job, it will be a change from London.'

'Aye, and a damn sight safer.'

Flora spent all next morning with Joan, explaining all the details of the work of the office; to Richard's relief they got on like a house on fire. Flora spent the afternoon putting in bedding plants in the garden, making the borders up to the front door.

It was another lovely morning when he went to Birchnott and turned off the main road into the narrow lane which ran through the woods, uphill to the farm. He had driven about two hundred yards when he heard a roaring noise, over that of the car's engine, and then leaves and twigs flew everywhere. As he drove on he saw something flash in the sunlight, then the trees higher up the hill shook violently, and a plume of black smoke rose slowly into the air. At that moment the postman came pedalling furiously down the hill, but stopped when he saw Richard, who wound down the window of the car and asked, 'What's happened?' The white-faced man said, 'Seven planes were goin o'er an one's crashed through t' trees an inta t' brook o'er top of the 'ill. Branches came crashing down, but missed me. I'm goin; it's not bloody safe,' and he rode off. When Richard got to the farm cottage two people were staring up the road, but he drove past them on up to the farm. Two men were running up the road, so he overtook them instead of turning into the farm. They were Harold Fowler and his man and a breathless Harold panted, 'I've rung police, they wain't bi long; don't go further up, Mr 'olden, road's pretty bad.' Richard parked the car and joined them toiling on up the hill, and on the right some trees were leaning at various angles, and leaves and branches covered the road. They reached the top and were looking down at the brook where a badly damaged aircraft had crashed nose first into it, and was blazing fiercely.

'I'm not going down to yon, it ull likely blow up.'

'I agree, Harold, it would be crazy to go near.'

The big police car came roaring up in a low gear and stopped. An inspector, a sergeant and a constable got out and came across to the bewildered men.

'Mornin, who rang up?' asked the inspector.

'I did,' said Harold

'Did you see what happened?

'Nay, I didn't, there were this awful roaring noise, then crashing and a big bang as I came out of barn, then smoke started.'

'Did you see anyone bail out?'

'Nay, nowt came down, just twigs and leaves.'

'That means the poor devil is in yon mess, but we can't go near until the flames die down.'

The constable, who had been walking among the trees, shouted, 'Come 'ere sir, there's a lump of jacket.' The inspector went into the wood as an RAF truck came roaring up, and out jumped a fire-fighting crew.

'Hell, is it down there,' said the sergeant. 'Bring that tackle, it 'ull be burnt out soon.'

They set off down the hillside, as the white-faced inspector came back carrying a blood-stained piece of a jacket, and walked up to Richard and asked, 'Are you the vet?'

'Yes, I am.'

'Then would you come with me.' Richard followed to the spot where the constable was standing. 'There are bits of a body scattered here, would you please collect them; we can't.'

'What have I to put them in?'

'Oh, use the constable's cape.'

Richard found part of a hand, a bit of the shoulder area, a piece of lung and some bits of broken rib; and then saw something glistening among the leaves. It was a blood stained bracelet, and on it was a name, a number and USAAF. He put it in the cape, and took them all to the inspector, who at once gave the cape to a doctor who had driven up. Harold said that there was nothing more they could do, so they climbed into the car and went back to the farm where Richard treated the heifer which had wooden tongue. They then went into the house and drank mugs of tea, and talked about the miraculous escape they had all had.

The last person for surgery that evening was Mr Twining, and the surgery card showed that he had not been for nine months.

'Good evening, Mr Twining.' Both man and dog walked slowly into the room, and as Richard looked at the pug and its swollen abdomen he thought, its heart is packing up.

Its owner put the dog on the table and said, 'Mr Holden, will you tell me what is wrong with Tudor; he can hardly get around.'

The examination showed slight jaundice, then a large lump in the abdomen. Richard palpated it carefully and then, looking at Mr Twining, said, 'There is a great enlargement of his liver, and jaundice, which accounts for him being so thin. At his age it must be a tumour of the liver which will soon kill him.'

'In that case, will you painlessly destroy him?'

'Yes, now if you will go.'

'I will not, Mr Holden, I will stay with him to the end and then I will take him home to bury him.'

Flora squeezed the leg until the needle was in the vein, and then released the pressure as Richard rapidly injected an overdose of pentothal sodium. Tudor silently sank down on the table while Mr Twining was stroking him and died. He lifted the dog down and put him into the suitcase he had been carrying.

'Thank you very much, Mr Holden.' He put three one-pound notes on the table and then said, 'Goodnight, both of you, the drinks are on me,' and walked out of the room very quickly. Both Richard and Flora were profoundly moved by the old man's unflinching determination to be in control at the death of his friend and pet. Tears ran down Flora's cheeks as she closed the front door behind him. It was only later when Richard went to Jim Lord for bandages and Elastoplast that he learned that Mrs Twining had been killed along with her sister six weeks before in a bombing raid on the south coast. Richard felt profoundly sorry for the old gentleman.

The offices of MAFF in Droughton were in a lovely red brick late Georgian house, but Richard did not spare it a passing glance the morning he ran up the steps to keep his appointment with Bob Dawson.

'Yes, these test results from Arrowsmith's confirm the fears I had, that among all these big reactions was lurking the old devil TB bovis, so the twelve have to go. It does look as though this Dick Warburton brought the infection, so tell Arrowsmith to take more precautions against infection getting in; he may take the hint and get rid of the chap. You know the tale, it's no use having a closed herd if you let the germ walk in with boots on.'

'I like that; I'll tell him.'

'You do, and retest the lot in three months, he could have left the germ in other places.'

'I do hope not. Thank you very much, Bob, for your help; interpreting results is difficult when the owner is grumbling and shouting at you.'

'Don't I know it. Cheerio.'

Richard did not want George Arrowsmith to buy in infection, so that evening he rang Uncle Harry at Old Alresford to ask him if he could recommend a closed herd of pedigree Friesians, but he was more interested in telling him all the family news. Harry was now a Major and after the fighting in Southern Tunisia had been awarded a Bar to his MC. Ezra was in the Navy and Annie was expecting another baby. At last he asked his question.

'Aye, Richard, I know one not far from here; it's a Captain Loftus, his father came from up your way.'

'I bet he did with that name,'

'It's Manor Farm, Mattingley; they are full pedigree Friesians and he is TT; he was one of the first round here to be tested. He's a gentleman; but he has some funny ways, he even makes me wash my boots with Jeyes before he'll let me in, but I've never heard any complaints about his stock.'

'Thanks, Uncle, that's the sort of herd I want to find.'

'How's our Ted? I haven't heard from your father for two years.'

'Well, he only sends me a card at Christmas; as far as I know he is all right, except for a bit of angina.'

'That's good. Nice to hear from you. Give my love to your Flora.'

'I will, good night.'

Work the next morning began at 5.40 a.m. with a visit to a cow with milk fever at Bridge House at Higher Garden.

'She's in t' box, Mr 'olden; she calved late last neet, and as oo ad it last time, I got up fearing she'd be down.' She quickly responded to the injection, and when Tom Nuttall picked up the red bull calf to carry it out into another box, the cow quickly got to her feet to follow him.

'That's the idea, Tom, don't leave him with her; ration him for a couple of days.'

Richard rang Flora from the box in the village.

'I'm glad you've rung, there's a cow down at the Reformatory farm at Runfold.'

'Another one; I'm glad I put a case of bottles in the car last night. See you later.' He jumped into the car and was off at full speed to the farm which was five miles away.

The dour Scotsman who was the farm manager opened the gate to Richard who drove straight up to the cow in the yard. Two rough looking youths were propping the cow up, and another was holding her head with a halter. The Scotch voice pleasantly welcomed Richard, and then he shouted at the lad in an aggressive manner. 'Pull her heid round, mon, for the vet.' He did so with alacrity, and Richard injected 500 c.c. of solution intravenously, but the cow did not respond much, so he injected another 500 c.c.

'That's a big dose you've given her.'

'Yes, it is, because she was not responding. She was more unconscious than she looked; if you had left her she would have been flat out on her side.' As though to emphasise the point, the cow pushed the boys away, belched and passed a lot of dung. After she had prodded the boy with her horns, he quickly let go of the halter. The manager told the boy to remove it. Richard pushed the cow with his foot; she watched him, but did not rise.

A boy came running across the yard, a piece of paper in his hand, which he gave to the manager, breathlessly exclaiming,

'Matron says you've to give this message to the vet at once, sir.'

Mr Rankin handed the paper to Richard who read: 'Please go to a cow down with milk fever at Duckworth Hall, Underley.'

'That's a fair way, mon, frae here.'

'It is that, must be fourteen miles; if she's not up in two hours, let me know. Good morning.'

Bill Rigby must have heard him coming as he roared through Olton. He was holding the cows back, and waved furiously, but Richard, holding the wheel firmly, did not let on he had seen him. He turned up the old short road into Underley, and then into the Hall, where the gate was open. Bill Bainbridge was waiting and opened the car door and got in.

'Good morning, Richard, I was beginning to think you hadn't got my message.'

'I got it in Runfold.'

'Drive on, she's in the field. You've come a fair way, then.'

'I've driven a fair way already this morning; this is the third one,' and it was a bad one, so very slowly 1000 c.c. of solution was injected intravenously. They left the cow sitting up ten minutes later.

'I blame myself, she's only been calved six days and I milked her out last night, because I was afraid she might get mastitis. Come on and we'll have a cup of tea.' Doris and Emma the dog both welcomed Richard who was glad of the hot tea, though he refused to have breakfast with them. Doris excused herself to answer the phone, and came back quickly.

'Mr Holden, there's a cow in the field at Whitehouse in Carden; it's got milk fever.'

'Really, not another. I've never known a morning like this before! Thank you for the tea. Cheerio.'

Bill Rigby, halfway across the yard at New Church, saw Richard flying back in the opposite direction. Richard noticed him, and said aloud, 'I bet he thinks I've gone mad.'

Coming down the hill he could see a man standing at a field gate on the other side of the bridge, and he waved Richard into the field. Tom Greaves was holding a bale of straw under the cow's shoulder to stop her lying flat.

'Am I glad to see thee, Mr 'olden. I'm fair worn out 'olding her up.'

'I bet you are, but I've come as fast as I can, I was at Underley.'

'Tha's ad another this mornin?'

'No, this is number four. Pull her head around.' She responded quickly to treatment, but wouldn't get up, so they left her and, getting into the car, drove to the gate. When Tom got out to shut it, he said, 'Conta wait, Mr 'olden, bugger's gitten up. I'll bring her in while I'm 'ere.'

Soon Richard watched Tom and the cow walking towards Whitehouse and he shut the gate. When he looked at his watch it was twenty-five minutes past nine. He really enjoyed his breakfast. Later that week the message read, 'Six bullocks ill at Poolside, Shipton,' but when he drove into the yard it was deserted, so he went to the house and knocked on the door. Mrs Parkinson opened the door and said they would not be long, because they had taken the wagon down the road to bring the six beasts home. Richard passed a few minutes looking at the pigs in the nearest building, until he heard them coming back. When they had unloaded they were driven into the empty heifer shippon and tied up, offering little resistance. Their diarrhoea was profuse, and they were all quiet.

'Where have they been grazing, Bill?'

'Down out marsh, this side, not on t' river side.'

'Is there plenty of grass down there?'

'Aye, too much; if weather's good it 'ull be mown in a fortneet.'

'And what about water?'

'They drink at brook, it's clean.'

'Then they have plant poisoning; they've probably eaten one of the marsh plants.'

'There's no need for 'em to do that, but there's a fair bit of lush stuff at end, and it were plain they'd been in there.'

'Well, it's irritating their guts, and coming quickly through them, so put them on dry keep, and dose them once with this medicine. There are four doses in a bottle; there's another and then a powder twice a day in water. If they are not a lot better in the morning let me know and fence off that far end of the field.'

'Aye, I will, Mr 'olden; if they're not doin' I'll let tha know.'

At breakfast the next morning Flora remarked that the 'phone had not rung yet,

'Yes, I had noticed. Probably the mad rush is over, so I'll take Jim for his walk down to the beach.' Hearing his name spoken, the dog became excited, running round the kitchen.

'Come here, Jim, let's get your lead on.' The dog obeyed, and Richard and Flora walked out of the front door into the garden bright in the sunshine. The dog saw another in Victoria Road and growled.

'Now then, enough of that, behave.' While they were talking the dog suddenly sprang over the gate, ripping the lead through Richard's fingers. He shouted, 'Jim, Jim, come here!' opened the gate and ran after him. The dog ran into Victoria Road and there was a squeal of tyres but he was going so fast, he went under the vehicle between the front and rear wheels. There was a long drawn out yelp, and Jim came out behind the lorry, lying still on the road. Richard, with Flora close behind, ran to him and picked the dog up; he was still breathing but blood was beginning to drop from his nose. They both rushed back and laid him on the surgery table, where he died.

'Oh, Richard, has he gone?' asked Flora beginning to cry.

'Yes, he has. The silencer or back axle squashed his chest flat; it would only be a second. Don't cry, come on and we'll have a cup of tea.'

'Yes, let's; he's always been a tearaway, but I am going to miss him so much, he has been such a wonderful pal.' Richard was not far from tears himself.

That evening it was announced on the radio that the RAF had bombed three dams in the Ruhr and caused extensive damage and flooding. It cheered them both up a lot, so they both had a drink before they went to bed, toasting the RAF and our Jimmy and Norman.

George Waring from Beacon Farm brought two dead ram lambs into the surgery and laid them on a sack on the table.

'Mr 'olden, why have these deed?'

Richard examined them. The scrotal sac was swollen, and he could squeeze bright yellow pus out of two recent wounds.

'Who cut these?'

'Luke Rider.'

'Oh him, he makes me tired; he never uses any iodine or cleans his knife, and good lambs keep dying, yet folk still have him; I don't know why.'

'I'll tell tha, becos he's cheap.'

'He's not cheap when you are losing good lambs like these.' Richard did a quick post mortem on both lambs; they had died from peritonitis.

'George, they've both died from peritonitis, caused by a virulent germ getting in where they were cut.'

'I thowt it were; wilta come and cut 'em for me?'

'Yes, how many have you?'

'Mebbe a 'undred or so.'

A day was fixed and Richard was guided up the valley past the reservoir where the lambs had been penned having been separated from the ewes. With three men helping him, he crushed the lamb's spermatic cords with his small Bundizzo forceps, and had finished in a couple of hours. As he was returning, driving past the reservoir, the car suddenly did not respond to the steering wheel being turned, and before Richard could stop it, it ran off the road, scraping along the stone wall, finally being stopped by running into a small rock. He climbed across the front seat and got out of the passenger door, thankful that the car had not gone through the wall when he saw the fifty foot drop on the other side. Using his calving smock as a groundsheet, he slid under the car, and could see the reason for the accident. The drop arm had come out of the fitting on the track rod, so he got his tool kit out of the boot and, pushing the arm back into position, tied it there with baling wire twisted tightly round it. Though it took him a long time, he was glad to arrive safely at Gordon's Garage by one o'clock. The latter had the car roadworthy by four o'clock, when Richard drove off to try to finish his day's work, vaccinating sows against swine erysipelas at Alan Williams' farm at Pelham. He was the first pig breeder to follow Richard's advice and to begin having all his breeding sows and his boars injected with vaccine against the disease. Getting a lot of his clients to believe that 'prevention was better than cure' was an uphill struggle; nevertheless he was pleased that since February there had been fewer mastitis cases on the farms where the disease was rife, though on one it had had no appreciable effect. Another farmer said that lamb dysentry serum was a waste of money until the laboratory report showed that his big lambs were dying of worms and coccidiosis. Richard had to take Bumble to Billsborough's again when she started calling, and he asked Tom to try a different male this time.

The lovely dry weather continued and Richard's health improved again, but he did not feel completely well, because he became tired so quickly. Having lost cattle in the spring the voice was worried, 'Tha'll evta cum quick, Mr 'olden, there's summat very wrong wi' mi beasts down on t' shore,' said Tom Bolton. Richard picked up Tom at the farm and having crossed the main Sandhaven to Droughton road, drove down the Banks lane until they came to the Bank – a wide high flood barrier built to stop the river from flooding all the lower lying land.

Leaving the car they scrambled up and over the bank and walked along the shore marsh, to where young Alf was waiting with some cattle – heifers and bullocks. The two which were tied up were restless, and unsteady on their legs. The lack of reaction to the light from his torch proved to Richard that they were blind. The cattle slowly milled around, and then one staggered away from the others, fell onto its side and had a fit.

'What's wrong, Mr 'olden? That un's goin to dee.'

'I am sure they have been poisoned, probably by lead. Have you been painting anything along the shore?'

'Nay, there's nowt to paint.'

'Paint tins could have been washed up by the tide or even an old door; you go that way and look and I'll go this.' He had gone probably a hundred yards, and found only the usual flotsam and jetsam left behind at the high water mark when Tom shouted for him to go back. When he reached him he had collected together a good few empty one-gallon paint tins, and they both could see where the hard dried paint had been chewed and licked away exposing the shining tin.

'So that's it, it is lead poisoning. Tom, you will have to get them all home and drench them to neutralise the lead. Let's go back to Alf and see what the one in a fit is like.'

It was dead, so Richard had to go back to the car to get his equipment; he brought also three opening drinks for cows, each containing a pound of epsom salts. He made a blood smear and then asked Tom to go with him to the farm house three miles away.

'Will you get two five-gallon churns full of water and take them back to the shore. Drench each beast with half a packet of the powder I've left with Alf. Pick out the bad ones and do those first, and mark them; you have six doses there. Don't forget to get hold of Robson to shift them.'

At the surgery, the blood smear proved negative, so he put every pound drench he could find into the car and asked Flora to make up some more, then he rang Bob Whiteside. He scrambled up the Bank again and as he hurried along the shore he felt dizzy, so slowed down to a walk. At the pen all the cattle were dosed, but Alf was not there; Tom had sent him to Sands House to borrow the tractor from Leslie Howarth, so that when the dead heifer had been pulled there it could be dragged over the Bank for Whiteside to remove it. Leaving instructions for all the cattle to be dosed again that evening, Richard left. He had asked Tom to get Bob to cut open the stomachs of the dead beast to try to find flakes of paint.

'It's a bloody scandal, ships in t' river throwin their muck over t' side, an' it's weshed up 'ere killing beasts. Whiteside found lumps and flecks o' paint in that 'un he opened. 'E said Bill Parkinson lost some down t' river round Poolside a few year back.'

'The others look brighter than yesterday; are they eating?'

'Aye, some are goin for t' grass and t'others for t' 'ay.'

'That's a good sign; I'll take a sample from this one, and I hope it's the last to go.'

'I do too, Mr 'olden.' The latter hurried away.

'Good morning, George, more trouble?'

'Nay, it's only a cow scouring' said Mr Arrowsmith. When they walked into the shippon the cow was eating cut grass with relish, and her temperature was normal.

'There doesn't seem anything wrong apart from the scour, so I'll take a sample of her dung and examine it tonight.' The sample was Johne's disease positive.

'I've ne'er had one afore, so 'ow 'ev I getten it?'

'I wish I knew; did you breed her?'

'No 'er is one o' t' last I bought, an oo's bin a good milker.'

'Then she could have had the germ in her when she came, it takes a long time to develop. She'll have to go.'

'I'll see she goes tomorrow.'

'Good, and don't forget to scrub that trailer out with disinfectant, and your boots. By the way, Mr Dawson agrees, get shut of those twelve right away, and have the lot tested in three months; another thing he said – you are not taking enough precautions to stop the disease getting in.'

A small truck drove into the yard.

''Old on a minit, Mr 'olden, while I show him where them three calves are.'

Tom Walsh the dealer from Ryton got out and followed George into a box, and came out pushing a calf towards his truck. George came back to Richard.

'So that's what he said. Whorra got ter do then?'

'For one thing don't let trucks into your yard or people go walking into buildings without washing their boots or wellingtons. You see, you don't know where they have been, and what germs they bring with them.'

'So I 'eve to 'ev a bucket of disinfectant at gate an' a brush. They won't like that.'

'Maybe they won't but you're the one who will suffer if you don't. I've got two farms doing it after they had trouble.'

'Dick wain't like it, I con tell thee.'

'Well, if he doesn't, you know what to do.' Some weeks later, after a row, he did sack him.

Flora was rather quiet at lunch, so Richard asked what was wrong.

'Nothing's really wrong; it's just I'm so disappointed that nothing's happened to me while Isabel Lord is having another baby. I went in the shop this morning, and she came through and told me.'

'They will be pleased.'

'But I'm not, Richard. I think we should try something else, because I learnt something the other day when I was in the Market Café. I found out that Dorothy Marsh's little girl is adopted. They got her through an adoption society three years ago, and I think it's about time we did something similar.'

'I've never given it a thought, do you think we should?'

'Of course I do, otherwise I wouldn't have brought it up, would I? I'm thirty now; in a few more years we won't want a baby running about, will we?'

'I think we would.'

'Speak for yourself. I'd have to look to it, because you wouldn't have time; so I'm going to ask her how they got her, and then we can apply.'

'So you've made your mind up.'

'Yes, I have; I'm not going into hospital again to be scraped and blown up, it's done no damn good.'

'Very well, then, love, you find out because I would like a son to follow me in the practice.'

'Really, you and the practice: it makes me sick; I'm talking about our future together. We'd still have to be together if we had no bloody practice.' Flora left the table and walking out of the room, slammed the door. Richard continued to sit at the table, annoyed by his wife's parting remarks, yet reluctantly admitting that she was right.

'Mr Holden, I've made an appointment for Mrs Roberts from Sykes to see you at nine o'clock in the morning here in the surgery. If that's not convenient, will you let her know,' said Joan.

'I'm sure that will be all right. Did she say what she wanted?'

'No, she didn't; my father said the other night that he'd be surprised if she stayed there after having that slight stroke.'

'Yes, it could be something like that, I suppose.'

When Mrs Roberts, who was using a stick, came the next morning, she was accompanied by her sons David and John. Joan asked them to sit in the waiting room, but when Richard entered he invited them to go upstairs to the lounge.

'No, thank you, Mr 'olden, I've 'ard work getting upstairs at the moment; we'll do here.' Richard sat down and asked,

'Now, how can I help you, Mrs Roberts?'

'Well, it's this way; our Tom has 'eard that the tuberculosis test is going to be started again some time in t' near future. We've both med up our minds to go TT but can't expect our Tom to help very much at my place, he's got his own work to do. So I'd like you to help David and John, really keep your eye on them, and tell them all they've got to do on t' farm before t' Ministry will 'ave 'em in t' scheme.'

'I'll do that with pleasure, Mrs Roberts, don't you worry about it. If you'll excuse me, I'll go and get you a leaflet I have which outlines precautions you will have to take on forming a herd free from TB.' He brought one.

'Here you are, Mrs Roberts; it's quite straightforward. The making of a double fence is the biggest job.'

'Thank you, Mr 'olden. You see, David, and John are going to run t' farm as equal partners from now on, that's why I want thee to promise me you'll help 'em.'

'I most certainly will do that for you.'

'Then we'll go; we've a lot to do, and I expect tha' 'as.' She got to her feet and limped to the door.

'Goodbye, Mr Holden.'

'Goodbye, Mrs Roberts.' Richard shivered slightly, and at once sensed he would not see her again.

It was just after lunch when Harry Gardner from the packing station at Middleton rang the bell, and came rushing in asking, 'Is anyone in?'

Joan coming out of the office, asked him what was wrong.

'It's mi cat, its back leg's in a weary way, I want Mr 'olden, quick.'

Richard came from the dispensary.

'I heard that, Mr Gardner, what's happened? Come into the surgery and put her on the table.'

The big black cat offered no resistance as he unfolded the blanket and gently moved the leg, which was broken above the hock with bits of bone sticking out of the mangled blood-soaked skin.

'And how did this happen?'

'I don't know like, one o' t' girls comin into t' stock room found it lying near t' door about ten minits sin; I think a dog's 'ad old on it.'

'It does look like it, the way the leg is crushed, and you can see it's only the skin which is holding this part onto the leg. It will have to be amputated.'

'Wilta do it for me? It's mi favourite.'

'Yes, leave it with me, and I'll do my best. Ring up in the morning to see how he's gone on, and just sign this form first.'

With Joan and Flora helping, he injected 20 c.c. normal saline straight away, injected local anaesthetic and amputated the lower leg. The cat was then put onto a warm bottle in a basket, and then taken upstairs in the coach house. Later that evening Richard injected more saline, and was delighted and pleased next morning when the cat drank some milk. Harry left the cat at the surgery for a week, before he took him back to Brick House.

'I'll be callin' 'im "Shorty" from now on, Mr Holden,' said a very grateful Harry. Richard wasn't sorry to see him go, because the reek of the urine of the tom cat so very strong in the recovery room in the loft was intensified by the hot weather. That afternoon he brought Bumble home, which gave some solace to Flora, still grieving over Jimmy's death, but this was partly nullified by the news on the radio that night that the film star Leslie Howard was dead. She hardly heard the next item that the air forces of America and Great Britain had bombed the Ruhr for twenty nights running.

When he called at Harry Helme's, the horse was better, and had been doing light work for a few days. 'An 'ow long will he stay reet?' – Harry's last question had Richard beaten, he had to say he didn't know. But he really enjoyed his dinner that night, Flora had started digging up new potatoes – they were delicious.

'They'd taste better still with butter on them,' he said.

Flora replied, 'You can have your ration on them if you like, but if you do you'll have to eat dry bread till Friday.'

'I can't do that; I'll do without first.'

The weather looked threatening, and it turned into a very stormy day for June. As luck would have it, Turner's the coal merchants in Droughton wanted a visit to a horse, so he decided to go to Wilton at the same time. He rang Mrs Foster, and she asked him to go at eleven o'clock.

When he arrived at the coal yard, Mr Turner himself was waiting in the rain and wind.

'Good morning, Mr 'olden, nice to meet thee. Tha's always sin mi lad afore, but he's bin called up, so I'm short 'anded like, till I con get an older chap. Johnny, bring t' horse out.' Richard could see the lump on its near shoulder as it approached.

'And how long's that been coming?'

'Quite a bit, but e were workin all reet, until he must ev knocked it and it's geten raw.'

'It is a tumour, and unless I operate and cut it out, it will go on growing.'

'So that's th' answer is it? How old is 'ee?'

Richard looked at his teeth and said, 'I can't be definite, but he's an old horse, probably about twenty.'

'Then I don't think al ev owt done to 'im, ees not a good worker. I'll sell him to t' 'orse butchers frae Salford; they pay a good price, tha' knows. Purr 'im back, an I must 'ev some greasy leg dressing o' thine, it's good stuff, 'cos I 'ev one just startin.'

Richard gave him a two pound jar, and left for Wilton. On the way there he saw a flash of lightning which was followed by a rumble of thunder, and then heavy rain.

He sprinted to the front door, which the maid opened at once; she must have been watching for him.

'Good morning, Mr 'olden, please go inta t' morning room.' There he found Mrs Foster, and a young man who was the split image of his mother.

'Hello, Mr Holden; what a wet morning. I'd like you to meet my son John.'

'It's nice to meet you,' said Richard, shaking hands, 'and are you going to hold this wild dog for me?'

'Mr Holden, how could you say such a thing; she's my lovely darling, aren't you, sweetie? Up you come,' and she put the dog on the table; Richard soon finished examining her.

'All clear this time, Mrs Foster.'

'That's good, off you go, my pet. Now, would you like a cup of tea? I think we all need one on a wild morning like this. John, please press the bell.'

The china sparkled and the silver tea service shone on the tray which the maid carried in. She gave a cup of tea to Mrs Foster who asked, 'How many sugars, Mr Holden?'

'Er, two please,' he replied, thinking that Flora would like the fortnight's sugar ration which was in the silver basin.

'Do have a biscuit with your tea.'

'Thank you.' They were not home made and were very good. They had chatted for a few minutes when John said,

'A great friend of mine is a vet, we were at Epsom College together. He did his training at the London College, but I went to the University and did engineering.'

'Really, and what's his name?'

'Terry Wilson; do you know him?'

'No, I don't know him.'

'You should meet him; he comes about twice a year to see us, when he is on his way to see his mother – she lives in Seaton at the Moorings.'

Mrs Foster said, 'She is awfully nice; Geoff her husband who died two years ago was the managing director of our Wolverhampton factory.'

John resumed, 'He has told me that he would like to work in this area, and so be able to visit his mother more often.'

'I can understand that. It was the reason my wife and I bought the Sandhaven practice four years ago, though I had been assistant there for two years before that.'

'How interesting it all is, but we must go. You will be here next month?'

'Yes, I will. Thank you for the tea and biscuits, Mrs Foster.'

'Don't, it's nothing. Bye.'

Another brief thunderstorm began in the afternoon when Richard was on his way to an urgent call from Bill Parkinson at Pooleside.

'By gum, it's a rough 'un for June, Mr 'olden,' said Bill. 'Come on through there int' big fattening house.' The sickly smell of cold boiled swill hung about the corrugated-iron roofed buildings, and they walked into a large square pen which had a cement trough running across the whole length of the wall at one end; again this was made of corrugated iron. Not far from the trough two well grown fourteen-week-old pigs were lying dead. There were twenty-eight alive in the pen.

'And you say that when you poured the first buckets in, they all rushed in and two flicked over backwards in a fit and died there and then.'

'Aye, that's reet, Mr 'olden – it were as quick as that.'

'Drag those two outside, and I'll open them and see what I can find.' He couldn't find anything and asked Bill to put the light on so he could see better, but that didn't help, neither did asking questions about the swill: how hot it was; and how many knives, forks, spoons and bits of broken plates were in it.

'It's funny – I've drawn a blank Bill. Start feeding again and we may see what happens.'

'Reet, I'll go and bring some. Alf!' he bawled, 'Come 'ere!' Father and son returned carrying buckets of swill which they poured into the trough, and the pigs charged forwards fighting and squealing. It was then that Richard noticed one jump on top of the others and slide forwards, but before it could get its head into the trough, it touched the wall and sprang back, landing on its back, twitching. Richard and Bill ran forwards to knock the pigs back, and Bill to steady himself put his hand on the wall.

He yelled, 'Hell, it's mi arm, it's 'lectric!'

'Alf, turn it off quick!' shouted Richard, running to him, but Bill was all right. 'By gum, that ran up mi arm like fire – so that's it.'

Alf came back.

'Bring me some steps, will you Alf?' Richard recalled two dead cows in similar circumstances years before.

'Who put this cable up here, Bill?'

'Birtwistle from t' village; it's for t' 'ot water boiler.'

'He should have put it in a conduit. You see, the rough edge of the iron has rubbed the rubber away down to the bare wire over the years with the pigs banging against it. I'd claim something off him for this.'

Bill and Alf looked at each other. Bill said, 'I can't do that. We put wall up aye six month after. So it weren't lightning after all, it were t' 'lectric.' The pig was sitting up, still looking rather dazed, but it got up when it was prodded. 'It was lucky for you, Bill, you were wearing rubber wellingtons, otherwise you would have been dead.'

'By 'ell, I hadn't thowt o' that.'

That evening after dinner, Richard was telling Flora how Bill Parkinson got the electric shock, and survived.

'It's remarkable how near to death you can get and yet avoid it, though this last few weeks the animals haven't: a lot have died – even our Jimmy.'

'You are forgetting Mr Roberts, and Uncle Jack.'

'No, I'm not, but they both did have sons to follow them.'

'And so could we. I've got that application form from Dorothy Marsh today.'

'Let's see it.'

'I'll go and get it; it's in my handbag. Here it is. When she gave it to me, she said that it took them six months to get Louise, and then she wasn't theirs until six months later.' They spent a whole hour answering all the questions; and finally Richard walked to the Post Office and put it in the box.

On his return, Flora said, 'After two operations, I hope it is third time lucky.' Richard agreed.

The next morning the car's engine repeatedly stopped, so Gordon was summoned and found the petrol pump was defective.

'Then you'll have to put a new one on it now.'

'I will; get in and I'll tow you to the garage. I think I have got one there.' He had, and Richard waited until Gordon had fitted it.

He asked him, 'Do you think it is worth spending more money on it?'

'Yes, it's still a good car, but the way you drive it, things will wear out – you know, the clutch, dynamo and your brakes.'

'Then I will keep it, but I do want you to get one of these good pre-war cars you were talking about as soon as you can.'

'I can soon do that, I know where there is one. It's been laid-up over a year but I could have it on the road in a couple of days.'

'Well, before you do that, Gordon, we'd like to see it, if you can arrange it.'

'I'll do that tonight.' He pressed the starter button, and the engine of the Morris roared into life.

'There you are; away you go.'

At eleven o'clock the next morning Gordon drove them to the Manor House, Wyresham, and Mrs Bold's chauffeur-gardener showed them the car. It was a 1936 Rover 4-cylinder with overdrive; the body was black and the upholstery was dark red leather. It had been driven 10,900 miles and was immaculate. Richard and Flora looked at BOK 478 and both wanted it; they finally bought it for £210. The next question was where to store the Morris, so Richard asked Gordon if he would keep it and overhaul it bit by bit when he had the time, which he promised to do.

They found Bob Hall waiting in the surgery, and he had two two-day-old piglets in a box. Richard asked him into the consulting room, and he put one on the table. Its belly was very distended, and the reason was that it had no anus.

'Can you do anything for 'em, Mr 'olden?'

'I don't know, Bob, until I cut in under the tail; if the end of the tube is there, I may be able to pull it back and sew it into position.'

'Then let's 'av a go, they're no good like this, poor little devils.' Under local anaesthetic Richard was able to correct one, but the other was hopeless so he destroyed it.

'Tha knows, Mr 'olden, I've ne'er 'ad 'em like this afore I bought yon new boar. Dusta think he's brought it?'

'Yes, it's probably from in-breeding: you know, a hereditary defect.'

'That's a devil, will every litter be like these?'

'They could be, you'll have to wait and see.'

'Oh 'ell, that's profit goin, and another thing, when I were cuttin their tushes, two o' t' little boars were all swollen where the balls should be.'

'That means they are ruptured.'

'Four out of nine wrong, that's near on 'alf of 'em, and worra bout ruptures?'

'I could operate on them when they are about four or five weeks old.'

'Tha con, well, I'll have to 'ev it done.'

'Then bring them a month today, but don't feed them for twelve hours before; put them in a crate.'

'Reet, I'll bring 'em; what time?'

'Two o'clock, Bob. I'll see you then.'

Tom Priestley was bad tempered – 'If I'm away 'alf a day on War Ag. work there's always summat wrong when I come 'ome. John says they were all reet yesterday when he looked at them.'

'They were; all t' seven o' them.'

'Then what the devil has killed her, Mr 'olden?'

'I don't know, but I'll have to have a blood smear first.'

'Then ger it done, I'll be back soon,' and he hurried away. The blood film was negative for anthrax, so Richard had a good look at the stomach wall in front of the developing udder of the heifer: there were two ragged-looking wounds about a foot apart from which blood stained fluid and gas was escaping.

'I'm certain she's been over a sharp stump or something like that, John, and it's gone into her guts. That's why she is so blown up.'

Tom came rushing back, 'Well what is it?'

'I think its peritonitis that's killed her from those stab wounds. She's probably been over a sharp stump.'

'Don't be daft, there are none in t' field.'

'I'm not being daft. It's either that, or someone has stabbed her twice with a knife.'

'I've never heard of such rubbish.'

Richard's temper rose, 'Maybe you haven't, but I've had horses killed with being stabbed with a hay fork. You don't know what people will do to get their own back on folk they've had a row with.'

'Then how can we find out?'

'I'll ask Bob Whiteside to meet me here and open her if you agree.'

''Course I do; I'm not going all the way to bloody Southall.'

'Then I'll do that, and you can see if you can find the cause.'

When Bob arrived at four o'clock, Richard drove up the field behind him, to see John chasing away two sows with their litters; one turned and charged him but he drove her off with his stick.

'Having trouble, John?'

'Not really, but she's always nasty when she's getten little 'uns wi' 'er.'

'I wouldn't trust any one that had piglets with her.'

Bob soon opened up the heifer, which had an acute peritonitis, both wounds having penetrated the abdominal cavity. He spread the bowel out and though it was slimy and fragile, the place where it had been torn was plain to see.

'Once that tear had been made, she had no chance; it was her death warrant, Tom.'

'I con see that.' Tom hesitated and then said, 'It's not reet somehow, tha might be able to stab beast once, but how the hell could you catch her to do it second time beats me.'

Nobody spoke; then he exploded again.

'I'll heve the law on t' bugger that's done it, if I con find him. Thanks, Mr 'olden for comin, and tha'll get cleared up, wain't you, Bob. John here will help thee,' and with that he strode away, a very angry man.

It was Eric Vickers from Pleasant View on the phone, 'Mr 'olden, I've three stirks in t' little field by t' house and one of 'em's dead.'

'Don't move it then, Eric, and I'll come and take a blood smear about the middle of the morning.'

The dead animal was lying behind the hedge which bordered the road and as Richard opened the gate, Eric appeared, climbing a ladder which was propped up against the side of a large hole in the ground.

'What are you doing down there?'

'Mekin a new septic tank, a bigger un; th' old un's too small, and overflowed in t' spring.' Richard made his blood smear and also took a swab, because there was a little bloody froth around the nostrils of the stirk.

'Don't move it until I ring you.'

'Reet, it's a grand day; I'll just walk down and see if that hay's ready, I turned it this morning. Cheerio.'

Richard did one more visit, and returned to the surgery, and having fixed and stained the blood film, examined it and to his surprise it was an anthrax case. He rang Eric at one.

'That you, Eric? Now, the stirk's died of anthrax, so don't move it, and I'll ring the

Ministry.'

'But Mr 'olden, it's gone.'

'Gone where? Look, Eric, I told you not to move it.'

'I didn't. While I were in t' 'ay field, our Robert saw Whiteside passin' and got him to tek it. He were goin to Pelham.'

'That's torn it. I'll deal with it. Goodbye.'

Richard rang Bob Dawson and explained the position.

'Don't worry, Richard, I'll get the police in Pelham to find him and send him back to Pleasant View; I'll have my chaps there by then.'

Bob Whiteside was furious because he lost a lorry load of cooked dog meat he was taking to the pet shops in Pelham and Mereside; and to add insult to injury he also had to go to the hospital for injections.

Richard had finished lunch when the phone rang. It was Tom Priestley.

'Wilta gerrup ere as fast as tha con, Mr 'olden? One o' them 'eifers as bin mauled by yon owd sow.'

'Good Lord, has she? I'm on my way now, Tom.'

When he arrived at Beech Tree the six heifers had been brought in, and were tied up in the shippon.

'Conta see it, Mr 'olden, it's a bit under 'er in front o' t' stifle.' There was a wound with blood dripping slowly off the hair surrounding it.

'We'll have to put her down to find out how far that's gone in, so get her in a box and I'll get my casting rope.'

'Ger 'er across yard inta t' second box,' Tom barked at John and one of his men, Owd Fred. The heifer was quickly roped and cast. Richard washed the wound with Dettol and water, then inserted his finger into the hole. The wound had reached the abdominal cavity and as he withdrew his finger greenish brown fluid escaped.

'It's no good, Tom, her bowel's torn; the sooner she can be killed the better. Let her up.'

'Blast it, I waint ev any more pigs on t' shop. John go and git wagon, bring it 'ere. Tell 'em to cock that hay, they can load it when tha gets back.'

'Where are you going to send her, Tom, the nearest abattoir will be best?'

'To Seaton then.'

'Then can I go in and ring Dick Williams?'

'Tha do; come on, Fred, and we'll git them two bloody sows out o' yon field afore they do more damage. Where's mi stick; bring board an' all; come on, we 'avn't all day.'

Richard explained to Dick that the heifer had a stab wound in her belly and her guts were torn, so she had to be slaughtered at once when she arrived. Dick promised that a butcher would be there ready and waiting for her.

Mrs Priestley, always pleasant and polite, asked Richard to have a cup of tea, and chatted about the good weather it was for hay making. Richard was enjoying eating a piece of cake when Tom came in. Richard had waited to hear the story.

'Any tay, Mother?'

'Yes, Tom. You do look 'ot.'

'I am 'ot, tha would be; them sows had to be chased all ower field afore we ger 'em in, Fred were fair done up. Tha would na believe it, Mr 'olden, but we were going across field to help load in t' 'ay field, an he sees yon heifer grazing and gerrin nearer sow that were rootin about. They were verra near when t' sow runs under t' 'eifer and chucks 'er 'ead up. 'eifer bellows an' lashing out runs off, so 'e comes back to find me quick.'

''Ave your tea, Tom.'

'I think boars and sows are more dangerous in hot weather; it was this time of the year when I were a lad that a sow threw me over a half door. I was lucky not to be hurt.'

'Yer were that; yer'd 'ear about that chap at Underwood last year going to tek a boar for killin; and 'e goes in t' sty an it killed 'im. Police shot the devil.'

'Yes I did. Thank you for the tea, Mrs Priestley. I'll be on my way.'

The heifer was a grade one carcase. That evening, as though he had not had enough to do with pigs that day, he visited two sows with erysipelas. Richard took the opportunity to preach the benefits of vaccination, but stopped when Les Windsor said, 'Aye, I knows that, but that 'un wore done last year.'

'Which proves what I have been saying; have them done once a year.'

Richard left Bank End thinking that he had won there; but he had not.

July started with lovely weather, and the first case of distemper Richard had seen for some time. The dog started having fits ten days later, so he destroyed it. On the Sunday afternoon Richard's reading of the *Veterinary Record* was interrupted by the phone ringing.

'Holden, vet here. Who?'

'Raymond Hill, Mercer Farm, Newton, a horse in a pit.'

'Are you Mr Hill? You are? Now tell me, have you had another vet to your horse?' No, you haven't? Then I'll come, and it's the first on the left going down the road out of the village, so you're near School Farm. Yes, I know where you are. Flora, where are my old tweed trousers, will you get them for me; a horse floundering round in a stinking muddy pit won't be like the Vicar's teaparty I can tell you. I'll take my slings, and I've got my casting rope. So long, see you at tea time.'

The muddy grey Shire, surrounded by flies, was lying half on its side partly submerged in watery mud and rushes.

'Are you Mr Hill? Well, how long has it been there?'

'Sin two o'clock when John 'ere cum and told me.'

John Tomlinson grinned, ''Allo, Mr 'olden, I thowt I'd stop an 'elp.'

'Thanks, because we'll need more, and I was just thinking two very strong long ladders, some cart ropes and a tractor.'

'I've gitten one.'

'Then go and bring it, and the ladders and ropes quick before he sinks further in.' He and some men went off fast. By this time neighbours were arriving, among them Bob Hall from Pelham.

'Hello, Bob. I didn't expect to see you.'

'Didn't ta? Course, tha wouldn't know his mi cousin, an he give me a shout to come o'er.'

The tractor, an old Fordson arrived, then two ladders, and the ropes.

'Now, Raymond, I want to get those ropes under him, so two will have to be tied together, and one end taken this way round the pit, and the end of the other rope the other way, then pulling to and fro we can work them under him, and then the belly band. Got it? Good, now push one ladder up to his head, and another to his tail. There'll have to be a man lying flat on the end of each ladder to guide the ropes under him, and a couple of men standing on this end as a counterweight so he doesn't sink it.' It took a long time to accomplish this, and their efforts were punctuated by much wit and bad language, and the steel D of the belly band was tied to the ropes, and another horse on the far side of the pit slowly moved away, dragging the band into the mud and under the now prone horse. When it encircled him, the steel cross bar was hooked on and with ropes and chains attached to it, to the tractor.

'Are you ready, Raymond?' shouted Richard. 'Then take the strain, right now, very slowly ahead, stop.' The horse was thrashing about and throwing his head up and down.

'Put that ladder back, somebody, and loop a strong rope through his head collar, and hang onto it. You two take it, now get that ladder out of the way.'

'Go on, Raymond, very slow.' There was a loud bang as a chain snapped, but as everything else was holding, he went slowly ahead, and dragged the horse well onto the bank, the sightseers scattering to get away from the flying muddy water. When he was released and his head pulled up, he reared up and got to his feet. The crowd cheered and began to disperse, but Richard finished up in the farmhouse kitchen with Bob and all of Raymond's family. Mrs Hill brought in mugs of tea, and brawn sandwiches, which were eagerly accepted. Richard asked, 'Why did you send for me?'

'Well, I were in a bit of a stew; tha sees, our vet from Mereside's bin ill a bit, so Bob told me to get thee.'

'Thanks, Bob; and what's wrong with him?'

'I don't really know, but they do say he wain't work again.'

He didn't: as the result of his illness he went blind.

When Richard arrived home Flora was on all fours watching Bumble who now had two kittens and later two more, in all one male and three females. It made Flora's day, cheering her up no end.

Richard was not happy, however, his indigestion was chronic, so he found his old recipe and made up a bottle of the medicine. He took a big dose after eating his tea, and got some relief, so began to read the *Record* again.

Flora later found him sound asleep, so did not waken him.

Flora stroked the head of the handsome, smooth-coated red dachshund as it stood on the surgery table. Its owner explained,

'It weren't so good in June, it had a cold like for a fortneet, but sin then it's getten this 'ere twitch.'

'I must tell you, it was not a cold. It had distemper and this is a nervous after-effect.'

'Will it get better, wife wants to know?'

'I've never known one, it lasts for life, and often that isn't very long.'

'Then put 'im out; wife can't bear to see 'im like that all time,' and the man turned towards the door.

Flora blurted out, 'Would you mind if I have him?'

Richard stared at her. 'But Flora, he is an ill dog.'

'I don't care, couldn't you try and get him better?'

'Well, if you want him we could try,' said Richard, resigned to having to give way.

'Missus, if tha wants 'im, tha con 'ev 'im, I'll be glad to be shut of 'im,' and in a second the man had gone, without paying his consultation fee.

'Let him go, Richard; I've got a dachsie, I've always wanted one. I can have him, can't I?'

'I don't know yet, let me examine him. Let's see if he has a temperature.'

He hadn't; so Richard went and slammed the door, but the dog paid no attention, he was looking at Flora and those appealing eyes had captivated her.

'Obviously he is over the acute phase of the disease, and loud noises don't affect him, but Flora, listen. In the weeks and months ahead the chorea may become worse, his brain degenerate and fits occur; he could even become vicious.'

'Have you finished? I am having him.'

'Then the first thing you're going to do, my girl, is wash him – he smells so sour; and burn that collar.'

'I'll do it straight away.'

'You do, and use Neko soap, I hope he's the last animal we collect. This house is getting like a zoo with six cats and a dog, that's seven.'

'No it isn't, it's eight – you've forgotten yourself, you old monkey.' With the dog tucked under her arm a laughing Flora fled.

Mrs Foster was worried, and wanted to know if there was an outbreak of distemper in Droughton.

'Yes, there is: I have had two cases brought here from Droughton.'

'Oh dear! Will Poppy have caught it? She has been on her lead walking with me around Droughton while I've been shopping.'

'No, she will not have caught it, but she will have been in contact with the germ, so I think it would be advisable to give her an injection of anti-distemper serum, just to be on the safe side.'

'When could you do it? I am too busy to come to Sandhaven.'

'Would Wednesday afternoon be convenient, Mrs Foster?'

'Yes, it will; please come about three, will you?'

It was hot on Wednesday, so there was little work to do because every farmer was making hay.

After lunch Richard was feeling tired when Flora asked, 'Have you only Mrs Foster's dog to visit this afternoon?'

'Yes, why, love?'

'Because I'd like to come with you, and look round the market and shops in Droughton and then get some slack from Turner's, so I'll put an old blanket in the car.'

'Then be ready at two.'

His indigestion was making Richard uneasy as he was driving rapidly into Ryton, and suddenly he felt dizzy and his vision blurred for a moment. He stopped the car abruptly, and put his head in his hands.

'What's wrong, Richard? Richard, what's the matter?'

'Don't panic. I'm just feeling dizzy; it's this damned indigestion – I should have taken a dose of medicine after lunch.'

'Listen, I'm certain indigestion doesn't make you feel like that. Let's go back home at once, and I'll get the doctor.'

'I'm not going back, calm down. I'm already feeling better.'

'Maybe you are, but if we are not going back now, you are going to see Bill tonight.'

'How can I? Don't be daft, I've got the surgery to do, haven't I?'

'Of course you have and I'm not being daft. You are going. I'll make the bloody appointment for seven fifteen, and I'll see you damned well get there.'

'All right then, calm down, I'll go love.'

'Good; if you feel well enough, let's go.'

Richard drove off, and began to speed.

'Will you drive slower, we are not going to a fire in Droughton.'

'Oh I will, now stop nagging.'

'I'm not nagging, but you are driving even faster in this car with its overdrive. Coming into Ryton you were doing seventy.'

'Rubbish.'

'Don't be so damned rude, Richard, and I'm not talking rubbish; bloody well slow down when I tell you, I don't want killing.'

He drove more slowly all the way to Droughton Market where Flora got out, and also all the way to Mrs Foster's, thinking over what his wife had said. Of course I am driving faster, I have to ...

'Ger 'ere as fast as tha con,' meant just that, so he did. Yes, I do often feel rotten, but I'll be better in a week, these do's always die away in a week. I wonder what Bill will find tonight, whatever it is I can't let five year's work go down the drain, can I?

'Yes, Mrs Foster, I think serum now, and then next month, a preventative vaccination is the best course to adopt.'

Poppy whimpered slightly.

'Oh, you're hurting her, Mr Holden.'

'I wouldn't say hurting, but 10 c.c. is a big dose of serum, so it's bound to cause discomfort.'

'There you are, let me rub it better,' Poppy's tail wagged.

'Oh, what a brave girl. Thank you, Mr Holden and you will come next month, and vaccinate her again?'

'I will.'

'Then I'll say good afternoon.'

Flora was waiting. 'And how do you feel now?'

'Better, it's passed off. Had a good mooch round?'

'Yes, I got two tea towels without coupons.'

'So you're on the black market now are you?'

'Yes – let's get to Turner's and get some off-permit slack. I don't know why it is that Jim Worsley has never got any at home.'

Will Turner let them have two bags 'It's a bit better than sleck is this – it's sweepings off lorries, so there's bit o' coal in it, it'll burn weel. Gimme a couple of colic drinks, and jar of stuff for grease while you are here, Mr 'olden.'

At seven fifteen exactly, the maid ushered them into Dr McConnel's consulting room.

'Good evening, will you come in and sit here, Flora?'

'Open wide, Richard, good, suck the thermometer, I want your temperature.'

'Now what has he been up to this time?'

Flora described the events of the afternoon, after which Bill closely questioned Richard and obtained many answers which began to form a clinical picture.

'Give me your hand while I count your pulse. Did you run all the way here? No, I thought not; then get your shirt off, now get up and run on the spot.' Richard did so for a couple of minutes, while Bill read his notes.

'That's enough, stop now,' and he checked Richard's pulse again. 'Do you feel dizzy?'

'No, I'd say a bit light-headed.'

'So your heart rate is up to 160 beats a minute. Please sit down,' and after another examination Bill pressed his chest and then his stomach. Richard grunted.

'That's sore, isn't it?'

'Yes.'

'Listen, you have a heart rate which becomes very rapid after slight exercise; it's over double normal, and also you have an undulating fever which must be caused by the abortion germ. Coupled with this you have got epigastric pain – probably some ulceration. Get your trousers off and let me look at your legs.'

The left was more swollen than the right.

'This is a recurrence of the old trouble, and there is only one thing which will definitely help and that's rest, apart from some medicine for your stomach.'

'I'm taking some, at least when I remember.'

'What is it?' Richard told him. 'Then I'll give you one without ext. belladonna liq. in it; you know that will affect your vision, but you must rest.'

'Bill how can I? I am single handed, I am on the go all day.'

'And often half the night as well,' said Flora.

'I know that, but Richard, you will have to slow down, or Mother Nature will sooner or later do it for you. I'll treat your heart condition now; and I'll arrange for you to see Mr Forest the orthopaedic surgeon in Droughton about your knees. Finally, if you can't rest, or take things easy, have you considered getting an assistant?'

'Not really but Flora did suggest it a bit since.'

'I'd think about it, so I'll see you next week at the same time.'

The next afternoon Richard said, 'Hello, Bob, come on through. Is the other one OK?'

'Aye, it's fine, though it's always getten a dirty behind. Where shall I put 'em?

'On the floor; now, they haven't had any food?'

'Nay, I gi' 'em a lile bit o' slop last neet, and pur 'em in t' crates.'

'Good; put number one on the table.'

With a brick under his hind quarters the piglet was tied down, and anaesthetized with ether, Richard castrated the boar, then dissected out the hernial sac after replacing the intestines. The sac was tied off, and the wounds thickly dusted with sterile sulphanilamide.

'Tha' not going to stitch um up?'

'No, Bob, the wounds will soon heal; dust them with this powder each time you feed them, and keep them on clean straw.' Richard soon did the second piglet, and Bob said, 'Thanks, Mr 'olden, I'll be 'aving some more; there's two litters by yon boar, and some of 'em are brocen.'

'Then let me know when they are this size and I'll do them. Cheerio, Bob.'

When Richard arrived at Whitehead's at Far Parkside, there were seven well grown heifers standing about near the water trough in the yard, and one lying dead near the gate into the field.

'What's happened here, Vic?'

'I don't really know; they've bin in t' big paddock and were doin well. Bein in t' 'ay I even't sin 'em for two days, but afore dinner Tom saw this 'un fallin about, so he brought 'em up, and it fell in a fit and deed.'

'So, they've been on grass only – you've not fed them anything extra?'

'Nay, they didna need owt else.' Tom came up.

'Will you catch one for me?'

'Aye they're easy, they don't seem ta see thee comin'. Seetha.' Richard waved his hand over the animal's face – it was blind.

'Vic, it's poisoning, I'm certain – that one's blind and that had a fit and died, where do they drink?'

'They've drunk 'ere now.'

'And what about in the field?'

'There's a trough.'

'Yes, but in this very hot weather, it could be empty.'

'Tom, go and see.'

Richard made a blood film, and was waving it about to dry it, when Tom shouted, 'Dad, there's nowt in it.'

'When was it filled last?'

'Bert 'ull know.'

'Will you go and ask him?' It had been in the previous week.

'Then it must be leakin'; let's go and see.'

The old wooden trough had been well maintained, layer after layer of black paint outside, and white paint inside had been applied over the years. In the heat the boards had shrunk; the paint had cracked and peeled off; where the cattle had been trying to eat it, it was plain to see.

'Vic, I'm certain it's lead poisoning. They are just like some I had not long ago. Can I go to the house and examine this slide, and then I'll open that dead one?'

It was negative for anthrax, so Richard cut open the heifer, and in the first stomach were bits of white paint. Even after treatment, one died the next day, and another was sent for slaughter because it was blind.

It was on the last Wednesday in the month that George Duke asked Richard to go to his office. He told him that Standard Life would issue a policy, and would he now pay the first premium. Richard paid by cheque, and as he walked down Church Street he began to worry about his finances; he seemed to be paying out the whole time. There was now the secretary's salary; he had bought the Rover, and now this policy, and he had the garage and drugs bills and the mortgage to pay. He went at once to the bank to see Dick Harrison.

'Oh, you are still in credit, Richard, even after paying the premium – though the balance is small this month. You haven't paid in very much, you know.'

'I realise the farmers are too busy to pay bills at the time of the year – this is my big worry. Anyway, I'll see how things go, before I bother you again.'

'Richard, it's no bother; come in any time.'

As he stepped out of the bank, there was a rumble of thunder. Walking up Cross Street he said to himself – 'if it's not one damn thing it's another,' because a back tyre on the car was flat. He changed it and got wet through.

'What are you playing at, getting soaked; why didn't you send for Gordon? You know you are not well.'

'Because I was trying to cut down on expenses; the Bank Manager has just told me that my credit balance is small.'

'Now you are not starting to worry about money again, are you?'

'No, but I can't go in the red, can I?'

'You won't; don't forget I've got some money, love – it's yours if you need it.'

It could have been relief, or because he felt weary, but his eyes filled with tears. As he quietly said, 'Thank you, Flora,' she kissed him.

The sultry thundery weather continued, and the outbreaks of swine erysipelas became more numerous; some were very acute – large pigs were found dead, their skin a purplish red all over; other had diamonds and a high temperature. Two large bacon pigs were found dead with not a mark on them. He did a post mortem on both of them, and the only lesion present was a very large heart and pericarditis.

'It looks as though t' diamonds ev wrecked their 'earts, Mr 'olden,' said Bill Iddon at Launds Farm in Willington. As there couldn't be any other explanation Richard agreed.

Flora went with Richard to Bill's surgery and was cheered when he found Richard's heart rate had fallen and his temperature was normal. The appointment with Mr Forest was arranged for the following Tuesday.

Richard in the dispensary checking the stock position was annoyed at finding that there was little left of some drugs. He found a large sheet of white card and wrote across the top of it in capital letters, 'URGENT DRUGS TO BE ORDERED,' and underneath drew three columns headed: date; name of drug; and amount left. At the bottom he wrote, 'Everybody please complete this list when dispensing if necessary.' Then he went into the surgery, and was looking at the list of operations to be done, when John came in.

'Ev you 'eard news, Mr 'olden? Old Mussolini 'as resigned.'

'Go on, John, I don't believe it; whose leg are you pulling this time?'

'Nay, I'm not; it's true, it's on t' radio.'

As it was Saturday evening, Flora was intent on getting Richard away from work, and made him go with her to the Palace. He for his part was surprised that so much had happened on the war fronts during the last few weeks which he had not even noticed, or heard about.

He watched the Pathé Gazette showing the Allies landing in Sicily; then the night-time bombing of Hamburg which filled him with amazement. He stared intently at the screen, convinced that no one could have survived in that city after such a bombardment. On Sunday he and Flora finally drafted an advertisement which they sent to the *Veterinary Record*.

'Experienced assistant required in North-West England in mixed mainly agricultural practice. Permanency right man. Live out. Box number.'

Flora said she would go and see if Mrs Clunie, who kept the Meatham Guest House on Fairfield Road would be able to accommodate another paying guest in the near future, and Richard would check up on when the car would be ready. As for extra instruments, he would watch the miscellaneous column in the *Record*. They talked far into the night making plans with a confidence Richard did not feel, but he did not tell Flora.

So August came with warm showery weather, and all the seasonal troubles including 'August bag', and sore eyes in young stock at grass. With the former Richard usually saved the cow's life though never the udder, but he was defeated by the eye condition; many went blind in one or both eyes and were sent for slaughter. On Tuesday Richard, accompanied by Flora, had his consultation with Mr Forest; and was disappointed that he was not given any immediate relief from the pain in his knees. The consultant confirmed that he had a synovitis in both of his knees, and some arthritis in his left one, both conditions probably aggravated by infection with brucellosis. To make certain he took a blood sample from Richard for laboratory examination. Treatment consisted of a course of a new sulpha drug, the use of acetyl salicylic acid and anodyne tablets when required, but mainly rest.

'I think it was a waste of time and money,' said Flora as they walked to the car.

'I do too; he did not tell us anything we did not know, but this new sulpha drug might help. If he's the best chap to see, I'm not going to worry about my knees any more; obviously I've just got to put up with them. But I am going to use what the charwoman uses when she is scrubbing the Town Hall steps.'

'Whatever's that?'

'It's an old car inner tube, half blown up, folded over and into a sausage shape with string.'

'That's a good idea; you will get one from Gordon, won't you?'

'Two, you mean, then I can always have a clean one in the car.'

Back in the surgery Joan Collinson asked if she could have the next morning off to go to her godmother's funeral – she was also her Auntie May. May Gebbie was one of three sisters; the other two were Joan's mother Mrs Collinson and Mrs Isabel Walker from Fell Top, Icken. May's husband James had died a few years earlier, and as he had been a chartered surveyor and agricultural valuer, he had left her very well off indeed.

Richard, listening to this family history, realised that Mrs Collinson and Mrs Walker were very alike: always pleasant, friendly and unflappable – he thought back to the night when all the windows at Fell Top were blown out by a land mine and Mrs Walker was very calmly brewing tea. It was a case of 'the iron fist in a velvet glove'. Richard gave Joan the morning off, and longer if her leaving the funeral early would give offence.

Among cattle more abortions and retained placentas were taking place, so Richard went to Boots the Chemists, and bought six pairs of surgeon's india rubber gloves, even though they cost two shillings a pair. He had reasoned that by using them he would reduce somewhat the skin contact with the abortion germ, and its toxins, and as they were easily sterilised they would be cheap at the price. More cases of tuberculosis and Johne's disease were found among cows at grass – the truth of the saying 'Johnny Green either cures or kills them' was very evident. This year certainly he was activating latent infections which soon became killers, and the losses were great.

It was almost lunchtime and Richard was at Intack in Middleton talking to Jack Booth, when Bill Goodier from Hunter's Farm drove very quickly into the farmyard, and, stopping near to them, shouted, 'Mr 'olden, wilta cum quick; mi best cow's gitten milk fever an rolled inta t' brook.'

'By heck, I will that; follow me,' said Richard. 'And I'll come and help thee,' said Jack, and in seconds three cars were screaming up the main road to the village at seventy miles an hour. Richard slowed down harshly as he swung into Smithy Lane, and drove on down it quickly to where some people were waiting at a gateway and waving him into the field. He was closely followed by the other cars and drove right up the bank where Mrs Goodier was holding onto a rope which was tied round the cow's horns down below in the brook. This was helping her elder son Robin to keep the cow's head above water.

'Right, Bill, pull hard on that rope,' said Richard and pulled on his thigh boots. 'Mrs Goodier, hand me this stuff when I've got down to her, quick.' He slithered down the bank into two and a half feet of water.

'Keep pulling up there. Robin, hold this rope, while I get the needle in the vein.'

Soon the solution was steadily flowing into the cow.

'How did she get down here?'

'Childer comin out at school, saw her staggering and cum an told me. I gorra rope an mi bike, but as I pedalled through t' gate oo were on t' bank an fell in. I scrambled down an put rope on her 'orns, and chucked it up for t' kids to old, while I kept 'er eid out o' t' water. One ran and told mi Mum, and thi wife told Dad tha were at Intack.'

The cow's ears began to move, then she belched, but Richard continued slowly pumping in the second 500 c.c of solution.

'Ooo's comin to, Mr 'olden.'

'Yes, she is; it's lucky you were here in time, she would have drowned very quickly.'

Bill arrived driving a tractor with a trailer behind it. He stopped and began throwing spades out, shouting, 'Will you lot start digging bank away so oo con ger out?'

Willing hands seized the spades and began at once. When Richard removed the needle, the cow began to struggle. He handed his equipment to Mrs Goodier and, seizing the cow's tail, tried to pull her onto her feet. She began to scrabble about, feeling for her footing and soon stood in the middle of the brook. He took the rope off her horns.

'That were reet quick, Mr 'olden,' said Robin, then he shouted, 'Warra doin', Dad?'

'Diggin bank away.'

'Tha stop it; oo'll walk tu t' old ford now.'

Half the village had arrived, and the diggers stopped work, and watched as the cow was slowly coaxed along the brook for about a hundred yards. As she walked up the gravelly slope into the field there was a resounding cheer. Richard did not cheer; instead he emptied a gallon of muddy water out of each thigh boot.

'Thanks a lot, Richard,' shouted Bill, as he walked off behind his best full pedigree red shorthorn; from the teats of her huge udder milk was beginning to drip.

Richard went to Mrs Foster's at Wilton and revaccinated Poppy. From there he drove through Droughton to Ashfield to a new client at Far Pasture.

'Good morning. You are Mr Dobson?'

'Aye.'

'Have you had another vet to treat this cow?'

'Nay, there's not bin one on t' place sin afore last Christmas.'

'Good, where is she?'

'In t' box; follow me.' The new calved Jersey was feeding her calf. 'Oo calved last neet, and it's t' other back tit that's blocked like.'

Richard drew out one squirt of milk, but the teat did not refill.

'There's a skin across the top of the teat. I'll try and shift it. Nose her for me, will you?'

Being as aseptic as possible, Richard introduced the corkscrew instrument, and pushed it up to the top of the teat. The first time he pulled it down nothing happened, but at the second attempt the teat filled.

'Try that, Mr Dobson.'

'Ee, that's grand.'

Stan Earnshaw had come in.

'There y'are Victor, I told thee he'd do it.'

'Hello, Stan, I haven't seen you for a bit.'

'Tha reet, I've had nowt wrong for a twelvemonth, but I want some mastitis powders now, and a bottle of dressing for mi horse; he's gitten sore shoulders.'

'And Victor, are you any relation of George Dobson at Catley?'

'Aye, he's mi cousin – one tha got them dogs for.'

'That's right, I did.'

'Now, Stan an me want tha to do t' test for TB on our cows. That sees, we've bin buying TT cattle for two year, an as Ministry may start scheme again next year we want to be ready. It's time they were done, isn't it?'

'Yes, it is.'

'Well, conta do em next month when we are not so busy like?'

'Yes, I'll ring Stan then and arrange it.'

There were only two replies to the advertisement in the *Record*. The first, handwritten, was from Northern Ireland, from a member who had been qualified six years, but already had worked in five practices. He said that he could not ask his boss for a testimonial because he might get the sack.

'But why hasn't he got some from the other practices where he has worked?' asked Flora.

'I think he can't be much good, so they didn't give him one and sacked him.'

The second, which came at breakfast time a day or two later, was typewritten and the post mark was Ludlow. Mr T.A. Wilson had qualified at the London Royal Veterinary College in 1939, since when he had worked for one year in the Walsall practice, and been in his present post for two years. He was single, and would like to work in the north-west. If required he would be pleased to attend an expenses paid interview. The testimonial from his principal in Ludlow said that he was a good worker, cheerful and a good diagnostician and surgeon. He said that he could recommend him to any position of trust, but would be sorry to lose him.

'Read that, Flora, I think he sounds like our man. I know that name, but for the life of me I can't remember how I do.'

'That is a good testimonial; I'd write back straight away and enclose an s.a.e. for his reply.'

Richard got the message pad, and drafted a reply, describing the practice, prospects, accommodation and car. He invited him to come on the Thursday next week, when he could stay the night, and discuss things more fully, and see the surgery and the area. As soon as Joan arrived she typed the letter and took it at once to the Post Office.

Next morning he went to see George Duke, to ask him what salary and other conditions he should offer Mr Wilson; he received the reply from George the next day.

Later that week Richard diagnosed his first case of husk that year – and presumed that the larval worms had not been killed off in the previous mild winter. The August weather was becoming hot, and the harvest was proving to be a good one, which was pleasing Flora who was cleansing all her bottling and jam jars. A cow calving at Bill Harrison's Cross Roads Farm, soon had Richard on the scene.

'Aye, oo's bin bagged up for four days an oo's three days overdue now.'

Richard examined the cow. 'Billy, she's calved recently; she's empty.'

''Er can't be; there's no calf or cleaning an there's no sign in t' field.'

'And you've really searched it?'

'Aye, it's pit field, and me an Tom wi Whittaker frae next door, ev bin all ower it.'

'Have you any foxes about here?'

''Ave we hell as like, I shoots 'em.'

'I'm sorry, Bill, I can't help you; get her milked or she'll get mastitis, she's really badly over stocked.'

'Aye, I will; by the way did ta 'ear that skinny May Gebbie left nigh on forty thousand quid?'

'Good Lord, no.'

'Aye oo es, equal to each niece and nephew.'

'That's a windfall for the two Collinson girls.'

''Tis that, I'd be suited if it 'appened to me, by 'ell I would.'

'So would I,' said Richard fervently.

Bob Hall said that the first two pigs were doing well, so he had brought two more ruptured ones. Richard operated on them that afternoon.

He thought that all his hopes were dashed when on Monday night Terry Wilson rang up, but it was only to say that he would not need accommodation on Thursday night because he would be staying at his mother's house. Richard thanked him for ringing and asked at what time he would arrive on Thursday. He said it would be about two o'clock.

Richard went through to tell Flora, and then the penny dropped.

'I know why the name was familiar. John, Mrs Foster's son, said he had a pal, who was a vet whose mother lived in Seaton.'

'That solves the question of finding accommodation if he wants to live at home,' said Flora.

'Wait a minute, we haven't even seen him yet.'

When he arrived they were favourably impressed. He was a well dressed, dark haired man, about 5 feet 7 inches tall, who wore spectacles with rather thick lenses. He was cheerful, smiled easily and often, and took a very great interest in everything, asking many questions. He admired the consulting room, dispensary, and office – giving Joan a charming smile when they were introduced.

The three went upstairs to the lounge, and Flora produced tea. As they drank it they chatted until Richard produced the Contract of Employment which George Duke had written, and an assistant's agreement, which was a copy partly of the one he had signed at Holme years ago. Terry looked at them, and then asked if he could take them with him to read at his leisure, to which Richard agreed. He also asked if he could come to see more of the practice on the Friday morning, so Richard told him to come at 8.45 and then asked him how he had come that day.

'In my own car. I use it in the Ludlow practice, and they pay my expenses.'

'That's a good arrangement, but as I said in my letter I will provide you with a car.'

'I was pleased to read that, Mr Holden, because my old Austin 10 is dropping to bits – it's so bad I left it round the corner.' Richard laughed and excused him at four o'clock, because he said he had promised his mother to be home then, but would be back next morning on time. Richard and Flora both hoped that he would accept the post.

Joan Collinson, dressed in black, arrived next morning, and told Richard that her aunt's father-in-law, after being ill for a week, had died. He was Tom Walker's father, who in his youth had been a very well known fell runner. Richard at once wrote a letter of sympathy to Tom. Terry, wearing an old tweed suit, a cap and wellingtons, went with Richard on his morning round which took them across the practice. He said that he accepted the employment contract of £10 a week to live out, one weekend off in four and a week's holiday a year, with car and all equipment provided. He told Richard the idea of permanency was very attractive and that he would like to obtain the position and be near home, so he would like to know soon if he had obtained the job. Back at the surgery, Richard took him up to the lounge where Flora joined them. He then poured out three sherries, told Terry that the job was his, and they all drank to a successful future.

The Tuberculin test at George Arrowsmith's produced two doubtful reactors, which was a better result than Richard had expected. It really pleased George who had now put in place all the precautions against infection which were required. He said to Richard, 'Tha knows, Mr 'olden, av learnt mi lesson: cheap labour is damned dear in t' long run.'

Richard wished that more of his clients felt the same way, because the ignorance and imbecility of the labourers on some farms was dreadful. Driving home down Victoria Road he saw that someone had painted in large white letters, 'Second front now' across the railway bridge, and he was acutely aware that his own worries and ambition had driven the war completely out of his mind for weeks.

The riddle of the whereabouts of the missing calf at Billy Harrison's at Cross Roads Farm was solved that day when its carcase came to the surface in the centre of the pit. 'Oo must ev calved ont very edge and it an t' cleaning fell straight into t' water,' he told Richard, but the reason why the cow chose to calve in such a dangerous place remained a mystery.

He had been to Whyngate, and was driving down the lane to the main road when on the corner he almost collided with two ponies which were being ridden at full gallop abreast in the centre of the lane. He swerved and jammed on his brakes, but the car slid along the grass before it stopped. One pony, a bay, plunged into the ditch on his near side and splashed past, but the chestnut shied away and galloped on with the child grimly hanging on to the pony's mane. He was so shocked and annoyed, he turned the car round and drove after them, seeing them go into the farmyard. He followed them in and Bill Meadows came up to the car to find out why Richard had come back.

'Because I could have killed those damned kids down the lane, they were riding abreast in the centre and they had no bally control over their ponies.'

'The girl riding the chestnut is our Brenda.'

'Look, Bill, she doesn't know how to ride; she can sit on it and steer, but that's not horsemanship, neither of them had any control; if I'd been the milk lorry they would be dead.'

'Don't say that, Richard. I'll have a talk with her, but you know she thinks the world of that pony.'

Remembering how much as a youth he had loved Dolly, his anger evaporated, and he said, 'I can appreciate that, but Bill, before there is an accident take her to a riding school for lessons, so that she can ride properly.'

'I'll do that, Richard; thanks for coming back and telling me. Liz ull wade in to her when I tell her what happened.'

'I hope she does, and you could ask Colin Greenwood at Hill House to help; you know he's an expert rider – he was in the Lancers.'

'That's a good idea; thanks Richard; I'll ask him to teach her today.'

'I never thought in 1939 that this Friday morning we would be starting the fifth year of the war,' Flora said at breakfast. 'How much longer is it going to go on? It's worse now than last year – everything's in short supply, or rationed.'

'You needn't tell me, but I wish I knew, because though the Jerries and Japs are being pushed back, they're still fighting as hard as ever. I suppose we will have to bomb them to bits, no matter what the cost.'

Richard looked at the post mark on the envelope; it was from Skipton and he at once thought of Norman. The letter was from Norman's mother who quoted the official notification: 'Flt. Lieut. Norman Robinson DFC missing on operations on August 27th, is presumed killed.' After the massive air attacks on Berlin at the end of last month Richard was not surprised, yet he was intensely sad that the last close friend of his college days had been killed. He left the rest of his breakfast untouched. Flora, quickly aware that the news had distressed him deeply, kissed him and told him to take the dachsie for a walk, giving him the lead. In that still golden September morning man and dog walked along the Promenade, and Richard stopped and looked across the shining water admiring the beauty of the view. But it was no good, he suddenly felt that strange sense of unease and shivered, and at once hurried back home.

'Feeling better, love?' asked Flora.

'Yes,' lied Richard. 'I'll have another cup of tea.'

'And have you had a good walk?' Flora said to the dog which wagged his tail.

'You know, we will have to give him a name, we can't go on calling him Dachsie. Have you any ideas, Richard?'

'Not really, but he is a little brick; he never lets that twitching leg stop him going anywhere.'

'But we can't call him Brick.'

''Course we can't, call him Rock.'

'No, Rocky sounds better.'

'That's it, Rocky it is from now on. I'll go and write a letter to Mrs Robinson.' He had just finished, when he rushed off to his fifth milk fever case in four days. At milking time that afternoon Dick Smith from Meatham Hall rang and asked 'For t' vet to come 'ere quick, bull's gitten loose and es in t' yard.' Reading the message, Richard asked, 'What does he think I am? A matador?'

He got a new large bull ring and the nose punch from the cupboard. Dick was standing at the yard gate with a pitch fork in his hand.

'Where's your bull now, Dick?'

'T'other side o' yon muck cart; ees brocken his ring; what are we goin to do?'

'I'll tell you, catch him. Now, have you got a cow riding today?'

'Aye, we ad when we brought 'em up.'

'Right, you go in, and tie her up opposite the door nearest to where the bull is, and I'll bring my stuff.'

When this was done Richard and Dick stood in the feeding passage, and waited until Leslie had opened the door and got clear.

Richard had his long casting rope ready. 'Now listen, when he mounts her, I'll get this rope round his horns, while you stop him coming over the top with your pitchfork, and Les and I will tie him to the top rail.'

'Warra about us?' asked Dick.

'Dick, he'll be more interested in the cow than you, just be quiet and don't startle him.'

The bull cautiously walked in, and then quickly mounted the cow. Richard's doubled rope held him, the cow's tie was cut, and she was pushed away. A second rope was passed through his head chain and secured. Les held the double rope while Richard slipped the ring into the bull's nose and tightened the screw firmly. He threaded the chain through the ring and the bull blew slime all over Richard's face.

'Hold that chain, Dick, I can hardly see.'

'Ee doesn't like thee, Mr 'olden, since tha rung him years sin.'

Richard wiped his face. 'I'll tell you something; neither would you, Dick, if I'd stuck a ring in your nose.'

Leslie laughed. 'Tha reet there, though like bull I'd ev bin more interested in t' female. Like carry-on next door, 'asta heard?'

'No, what are you on about now?'

'Eee, I must tell thee. They git two o them Itie's – that knows, prisoners o' war – next door last May, an one of 'em is a big black 'aired fella an our Les sez he talks English. I thinks he musta bin an officer. Any road, many a day he were in t' house wi Ada, and t' other chaps slaving away outside.'

'Dick, you are a real scandalmonger.'

'Nay, I'm not; nature will out. Oo's bin short of a fella sin 'er Bert died. I've seen 'er looking our Leslie o'er once or twice.'

'Well, she could do a lot worse.'

Leslie blushed furiously, but said nothing.

'Mebbe; but to cap it all, they're goin to get wed soon at St. Peter's. Father's bin up to give 'er lessons, but what for I don't know; I don't think oo'll need any.'

As Flora remarked, there was husk every day, interspersed with milk fever cases and cows down. The grumbling was continuous:

'What's keeping 'er down?'

'Why won't she gerrup?'

'It didn't use to be like this.'

'Can't ter do owt else?'

Richard repeated 'shortage of minerals' all the time, and began to sell so much that he bought it in 1 cwt drums and dispensed it in 2 lb packets. Later that week, one evening, he switched on the radio to listen to the six o'clock news, and was just in time to hear that Italy had surrendered before the first client came for evening surgery.

When he pulled up at White Gate in Wilton, there was a magnificent sports car outside the house. Richard was fascinated by it – it was a red Cord which had large gleaming chromium exhaust pipes coming out each side of the bonnet. These ran down both sides of the body and over the rear mudguards. He was still admiring it when a tall distinguished looking man, immaculately dressed in a dark suit, came out of the house.

'Good morning. You are Mr Holden the vet aren't you?' he asked.

'Yes, I am.'

'I am Frank Foster, it's nice to meet you,' and they shook hands. 'I notice you like my car.'

'I do, I've never seen one like it before.'

'You won't have; not many have been made: I've bought it because I can get around the country very quickly driving it. But I mustn't keep you because Doris is waiting, so I'll say good morning.' He got into the car, and with a deep roar from the engine, he drove away quickly.

Poppy was very welcoming and in perfect health. She had not had any reaction to the vaccine last month. Mrs Foster was curious.

'John told me that his friend Terry Wilson is coming as your assistant soon. When will he arrive?'

'In a fortnight's time; I am looking forward to his coming to join me.'

'I expect you are, and it will be nice for Norah his mother to have him home again, because though she is a great poker and bridge player she has been rather lonely this last year or so. I do hope he will like the area and settle down.'

'I do too; I would not like him to be here for say a year, and then leave. Farmers don't like it; once they get to know you they are very loyal and don't like changes.'

'I can understand that; I don't either, so I hope to see you next month.'

'Yes, Mrs Foster.'

'Goodbye for now, then.'

As he drove away he was doing mental arithmetic, adding up how much Mrs Foster had spent on Poppy already, just to be assured that the dog was well. With Terry as assistant he would be able to do more small animal operations and take a greater interest in the health and fitness of dogs and cats. He promised himself that as soon as the war was over he would have an X-ray machine, and a new operating theatre away from the consulting room. Looking at the *Veterinary Record* that evening he saw that a general meeting of his division of the NVMA was going to be held in the café in Droughton where he and his parents used to have coffee on Saturday mornings so many years ago. The discussion would be: The scheme proposed by the Ministry of Agriculture for the vaccination of calves against contagious abortion. He said to himself, I will be able to do that because Terry will be here then, so he wrote the date and time in his daily diary.

The next morning Joan Collinson was not her usual beautiful smiling self, and Flora asked her what was wrong.

'Haven't you heard the news, Mrs Holden?'

'No, whatever has happened now?'

'My mother was so upset when she got home at tea time yesterday. A dreadful thing happened at the WI meeting. Mrs Roberts, you know from Sykes, collapsed and died there and then, and another lady was so ill with shock she was taken to hospital. It's the third death recently.'

'Dear me; how sad for the children: I'll go and tell Richard now.'

He listened, feeling dismayed that a premonition had come to pass. 'Flora, I am certain that she had a foreboding when she came that morning and asked me to look after the boys.'

'It makes me think that somehow she knew. By the way, I am going on the allotments today, to swap stuff with Dick, and some of his friends, and I want to get apples to put in the loft and more fruit to bottle.'

The good harvest was steadily getting better, to which the increasing amount of brown stubbles bore witness. Richard was cheered by the sight, saying to himself, if the farmers are doing well it is good for me. Terry arrived at a quarter to nine on that third Monday morning in September and soon he and Richard were away on the morning round. They talked as they drove along, and Terry said his mother was very well, pleased that he was home, because it helped her food ration a lot, and she was hoping he would be able to bring extra food home from time to time. Richard told him that the farmers were helpful, but never to put himself in a position where later they could almost blackmail him. They decided to make an inventory of all the drugs, instruments and equipment which Terry had brought in the afternoon.

Introductions were made to George Meadows at Boundary Farm, then at Whitesides, Seedhill. Terry removed a retained cleansing from a cow at Bill Rigby's at New Church Farm, Olton.

At Duckworth Hall Bill Bainbridge told Terry that he was pleased to see him, because in his opinion Richard was killing himself by working so hard. Richard said in that case Terry could examine the cow which had only been calved a few weeks, but was now eating poorly, and her milk yield was dropping steadily. He quickly asked Bill about the cow; and then did a very careful clinical examination of the animal. Terry told Bill that in his opinion it was a case of false slow fever, where the cow's liver was diseased. Richard at once examined the animal and came to the same conclusion. Bill said that she had been very fit when she calved, but soon gave less than the seven gallons a day he expected. Richard told him that her chances of recovery were about evens, but Bill still wanted her treated, so he was advised to increase the starchy part of her food; glucose solution was given intravenously, and alkaline glucose powders and minerals were left with him.

Richard – carrying his new bowler – and Flora were part of the large congregation at St. Nicholas, Middleton. David Roberts and the two other children, with Tom Lee and Mrs Walker with their respective partners, led the procession into the church. Richard was troubled because his unease over Mrs Robert's request had proved correct. He was vaguely aware that two faceless male figures had entered his thoughts, but quickly dismissed these and turned his attention to the service. When the coffin was being lowered into the grave, Flora and many other ladies were in tears, and then the crowd quietly dispersed. Tom Walker thanked Richard for his letter and said that after three funerals in as many months, he hoped there would be no more for years. Richard agreed with him.

When the phone rang early on Wednesday morning Richard was surprised to hear Mary's voice, and gave the instrument to Flora, who learned that when her sister had arrived home last night on leave she had found Jean to be ill.

She had at once got the doctor, who had diagnosed gall bladder inflammation probably caused by gall stones. He was annoyed because Jean had not sought his help earlier, and prescribed a medicine to ease the pain. Mary was now very worried because Jean had spent a restless night, and had just vomited some blood, and wanted Flora to go and help. She said that she would catch the first available train to Holme.

Returning from the station, Richard found Joan and Terry in the dispensary, and she was apologising for not knowing where the various drugs and instruments were kept, saying that she had been the secretary for only two weeks.

The two vets spent the morning doing the first Tuberculin test of the cattle of Vic Dobson and Stan Earnshaw at Ashfield. Terry remarked that the farms near to the steelworks and coal mines reminded him of the Walsall practice, which he had been glad to leave.

Both Richard and Flora were very tired when they met at the station late that evening. Jean had been admitted to hospital for further tests because her doctor took a serious view of her condition as she was very anaemic. Flora said she was certain that the specialist would advise an operation, and after this had been done where would Jean go? They decided that she would have to go in a nursing home for a fortnight, and then come to Sandhaven.

The record harvest was almost finished, when farmers began to come to the surgery to obtain supplies of braxy or lamb dysentery vaccine for use in their flocks. Flora for her part had more fruit and vegetables stored than ever before, though she had given plenty to John as part payment for all the hard work he had done in the garden, and he also got one of Bumble's kittens.

Vic Dobson had a very good test, so Richard told him to take all the precautions required to prevent the reintroduction of infection. Stan Earnshaw had five animals fail the test, three of which were recently purchased young stock, and he was very annoyed.

'I'm not buying 'owt else after this. What the hell conta do if tha can't trust a well known breeder? I sez he's a rotten devil. Thee gimme a Certificate, Mr 'olden, to say they've failed, I wants mi money back. I'll go and dump them on his bloody doorstep, I will that.'

When he had cooled down a bit, Richard told him that for a first test it was a good result. He had to return the three yearlings at once, and afterwards disinfect the lorry and the box where they had been. The two cows could be sold, and then a double fence would have to be made between the farm and its neighbours. The next test would have to be in March the next year, by which time the Ministry could have announced its intentions with regards to the Attested Herds scheme.

As they were driving along the main road at Marhey they saw that Harold Briggs had felled a huge dead beech tree in a field near the road. Richard stopped the car, and after he had introduced Terry to Harold, asked if they could have some logs for the winter.

'Aye, course tha con, Mr 'olden; tha come here in a couple of weeks, I'll ev sawn it up bi then.' Richard was pleased that he would get some, because when Jean came to recuperate after her operation she would need to be kept warm. Terry said they would be a blessing for his mother, who had a very small fuel allocation.

When Gordon brought the Morris car, it was obvious that he had done an excellent job – it looked and drove like a new one. Terry was very grateful that he had been provided with such a good car, because his own was in a deplorable state. He spent a long time filling the Morris with all the drugs and equipment he needed. Richard gave him a short list of farms to visit the next morning; this would allow Richard to go off early to do herd examinations.

When he went to Duckworth Hall and re-examined the cow, she had not responded to the treatment given, so he had to agree with Bill that she should be sent to the abattoir at once. To satisfy his curiosity, he wanted to see the cow opened up after she had been slaughtered, so asked Bill to send her to Seaton. At the post mortem the cow had a large fatty liver, an incurable condition, so the organ was condemned, but the carcase was passed fit for human consumption. Later that week, after a cow had been treated for milk fever and got to her feet, she suddenly collapsed and died, as she was walking about.

'That's a devil, Mr 'olden,' said Harry Allen. 'What the hell caused it, oo were as right as rain as oo walked round the box.'

'I think probably heart failure, Harry.'

'Dusta now, tha knows, tha doesn't think of cows evin 'eart trouble like we do.'

'No, it's not common; now I'll take a blood film and then I'll ring Whiteside because I'd like to see her opened up.'

'So would I.'

The post mortem showed enlargement of the right side of the pale flabby heart. Two cases of fog fever were found; one was dead, but the other at Hillcrest at Catley was in the field sitting up breathing very quickly, and blowing froth from her nostrils.

'Oo looks in a bad way,' said Bob Whittaker.

'She is. I am going to inject her with atropine to try and stop her making all this froth in her lungs and drowning.' She died about five minutes later. Richard, as he drove away, considered it was his most unlucky farm; every case was an emergency and they always died. He thought back to the morning when young George was drowned in the Canal; everything had gone wrong since then; surely his luck would turn soon.

Jean Dickenson had her operation early on the Wednesday morning, so Flora at lunch time went by train to see how it had gone. She had not recovered consciousness, and was being given a blood transfusion. Mary was on compassionate leave, so the sisters went to Hill House for tea, but Flora declined the invitation to stay for the night. Next morning when she phoned the hospital, she was told that her mother's condition had improved, but she was still unconscious.

'There's really no point in me going over today, as Mum is still flat out. Do you think she will recover?'

'Of course she will, Flora, it's barely twenty-four hours since she had a major operation; you're expecting too much.'

'You really think so; well, I'll go tomorrow to see her, and I want you to go with me.'

'Of course, we'll go together. Terry can take us to the station: I am certain he can manage for a day or two on his own. In case there is something urgent, I'll give him the hospital's and your Holme telephone number.'

Next morning at the hospital, a nurse led them into Room 8, where all they could see of Jean was a very pale face, and two white arms. A clear solution was slowly dripping into a vein in her left arm.

'Mrs Holden, Mr Duncan has instructed me to tell you that your mother is doing well and is almost out of danger this morning. Now, would you both like a cup of tea?'

'Oh yes, please, that would be nice.'

In spite of the nurse's remarks, it was a rather despondent Flora who went over to the bed, kissed her mother, and said, 'Hello, Mum, it's Richard and me, can you hear me?'

Nothing indicated that she had, for apart from her breathing she was motionless. The nurse returned with two cups of tea, and told them that they could come back at any time after four o'clock that afternoon. Half an hour later they left and went to Hill Cottage because Mary was expecting them for lunch. When she told them that Bill would be arriving about four o'clock, Flora began to cheer up. When he arrived at that time, he looked huge because he was wearing his greatcoat, and he swept both his sisters into his arms and hugged and kissed them, making it into a great reunion.

They had tea and then decided that Richard and Flora would go first to the hospital at five o'clock, so that they could catch the early evening train to Sandhaven.

It was a different nurse who led them to Room 8, and before she left them, she said that Mrs Dickenson's condition had improved all day. Flora kissed her mother, but again there was no response, so they sat down on chairs beside the bed and, while watching the patient, talked quietly. When it was time for them to leave, Flora went and gently stroked Jean's hair, and said, 'Mum, we are going home now, but I'll be here tomorrow.' To her utter amazement the first two fingers of her mother's right hand twice gave the V for victory sign.

'Oh Richard, she can hear me,' cried Flora and began to sob with relief, then she kissed Jean repeatedly. On the train, an excited Flora said, 'Richard, do you know you've been really well today?

'It's been just like old times.'

'You're right, I do feel well again. You know, I did not think much of Mr Forest in August, but I must say that after taking this new sulpha drug, I've very little pain in my knees, and I've not had a sweating attack for weeks. So his treatment is working, and I now wish I had seen him a year ago.'

'So do I, love,' said Flora.

'But you know, Terry has contributed to me feeling better – his just being here has lightened my load of work, and let me take things a bit slower.'

'Richard, I'm sure it has already, and besides, with him sharing the night work you have less strain driving in the damned blackout.'

'That's true, but to crown it all is the non-stop worry over rationing, everything unavailable or in short supply, it jades and wearies you so much.'

'You needn't tell me anything about rationing getting you down, it's worse than ever. You should hear some of the language women come out with when they are queuing in the rain outside the Field's or Dick Heye's – it's really dreadful. The young ones must pick it up at work off the men in the Dock Road factories.'

'Don't you mean more likely off the Yanks?'

'Some of them, definitely, the way they carry on with them at night.'

The next day Flora was overjoyed to find Jean sitting up in bed drinking tea.

'Oh Mum, it's marvellous to see you're better.'

'I don't know about better, you pour me some more tea; I've not had any for three days; I could drink a bucketful.' Soon Mary and Bill arrived and it was a very happy and relieved group of people which met there in Jean's room. Mr Duncan had told Jean that all being well she would be discharged in ten days' time. He had made her get out of bed, and assisted by two nurses she had walked round the room.

'Mum, you really are remarkable,' said Bill, 'but where will you go when you are discharged?'

'To Hill Cottage, my own home; there is nowhere else I would go, and besides there's Margaret next door. When I leave here, Mary or Flora can come and stop for a few days until I get stronger.'

'Richard and I wondered if you would like to come to Sandhaven for a short time?'

'That's a nice idea, but not at the moment, Flora; I'll come in two or three weeks' time.'

When Richard walked into the surgery Joan came running after him.

'Mr Holden, a Mr MacDonald from Southall wants you to ring him as soon as possible. The number is 148.'

'I wonder what's wrong.'

'He didn't say, but it is very urgent.'

'Then get him on the phone, Joan, at once.'

It was quickly done and Richard said, 'Hello Bill, how are you? I've only just got in, what's the trouble?'

Bill said he was very well, but he wanted Richard as a second opinion to go with him to examine a herd that afternoon.

'I can be at your place at three thirty.'
'That will do fine, Richard.'
'Good, I'll be there.'

He was there just before the appointed time, and Bill told him that two cows had been bought at the auction on Thursday. One became ill on the Sunday and developed pneumonia, and acute diarrhoea, and the disease had spread rapidly. The cow had died in the night, and nine others were ill, and he thought the condition was transit fever.

'Right, Bill, let's go. I'll leave my car here.'

It was about five miles to the large dairy farm, and as they drove into the yard, they saw the dead cow lying outside the shippon door.

'Bob Whiteside will be here about four, and will open that one for us.'

The farmer came across the yard to meet them.

'Mr Butler, this is Mr Holden who has come from Sandhaven to give the second opinion you asked for.'

''ow do you do, Mr 'olden, it's good of thee to come at short notice. Badly cows are in t' big shippon, and it's going up one side; nine of 'em are ill now.'

'Very well, Mr Butler, I'll start here.'

'Thee do, I'll be back in five minutes.'

Suddenly Richard remembered that he had seen this disease years before in Cheshire – cows with a high temperature, pneumonia and diarrhoea followed by death within 24 to 36 hours. The cause of the trouble had been newly purchased cows being brought into the herd.

'Bill, I am certain this is the same type of pasteurella infection I've seen before.'

'I agree with you; it's like a transit fever.'

'It is, and very virulent.'

Mr Butler came back and asked, 'Dusta know what it is, then?'

'Yes, the new bought cows brought the germ with them.'

'Arta certain o' that?'

'Yes, I am.'

'Well, what arta going to do?'

'I'll tell you; first open all the windows and doors, and turn all the healthy cows out.'

'Nay, not in this cold weather.'

'Yes, in this weather. A famous professor advised it last time I saw the disease; he said that fresh air was more than half the treatment. You can let them lie in at night, but leave all the doors and windows open if you do.'

'Is that the lot, then?'

'No, the ill ones will have to be given a new sulpha drug and all the cattle must be injected with anti serum.'

'I'll do owt tha sez. I've lost one already, and them two there won't last long.'

'I'm certain they won't, Mr Butler; what do you say, Mr MacDonald?'

'There's no doubt about it, they will die soon. I came to the same diagnosis as Mr

Holden, so I ordered serum at lunchtime.'

'If tha both thinks that's what I should do, I'll ger on wi' it, and let 'em out.'

'You do, and we'll treat these ill cows.' Richard helped Bill and they had finished when Bob Whiteside arrived. He soon cut open the cow, and brought out the lungs and intestines, and they showed Mr Butler the pneumonia in the lungs, and the enteritis in the intestines. He thanked Richard and paid him his fee; so both the vets disinfected themselves thoroughly and left.

As they drove away Bill said, 'I am really grateful that you came, Richard, because Dick Butler can be an awkward old cuss. You see, he's a great talker and knows everybody, being the Chairman of the local branch of the NFU. He can make life pretty uncomfortable for you if anything goes wrong. When he left Bob Townsend and came to me, Bob said that he was glad to see the back of him, but so far I've been able to manage him. By the way I am getting married next year.'

'That's great, and about time too. Who's the lucky lady?'

'No one you know, she is a doctor in Edinburgh. This is just an advance notice of the wedding which will be held in March next year, and you've got to be there – and that's an order.'

'I will, Bill, thanks for the invitation. Cheerio for now.'

The next morning Marjorie sent a message to let Richard know that her father had been taken to the Memorial Hospital because his condition had worsened during the night. Richard felt somewhat ashamed because he had not been to see Mr Parsons though he knew that he was ill. He rang the hospital to find out what time visiting was allowed that evening, so that he could go and see him. Joan came in to the office, and Richard noticed that she was very smartly dressed and everything about her was immaculate. At lunchtime Flora said, 'I don't know what's got into Joan; lately, she's coming to work dressed up like a fashion model. I'm beginning to think that she has got designs on Terry.'

'Don't be silly, Flora, he's hardly been here a month yet, and why shouldn't she look smart; she'd have to be in a London hotel.'

'Maybe, but every time he comes in, she can't take her eyes off him.'

'Well, we can't stop it, and he could look a lot further and do a lot worse, because Bill Harrison told me that their Auntie May had left nearly £8,000 to each niece and nephew.'

'As much as that? Then she can afford to dress well, if she's got the coupons.'

'Anyway, don't worry, it may only be a passing fancy; time will tell.'

After Richard had visited Mrs Foster's peke, he went on to another new client at Cuthbert Hall, Wellington. Michael Winder, the owner, was the brother of Leslie at Bank End, Pelham. Richard was pleased to have him as a client because he had a big Friesian herd in buildings on one side of the road and kept pigs and poultry on the other side.

'It's nice to meet you, Michael, your Leslie said you would be ringing up.' With help

Richard took extra setts off the udders of eight heifers, and treated another which had wooden tongue.

'That's it for today, Mr Holden; now I must tell yer afore that goes. If tha comes t' other buildings after dark, blow yer car horn, and wait for me to come because mi two guard dogs ull be loose.'

'Thanks for telling me, I'll remember it.'

That evening, Richard was about to lock the surgery door at seven o'clock, when a wild-eyed, badly dressed man walked in coughing vigorously, and asked loudly in a broad Irish accent, 'Are you the vetenry?'

'Yes, I am; what do you want?'

'The saints be praised I've found one. I want some horse 'lectuary for mi cough – it's real cruel.'

'I'm sorry, I can't give you that; it would poison you.'

'Now, you're not refusing a poor sick Irishman a drop of medicine, are you?'

'No, I'm not; I'll let you have a bottle of cough medicine I make up for farmers.'

'Is it strong?'

'Yes, it is, you must take it diluted with water.'

'Then, I'll have a bottle.'

Richard brought a ten-ounce bottle of undiluted Mist. bronchialis from the dispensary.

'Here you are, that's half a crown.'

The man produced a ten shilling note.

'Thank you; I'll go and get your change.'

He was getting this in the office when he heard the man coughing again, and as he walked into the consulting room, he was taken aback to see him drinking the medicine straight from the bottle. He took the bottle from his lips and gulped. 'Holy Mother,' he gasped. 'That's strong.'

'I told you it was; I'll get you a glass of water.'

'Don't bother, Sor,' said he as he pulled a half-full bottle of whisky from his coat pocket and took a long drink from it. Richard gave him his change, and was thanked most effusively for stopping the cough.

When Richard arrived at the hospital he found Mr Parsons in bed in a large medical ward. He was very pale and thin but he was genuinely pleased to see Richard. They talked for half an hour, when Marjorie arrived, late and flustered, and was told off quietly by her father. As it was almost the end of the visiting time Richard excused himself and left. The next morning Bill McDonald rang to tell Richard that the pasteurella outbreak at Mr Butler's farm had stopped spreading and that the cattle seemed to be over the worst.

When George Duke came on Friday morning to make the half-year audit, he explained to Richard the alterations being made to the PAYE regulations. When he had finished his audit in the afternoon Richard asked him for guidance in making Terry a salaried partner in December, because by then he would have worked in the practice for three months. He said that they got on very well together; he was an efficient and capable veterinary surgeon, and he would like Terry to become permanent in the practice when the three months probationary period ended.

George said he thought it was an excellent idea, and a good incentive for a young man to give of his best, because it would have to give details of progression to a partnership later, and the amount of finance needed when that position was reached.

The letter in reply to their application to the Adoption Society annoyed Flora because it was a refusal, on the grounds that they were unsuitable to adopt a child because of their ages, especially Richard's.

'I've never read such rude rubbish,' said Flora, 'for here we are with a lovely home, you are a professional man, and I can spend all my time bringing up a child, and they bloody well refuse us.' Tears ran down her face.

'Don't cry, love; they know all that from that damned questionnaire we had to complete. It's me, it's just my age, but Tommy Bishop is the same age as me, and he is bringing up a baby famously. I suppose if we were a couple of scatterbrained twenty-year-olds with not a penny in the bank we could adopt one tomorrow. It's plain bloody silly.'

'I know it is, Richard, but that is not what is bothering me. What are we going to do now?'

Her simple question stopped Richard dead in his tracks, and after a pause, he said, 'I don't know, Flora; I was certain we would be allowed to adopt a child.'

'So was I,' and she began to cry again. In a flash Richard knew that Flora had staked all on this Society, and she was now a very pathetic, heartbroken person – the barren wife.

He quickly sat down beside her and took her into his arms. 'Listen to me, darling, this is not the only adoption society in the country, there will be others, and you can adopt privately.'

'Yes, I know, but why are they looking for parents for all these babies, even more so now the girls are having them by the Americans, and then refusing people?'

'Well it could be that the managers of this religious society are very cautious, and others may not be so strict. I know what I will do, I'll go and see Tommy Duke. Solicitors have to deal with adoptions to make them legal, and even Bill McConnell may know of a baby for adoption privately.'

'That's a good idea, you go and see Tommy first, and then we can go together so see Bill.'

Because the weather was so wet and windy, Terry asked when the logs would be available, because they were very short of fuel at The Moorings, and had stopped using the central heating. Richard was going that way in the afternoon and said he would ask Harold Briggs if they were ready. They were, and had been cut into chunks of wood which were easy to handle. On Sunday he and Flora emptied the car, covered the seats and the floor with sacking, and then went to the farm. They filled every bit of space in the car with the logs, and paid Harold the thirty shillings he charged.

'If tha gets short, Mrs 'olden, thee tell thi old man to call. I allus 'ave some, 'cos there's lots of dead trees in Underley Wood.'

Flora thought the logs were a bargain at the price. At the surgery Richard and Terry divided the logs equally between them, and the latter paid fifteen shillings for his share, saying his mother would be delighted with them. Flora said she was tired and did not feel like going to the hospital that night; Richard did not go either, because it was so wet and stormy, saying he would go tomorrow.

It was the next Monday morning when Marjorie came to the surgery, and told Richard that her father had died suddenly last night, owing to heart failure brought on by chronic kidney disease. Richard thanked her for coming, and said how sorry he and Flora were at the news, especially as her father had had such a short retirement. Marjorie said the funeral had been arranged to take place at 9 a.m. on the Thursday morning at St. Peter's Church. It was very cold, and barely one-third full for the service, after which they followed the coffin and the mourners into the graveyard. Two shadowy male figures again came into Richard's thoughts and as the coffin was lowered into the grave, one disappeared.

He shivered; Flora asked if he were cold, and he replied that he was. This was a white lie to cover his sense of dread. They went and offered their condolences to Mrs Parsons and Marjorie and then hurried back to their car, to get out of the very cold wind.

'You know, Flora, I am really sorry he has died, after such a short retirement. Without his help we would not be where we are today.'

'That's right, and though they had such good intentions, they were never really friendly towards us.'

'That's true, but they were like that with everybody all the time, which probably accounts for so few people being in Church just now.'

At 2.15 p.m. the next day he walked up the carpeted stairs into the café in Droughton, and was surprised to find the room already almost full. He put his trilby and overcoat on a chair, and looking round saw Bill McDonald, who told him that the outbreak of disease at Butler's farm was over, and that only one more cow died. Alistair Duncan from Lindley came up, and greeted him warmly, and said how nice it was to meet again. Richard made a similar reply, but reserved his judgement on the friendliness of this man who had proved to be so sharp and cunning in his business affairs, even though he said that Lewis had retired and was very ill. Campbell Morrison and Bob Dawson came in together, followed by the Secretary and the President; the latter at once called the meeting to order and at 2.30 it began.

The main item on the agenda was the scheme proposed by the Ministry of Agriculture for the vaccination of calves against contagious abortion. Campbell Morrison spoke first giving a description of this American S19 vaccine and its method of use. He said that the payment of one shilling would be made to the practitioner for each calf vaccinated, and the Ministry's whole-time staff would also do this work. These remarks lit the fuse which caused the meeting to explode into a furious verbal battle. The Ministry were accused of encroaching on private practice, by using whole-time staff. Others said that to accept the paltry fee of a shilling per head would be to prostitute the profession. A lecturer in bacteriology advised caution, saying that any modified bacterium had the ability to revert to full virulence suddenly and the result would be disaster. What would be the effect of vaccinating an already infected calf, would it became a chronic carrier? Another wanted to know what effect the modified germ would have on the practitioner or a farm man who was accidentally injected with S19. When the meeting was finally closed, it appeared to Richard that only about fifty per cent were in favour of the scheme. He had enjoyed the stimulating effect of discussion with professional colleagues, and was determined to be a regular attender in future.

It was after evening surgery, when he had to go to Michael Wilding's at Wellington to a sow which could not farrow. It was a very wet cold night and the heavy rain and poor headlights made driving tiring and difficult. When he arrived at the farm, he drove up to the buildings on the left hand side of the road. In the light from the car the gate had just come into view, when behind it appeared two very big English bull mastiffs barking furiously.

'I'm not going near that gate while those two are loose,' he said to himself and blew the car's horn repeatedly. Suddenly the dogs ran away, and then Michael, with a gun under his arm, opened the gate and waved Richard in. The piggery was warm, and Michael was intrigued when he saw Richard's kneeler and said he would make one for his own use.

After he had extracted a large dead piglet which had been wedged across the sow's passage, with her assistance he rapidly delivered ten live piglets. He put two pessaries into the uterus and then gave the sow an injection of oxytoxin.

'That's a good do, Mr 'olden; you see she is a pedigree large white, and I had her mated with Carden Conqueror – that one of George Bamber's – dusta' know him?'

'Yes, he's a good client of mine. So you're making a pedigree herd, are you?'

'Aye, good stuff sells well, an' it will be wanted more when t' war's over. Let's go an 'ev a cup of tay.'

'I will, thank you, it is a shocking night.'

In the warm farm kitchen, Mrs Wilding served them with tea and cake. Michael then explained that he had bought the dogs to try and prevent the serious losses he had been having through thieves robbing his turkey houses and his laying hens and eggs, a year earlier, before Christmas. Mrs Wilding said they had been bought so that she would not have a heart attack. Michael, laughing, said that before he kept a loaded gun by the bed, and when he was disturbed, he would quickly open the window, and fire both barrels of the twelve-bore blindly into the night. It didn't do any good, and startled Mrs Wilding, she being rudely awakened by the crash of the gun being fired. When he investigated later he always found that a vehicle had been backed through the hedge, and a cabin emptied of birds.

'They've only tried it twice since I got dogs, and first time they took nowt, but last time dogs 'ad 'em, there were bloody torn clothing up there next morning, where t' dogs had 'ad a go at 'em. They've not bin back sin then.'

Richard thanked Mrs Wilding for the tea, and Michael went with him back to his car, and closed the gate. As he backed away, he saw that the dogs were already on guard in the yard, as Michael walked away with the gun under his arm.

Early in November Richard had received a letter from a Mr Keith Barrett, a third year student at the Royal Veterinary College in London, who asked if he could come and see practice during the Christmas vacation. He wrote that his father had been transferred by the company for which he worked from Southampton to the office in Mereside, and that his family now lived in Pelham. When Terry read the letter, he said that he did not know Keith, but thought that he could be useful. Richard replied that he would be pleased to let him see practice, if he came for an interview first, and agreed to signing the usual binding out agreement.

Jean came to stay on the first of November having made a good recovery from her operation, but she was still weak. Flora said that this was because the operation had aged her mother a lot. On the odd nice day Jean would take Rocky for a short walk along the Promenade, saying that the sea air was as good as a tonic, but usually she spent the day in front of the lounge fire reading the paper or doing embroidery. Nevertheless, she helped Flora by making her own bed, dusting, washing up and preparing food, but she tired very quickly. She was reading the *Evening News* when she called Flora, and showed her a report which said that five RAF personnel had been smuggled out of France under the noses of the Germans, and had finally reached England. Among the list of names was that of Flight Lieutenant Norman Robinson DFC. Flora snatched the paper from her mother's hands and ran downstairs two at a time calling, 'Richard, Richard, come here quick!'

'Whatever is the matter, Flora?'

'Look here, it says Norman Robinson is alive and has got back home.'

As he read the story his eyes filled with tears, he was so overcome by the news that his friend was alive.

'This calls for a drink,' he said, and upstairs a toast was drunk to 'Norman Robinson, may God preserve him.'

After he had finished the surgery, he wrote a letter of congratulation to Norman, and invited him to come and stay with him. This was possible because Jean said that she would go and stay in the Porter Arms for a few days.

Richard had told Terry all about the heated discussion at the meeting of the Lancashire

Division of the National Veterinary Medical Association, and how opinion for and against the scheme appeared to be equally divided. Terry said he was in favour of it, but did not know enough about the vaccine. He asked a question which had not been answered in the meeting. It was this – if you vaccinated an already infected calf did it become a carrier, and which germ would it excrete? Richard did not know the answer, but he was against introducing the live abortion germ onto a 'clean' farm. They decided not to use the vaccine, but to wait and see how the scheme progressed. However if a farmer asked to have his calves vaccinated, they would do it for him.

It was a very cold, wet and windy day when Richard went to Intack farm at Middleton. Jack Booth and his son Richard went with him across the yard and into the warm old shippon.

'I've brought 'em in, 'cos they're nearly ready for t' Christmas Fat Stock Show. It would be daft leaving 'em out swealing away in this cold.'

'It would that, Jack; what's wrong?'

'This 'un's gitten a bad eye.'

The two Friesian cross Hereford bullocks must have weighed at least thirteen hundredweight each, and there was very little room to get in between them in the double standing. The one with the bad eye was standing on the right and would not move over.

'Cum o'er you stupid devil!' shouted Jack as he thumped the beast with a stick, and the two Richards struggled to make the animal move. It did a little, and Richard was pushing as hard as he could to get in between the two, when it trod on his foot, and then put all its weight on it.

'God, my foot, Jack, get him off my bloody foot, he's breaking it!'

Jack who was wearing heavy clogs kicked the bullock hard, and it moved over, releasing Richard's foot.

'By jove, that hurts, that beast weighs a ton.'

'Aye, it 'ull be sore, they're not light weights; Richard, let that 'un out in t' next boost, then reach o'er and loose this 'un.'

Finally the huge animals were driven out and the vet limped up to the bullock's head. By the light of his torch he could see that there was a chaff on the cornea, and as soon as Jack had nosed the beast Richard quickly washed it out under local anaesthetic. His foot was very badly bruised; swollen, and the skin discoloured black and purple; it was very painful, making him limp for a week.

Mrs Foster was very worried because Poppy was passing maggots in her motion.

'Mr Holden, will they harm her?'

'Before I answer your question, can you describe these maggots?'

'Yes, they are little cream oblongs and they move slowly.'

'I thought so, they are tape worm segments, I'll come and see her today.'

'Please do, I don't like her to have anything wrong.'

The gardener showed Richard some motion on a shovel, and it contained segments.

'What do you do with the dog's motion?'

'I sweep it up, and burn it in the green-house furnace. Mr Frank says I have to.'

'He's right; burn anything she passes. The worm, Mrs Foster, can be long, up to say three feet and the segments break off the end and so are passed.'

'You can get them away?'

'Yes. This is a dose of Tenaline; follow the instructions, and the tape worm will be expelled about half an hour after the dose has been given. The gardener is right in burning everything she passes. Apart from this, you are very well, Poppy.'

'Thank you, Mr Holden, and how is Terry getting on?'

'Very well, and he gives the impression that he likes the practice and this area.'

'I'm so glad. Norah said it is nice to have him home, but I mustn't keep you, so good morning.'

It was after dinner that evening when the phone rang and Richard picked it up and said, 'Holden, veterinary surgeon.'

'Richard, it's me, Norman.' He used the same words and quiet voice as he had that morning at the front door after the bombing of Liverpool three years before.

'Norman, where are you, do come over and stay, how are you?'

The reply was lengthy, and finally he apologised for not being able to accept Richard's invitation.

'I have so much to do, and so many people to see that my leave is half over, and soon I will have to rejoin my squadron. It's been like old times talking now, and I am glad things are going so well. I'll say best wishes for the future to Flora and yourself, and cheerio.'

Richard replaced the receiver, but had an uneasy feeling that he would not speak to Norman again.

'What is it, Richard?'

'Nothing, but he sends you his best wishes, and he is sorry but he is too busy to come and stay.'

'That's a pity, it would have been nice to see him again.'

'It would, but it's not to be; so you can tell Jean she has no need to pack.'

In his reply Keith thanked Richard for his letter, and wrote that he would come for an interview on Saturday 18th December, but would phone first to see if it would be convenient. With Terry living in Seaton, Keith in Pelham, and maybe Mr Campbell Morrison in Seaton, the area was going to be well supplied with representatives of the veterinary profession. In the dispensary Richard wrote out a long list of drugs on the order form so that the hampers would arrive before Christmas. He put Rocky on his lead, and took him for a walk down Victoria Road and High Street to the GPO. He then began to retrace his steps and noticed that a couple walking arm in arm had crossed to his side of the road, a little ahead of him, and that there was something vaguely familiar about them. In the light from a passing car he recognised Terry and Joan, so he walked slowly until they had crossed Victoria Road, and then hurried home.

'You won't believe what I've just seen, Flora.'

'Why not, what was it?'

'Terry and Joan walking arm in arm down High Street.'

'Well I never, so I was right after all. I told you she had set her sights on him, and you said it was rubbish.'

'It was then, but that was weeks ago.'

'I wonder if it's serious, because if it is, it will be a big wedding.'

'Flora, don't jump the gun, they are only walking out together.'

'Maybe, but one thing leads to another. I'll have to try and find out somehow.'

'Knowing you, you will that.'

But she didn't, because in the surgery neither of them betrayed the fact that there was a blossoming romance between them. The practice was busy, and Terry was having to do more of the emergency visits and operations because Richard had a long list of herd inspections waiting to be done, and visits under the Panel Scheme. Even when he was not on duty he often spent the evening sitting at his microscope looking for the germs of tuberculosis, mastitis, Johne's disease and contagious abortion. He found them regularly.

Towards the end of the month, one wet wintry night, Bob Whittaker rang quite late wanting a visit because he had a cow with a prolapsed uterus. Richard, being on duty, soon arrived at Hill Crest at Catley. With the help of Bob and his men the cow's hindquarters were soon raised, the uterus replaced, and the strappings applied.

When they lowered the cow's hind legs, it was obvious that she had milk fever, so Richard treated her with 500 c.c. of solution, and waited to see if that was sufficient. Next morning when he went to remove the strappings, the cow was up and eating normally. Driving away from the farm, he realised that it was the first animal which had lived after treatment there ever since the son was killed more than two years before. He said to himself – at last my luck has changed!

In spite of Flora's protests, Jean decided to go home, to see – as she put it – if her house was still there. She promised to come at Christmas, because both Bill and Mary would be due for leave then. That evening Richard and Flora had an appointment with Dr Bill at eight o'clock, and they told him that it if were possible, they would like privately to adopt a baby. He listened to what they both had to say, and then in his relaxed quiet way began to explain the difficulties which might arise, and the length of time it would take. At that time he did not know of any pregnancy which if it were successful would later be available for adoption, but he would inform them at once if one came to his notice. He then began to talk about the treatment of infertility, and advised injections of gonadotrophin eight days after the last menstrual period. He said that he had been discussing Flora's case with Mr Graham, and he had suggested it, because it would make ovulation occur, which should increase the chance of conception taking place, any time during a trial period of six months. Flora asked what other effects the treatment would have, and Bill replied, none as far as he knew. Flora said that she would like to have the treatment as soon as possible. Bill asked questions about her last period, and then said that she would have to come for an injection on 14th December and then at monthly intervals.

As they drove home Flora said, 'I do hope this new treatment will work, because I wouldn't want anything else if I had you and our own baby, not an adopted one.'

Richard thought for a few moments and then said, 'I feel the same; I would be completely happy and satisfied if I had you, and our own baby son or daughter, it wouldn't matter which it was.'

'You're right, Richard, it jolly well wouldn't matter.'

The dreadful weather continued, and it must have contributed to the rapid spread of an outbreak of flu making a lot of people ill. Mavis could not come to clean for three days because her mother was ill with it, but in spite of her arthritis she recovered slowly. The 'Notice of Deaths' column in the *Evening Post* was much longer than usual for some weeks.

George Duke sent Richard two documents to read; one was an outline of the salary scale for a salaried partner, and the other was the legal agreement drawn up by Tommy the solicitor. Flora and Richard read them carefully and after some discussion provisionally accepted the details in both documents. Richard decided that the practice could afford the increased expenditure, because it was steadily growing, this fact being reflected in the increase in the amount of money he took to the bank each Monday morning. As the three month period would be up on Sunday 12th December, they thought it would be nice to give them to Terry the following day. As neither he nor Joan Collinson in any way indicated that anything out of the ordinary would happen, Richard hoped that this would cause him to reveal his plans. Terry was never at home when he was off duty, and had volunteered the information that he was having a new suit made. As he had plenty of clothes, Richard wondered why he wanted another suit, but Terry kept mum.

It was a bright cold Saturday morning, when Richard drove past Whyngate on his way to Town End at Mereside. In the field next to the road he noticed Coln Greenwood and Brenda Meadows cantering from corner to corner. Brenda was riding to attention, and going with her pony beautifully. This pleased Richard – his warning and advice had been taken seriously. At the farm Bill Tomlinson had three cows to be treated, and when he had finished he went with Bill into the house for a cup of tea. It came as a surprise when Bill told him that as soon as the war ended he would be leaving the farm.

'But why, Bill?'

'Well, you see I am a tenant, and so is Alder Heys, and we've both had a letter from Mereside Council that they will need our land for new houses and an extension to the hospital.'

'I'm sorry to hear that, but what would you do?'

'I'd try and get a County Council place to rent, or a smallholding. I couldn't retire and give up work.'

'Come to that, neither could I, Bill.'

Driving along Richard thought about this, and decided that if Mereside Town Council already had plans for post-war building, then Seaton, Droughton and Wyresham would have them as well, which meant that in a year or two's time he could lose a lot of farm clients, and Ministry work. If that happened would there be enough work for the two of them, and how would he replace the loss of income? He was still thinking about this that evening.

'What's the matter, Richard, you are very quiet?'

He told her. 'But you've nothing to worry about, you've got ten farms in four and a half years, and there are many round Runfold and Goswick that could become clients.'

'I suppose there are, but it came as a bit of a shock to learn that four Town Councils could take away a lot of our income overnight, so I'm not going to mention it to Terry, it might unsettle him.'

'Neither would I; but things are bound to change, and we will have to plan to adapt to them; you could even open a branch practice.'

'I hadn't even thought as far ahead as that, but you are probably right. Anyway, let's have a drink; it's bed-time.'

The last day of the month brought two events which had opposite effects on Flora. The first was that Isabel Lord had given birth to a baby girl, and the second was an invitation from Tom and Alice Collinson, Park Hall Farm, to a party on Saturday 11th December. The birth of the baby depressed Flora, but the invitation propelled her into frantic activity; in minutes she was going through her wardrobe trying, as she said, to find something to wear. Richard said that he would wear his new suit, because he had only worn it a few times since it was made.

'Yes, that will do for you; but what about me? I'll have to go to Droughton and find a party dress.'

'But you said that you hadn't any coupons.'

'Did I? Well, Mum and our Mary both know how to get them, so I'll have enough. I must go on Monday in the morning because Terry's mother is coming for a cup of tea in the afternoon.'

'Look, before you do anything else, will you write a formal letter of acceptance to Tom and Alice, and we'll have to think what we should take them – a present of some kind, maybe flowers or chocolates.'

'Flowers are over for this year; I think a bottle of sherry or whisky would be more welcome.'

'Good idea, I'll get a bottle from Jim Lord or Ben Belcher.'

'And I'll have to go and see Isabel this afternoon.'

'By the way, when do they want that kitten they asked for? If they don't take it soon it will be having kittens itself.'

'I'll see what Isabel says, but I think she will be too busy at the moment.'

The weather at the beginning of December was a continuation of November's cold wetness. On the Monday Richard had lunch in the coffee shop's café, and then did a round of visits which he finished as darkness fell. Arriving home, he went up to the lounge and there found Mrs Wilson and Flora having tea. Terry had brought his mother that afternoon from Seaton to have tea with Flora. Richard was pleased to make her acquaintance, and join in the conversation as he was enjoying his cup of tea. Norah Wilson told him that she knew about Joan, because Terry had taken her to The Moorings for lunch.

'I think they spend all their spare time together, Mr Holden,' said Norah.

'I am sure they do, because I've seen them out walking when he's off duty.'

'I haven't met her father and mother yet, have you?'

'Yes, I have; he is a client of mine. It is a nice family, there are two boys and two girls.' Flora, taking the bull by the horns asked, 'But you are going to the party next Saturday, aren't you?'

'Oh yes, I am looking forward to it so much.'

'So am I. I went to Droughton this morning to find something for the occasion.'

'And what did you get, or is that a state secret?'

'It is very much a secret.'

At this Richard excused himself, saying that he had a lot of herd inspection certificates to complete and then post. After he had filled in the account form, he wrote a letter to Bob Dawson asking for Terry to be appointed a Panel B local veterinary inspector of the Ministry. That evening when he asked Flora what she had got on her shopping trip, she told him to wait and see.

On a frosty morning, later in the week, he went to Wyresham to see a dog which was 'poorly'. He had to ring the door bell three times before the door was opened by a woman who was wearing a dressing gown.

'Good morning, are you Mrs Travis?'

'Yes, that's right.'

'I am the vet, Mr Holden.'

'Do come in, then; my dog's in the living room, in 'ere.'

It proved to be a bitch which had three newly born puppies, one very swollen mammary gland and a temperature of 105°F.

'When did she have her puppies?'

'Last night at bed-time.'

Richard examined the animal's abdomen, and found that parturition had been completed.

'She has no more puppies to come, but she has this inflammation in this gland, it's a bad mastitis.'

'Will she get better?' said a male voice. Richard turned round and saw a fully dressed big man standing there.

'I will be able to tell you that when I come tomorrow.'

'I'll go then, luv,' he said to the woman, and left.

'Now, Mrs Travis, watch me, as I give her these three tablets like this. I want you to give her two at five o'clock, and one at ten o'clock and then one first thing in the morning. Let her have plenty of water or milk to drink.'

''Er likes sweet tay.'

'Then let her have plenty and I'll come and see her about this time tomorrow.'

As he left he thought her husband did not show much interest in their dog. The next day he was a little earlier and again after a delay Mrs Travis, wearing her dressing gown, opened the door and let Richard in.

'I think oos gettin better, Mr 'olden.'

He found her temperature was down to 103°F, and the puppies must have got some milk because they were quiet. A man came down the stairs, shouted, 'Tara luv,' and the front door was noisily shut.

'Has she eaten anything?'

'Aye, bread and lights an oos ad plenty of tay.'

'That's good; she is improving, now here are more tablets, give one now, then at five-hour intervals; I'll call tomorrow morning.'

On the Saturday morning Mrs Travis was fully dressed; the room had been tidied up and the furniture dusted. A very pleasant man had admitted Richard and held the bitch while he examined her. The bitch wagged her tail, and was almost normal. 'She is better today.'

'What was wrong wi 'er?'

'Inflammation of this milk gland – you can see it's still a little bigger than the others, but it will go down.'

'That's a good do, so I'll pay yer.'

As he was opening the door to let Richard out, he asked, 'When tha' came yesterday, an t' day afore, were there anybody 'ere wi t' wife?'

Richard thought quickly, and lied, 'No,' and hurried to his car. It was a week later when Joan asked, 'Mr Holden, do you know anything about this postal order for a pound? The post mark is from Wyresham but there is no account with it, and I can't find one for a pound in the small animal ledger.'

'Yes, it will be from some people who had not enough money when they paid in cash. Just put it with the cheques.' That night Richard told Flora the story and she commented, 'I think she is a dirty double crosser. Don't you or Terry go there again.'

'I'll see that he doesn't, because her husband smells a rat, and I don't want him to belt me to find out what I know; he could half kill you.'

Bob Dawson rang and asked if Terry would be available in the surgery about 10 a.m. because Mr Campbell Morrison wanted to see him. When he and Bob arrived he introduced them to Terry and then went in search of Flora to ask her to make some coffee. Carrying a plate which held slices of cake, he followed Flora into the room. Bob said, 'We have just about finished. This is very acceptable, Mrs Holden; we are all ready for a cup of coffee.'

Campbell Morrison continued, 'Yes, it really is very welcome and it has been nice meeting you, Mr Wilson. With your experience you will be appointed to the Panel B list of Inspectors quite soon, which I know will help Mr Holden, who has a lot of Ministry work to do.'

'Thank you very much, sir,' said Terry, 'and I will do my best to help with the Ministry work.'

'I'm sure you will, but we must be away, because I have an appointment with an estate agent. So good morning to you both, and you will thank Flora for the drink and cake.'

'Yes I will, sir, and goodbye for now.'

'I was surprised that both Mr Morrison and Mr Dawson were so nice and friendly,' said Terry.

'Oh, were you? Why, Terry?'

'Well, in Hampshire everybody was frightened of the SVI and the DVI.'

'You are not in Hampshire now, my lad, we are Lancastrians, well known for the warmth of our welcome. Our two are OK, but they will give you a lot or work to do and then thank you for doing it. Later they will grumble that the valuations you made were too high. I wish they would send guidelines out each month along with the lists of herd inspections.'

'I'll be able to help you with them soon.'

'I hope so, what with doing them, the Panel Scheme, and preliminary Tuberculin tests, before long I won't have time to do ordinary work.'

'I had noticed how much busier it has been lately, Mr Holden.'

'And it's not showing any signs of easing off, so we must go, we can't stand here talking all day.'

It was very frosty on the night of the party, and as he was on duty Richard asked the exchange to re-route any calls to Park Hall Farm. He put a thick rug into the car, and the bottle of sherry – the present having been neatly wrapped in red crepe paper. When he went back into the house, Flora was in the hall and was wearing a blue and white floral jacket and a dark blue skirt. She was putting on a white hat which had a blue and white ribbon sewn round the crown.

'Darling, you look stunning, I really like that outfit. Are you ready?'

'Yes, I am now.'

'Then I'll lock up; I've put a rug in the car because it's freezing.'

It was only a few minutes drive to Park Hall, and they followed other cars in, and parked in front of the house. When the door was opened, they stepped inside into the vestibule and slipped through the thick curtain into the hall. They were warmly welcomed by Tom and Alice, to whom they gave the present, while John the younger son took their coats and hats, and told them to go into the lounge. There they were met by George the elder son and his wife Mary who were in charge of the bar, and gave them the drinks for which they had asked. Flora, turning round, began to talk to Norah Wilson and introduced her to Jack and Mrs Booth, and then to George and Mary. They all waved to Granny Collinson who was smartly dressed, and was going in and out of the dining room, putting finishing touches to the buffet.

'No one would think she was eighty-two, would they?' said Jack.

'They wouldn't, she is remarkable for her age, she misses nothing,' said Mary. Doris and Joan Collinson joined the circle, and then Bill McConnell and Terry. The very large room soon filled as more guests arrived, among whom were Dick and Betty Heyes with the Harrisons from Bank House. The two Collinson girls and Bill and Terry excused themselves and left the room. Soon Tom and Alice came in and walked into the centre of the room, and Tom in a loud voice said, 'Hello, everybody, are all your glasses full? Come on, George and Mary, get 'em filled up quick.' As soon as this was done Tom continued, 'Alice and I 'ave asked you all to come 'ere tonight to celebrate a unique event, which has been sprung on us just o'er ten days sin.'

At that moment Joan, holding Terry's hand, and Doris, leading Bill, came into the room.

'And I have the pleasure to announce the engagement o' both mi daughters.' There was a big gasp of surprise, and some talking but Tom continued, 'So we want you all to raise your glasses, the toast is to "The happy four". The first toast is Doris and Bill,' everybody drank, 'Now Joan and Terry,' everyone drank again, and then began to cheer, and crowd round the four happy people and congratulate them. It became a free-for-all with all the ladies wanting to see the engagement rings, and the men to kiss the girls and shake hands with Bill and Terry. Cyril Johnson, the High Street photographer, came in and set up his tripod and camera. He took photographs of each couple, then others when their parents and relations had joined them. Finally all the guests went to one end of the room and a group photograph was taken. Then Tom announced, 'Will you all please mek your way inta t' dining room, and 'elp yourselves to t' buffet.'

Obviously the senior members of the Collinson family disregarded rationing, for the table was groaning under the weight of food lavishly provided with typical farm hospitality. After supper the lounge carpet was rolled back, and the big radiogram was switched on by Joan and Terry. The sound of Joe Loss and his band playing 'In the mood' filled the room; couples crowded onto the floor, and the party began to go with a swing. All the songs of the war were played, and then the evening's dancing ended with Vera Lynn singing 'We'll Meet Again'. They all made a circle round the room and 'Auld Lang Syne' was sung with gusto. After thanking their hosts they said their goodbyes, and drove home through the frosty night.

'Gosh, that was a good party,' said Flora. 'I still feel a bit tight. I'll go and make a cup of tea.'

'Oh no, you won't,' said Richard, 'you'll give me a kiss first, I've not had one all night.'

'Here you are then, love,' said Flora, and she flung her arms round his neck, and passionately kissed him.

'That's better, now, where's the tea?'

'I didn't think you would want any after that,' and laughing uproariously she went into the kitchen.

Terry was on duty on Monday night, and when he had finished evening surgery, Richard asked him to come upstairs to the lounge. Flora had made some of her well known milky Camp coffee, and when they were seated Richard said, 'I presume I needn't tell you, Terry, that you have been here three months today, and I suppose after Saturday it's been a pretty good three months for you.'

'You're right, Mr Holden, it has been great. I do like being here; for me everything's going on so well.'

'I must say I reciprocate those sentiments, and also now, Terry, I think in private you must call me Richard, but I do like us to be addressed as professional men in public. The reason I have delayed you is to give you these two documents which are self-explanatory, and underline the fact that we would like you to be permanent here.'

'Thank you both very much – that's great. Joan and Mother will be pleased, though Joan did say that she would go with me anywhere if I was not suitable here.'

'Not suitable, what utter rubbish, Terry. Really, I feel it's for me to be grateful to you for staying, because my health and temper have both improved a lot this last three months. So will you, or all of you, read them, and let me have your reply soon.'

'I promise I will do that this week, Richard, so if you will both excuse me, I'll go, because Joan is waiting at Park Hall, and we can read them together tonight.'

On Tuesday evening Mavis arrived to clean the surgery, because John had now got flu, and she had told him to stay in bed while she came to do his work for the next few nights. Flora thanked her for coming and, accompanied by Richard, went to the doctor's surgery. She was feeling a little nervous, when Bill gave her the injection which she hoped would end her infertility. Doris Collinson, wearing her dark blue Sister's uniform, held her leg firmly and then said, 'There you are, that didn't hurt at all, did it, Flora?'

'No, it didn't, thank you.'

'Good, then come for the next one in a month's time.'

'I will, Bill, thanks; and thank you, Doris, too, for being here.'

'Oh, she's got to be here now – I am starting her off on the right foot.'

'Really,' said Doris, 'that's news to me. Flora, don't men get some strange ideas?'

'They do, Richard is an expert at it,' and they all burst out laughing.

The large buff coloured envelope which arrived for Terry the next morning, confirmed that he had been appointed a Panel B local veterinary inspector. As he had never worked for the Ministry before he was very pleased.

The phone call for Mrs Holden made Flora run down the stairs, and she stumbled and lost her shoe at the bottom.

'Damn it, Richard, when are you going to get a bloody phone put upstairs, or do you want me to break my neck?'

'Of course, I don't; I'll get it done, are you all right?'

'Yes,' she shouted and ran into the office and seized the receiver.

'Hello, yes, Mum, are you all right? . . . Yes, well what's the matter? . . . Our Mary's very ill, and in hospital in Bromley in Kent. You're going tomorrow morning; then I'll go with you, and meet you at Droughton for the eight forty-five, and stay the night. Yes, Mum, I've got that, I'll be there; see you in the morning,' and she replaced the receiver.

'I'm sorry to hear that, what's happened to Mary?'

'She caught flu after getting soaked driving her truck, and it's turned to pneumonia, so she was taken to hospital in Bromley last night, and they've just let Mum know.'

'Then I'll ring Mrs Foster and go to see her peke early in the morning – that way I can drop you off at Droughton Station. You'll be back Friday night.'

'Yes, that's what Mum has arranged already.'

That evening news announced that Mosquitoes of the RAF had been bombing Germany, and Richard secretly prayed that Norman would be safe, and especially Jim if he were flying again.

Next morning Richard parked the car outside the main entrance to Droughton Station, and bought a platform ticket for himself and a Sandhaven to London return for Flora. They met Jean on the platform, and both remarked how well she looked. The very long train was fairly full, but both women had got a seat when he waved them goodbye.

Mrs Foster wanted to know all about the engagement party, and it was a good few minutes before he found that Poppy had passed the tapeworm, much to Mrs Foster's relief. A message came for Richard to go at once to Dunthwaite Underley to a horse with colic which proved to be a spasmodic one, so the usual treatment was quickly administered via the stomach tube, and then the horse was walked about. Arthur Gardner told Richard that he would want a two-year-old colt cutting next spring, but he wanted two six-month-old foals docking as soon as possible. Richard made a note, and after giving him a packet of worm powders re-examined the gelding. It was recovering from the attack, so after taking a dung sample he left.

That afternoon he went to see John Greaves at Foxlands, Waterford – another new client and Richard was curious to know why he had rung up when he lived two miles from the nearest vet.

'Well tha sees, Mr 'olden, I 'ad Woods from Mereside, but he's gone blind, an' 'is lad's a quack; he never got through College. So I tried Captain Richardson in Runfold, and when he turned up he was drunk. Sow t' wife got mi to ring our Raymond, an ee told me to 'ave thee. Tha knows place, we'd ta got th 'orse out o' t' pit i summer. Mercer Farm.'

'Yes. I remember that very well.'

'Tha' sees ee's wife's brother.'

'By jove, you are all related round here, I'll have to watch what I say; anyway, it's nice to meet you. Now, what's wrong?'

'Nowt; I 'ev four calves I want cutting clean, 'cos Woods used Bundizzo and two fat were graded as bulls so I lost some brass. Tha' sees, one o' their stones hadn't shrivelled away.'

'I know, it can happen. Where are they? Let's get on.' The calves were big but Richard soon injected plenty of local anaesthetic and castrated them.

'Now, you've seen their testicles removed, Mr Greaves. If there is any argument in future let me know, because I'll take a description of them.'

'Tha do, an I'll gi thee t' ear numbers, they cum frae a pedigree 'erd an they're marked.'

'That's good; and here is your dusting powder, put it on the wounds twice a day until they are healed.'

That night the mist was thickening slowly when he drove to Churchlands at Underley.

''Ello Mr 'olden, tha's med good time through t' fog.'

'Yes, I have but it was only mist as far as Marhey, it's got worse this last five minutes.'

Stan Rainford was a powerful big, black-haired man, and as soon as Richard had corrected the malpresentation, pulling the head into the correct position, he heaved the calf out very quickly.

'It's a 'eifer an' wick; I thought it came easy. Like a cup of tay?'

'No thanks, Stan, I'll be off back, before it gets any thicker.'

It did, and Richard had to drive very slowly, which was fortunate for him because he met the Viking bus on the narrow humped-back canal bridge in Marhey. They had both stopped at once, and the bus driver came and guided Richard back, after which the bus and two Army lorries drove past, leaving the road to him to continue his journey home, which took almost an hour.

The news told of the illness of Mr Churchill, who had a bad cold which had turned to pneumonia, but he was beginning to improve.

Though he had forgotten to put a hot water bottle into the bed, he was soon asleep. On the Friday at Ryton Grange, Will Turner had a sow which could not farrow. After putting on his overall, Richard placed his kneeler behind the sow.

'Is that thi kneeler?'

'Yes it is.'

'I bet tha don't tek it to church, 'cos Vicar won't like it, all covered with pig muck and stinking like hell.'

'I know he wouldn't, seeing he's a relative of my wife's.'

'Ee is ee? Any road, it's a good idea. What's wrong wi 'er?'

'Nothing, they are just packed in so tight, they are like sardines in a tin. She's blown up with piglets.' Richard delivered fourteen alive and two dead.

'It's lucky she has twelve good tits, so I con put two on one that's only got six alive. Mr 'olden, what meks 'em ev half a dozen dead?'

'There's no straight answer to your question, Will; I think it is disease usually, but also bruising or injury could cause it, even something wrong with her ovaries.'

'Then she'll ev to go fat when she's reared these eight, there's a good trade for fat uns tha knows nowadays.'

At nine o'clock Flora rang from Droughton, to say she was catching the connection for Sandhaven and would be home in half an hour. Richard met her, and though she was tired she was in good spirits because Mary was recovering steadily, having been at her worst on Wednesday.

'I'm glad to hear that, and how was Mum?'

'She's OK; she wasn't tired at all, she was never still just like she used to be. Is there any news?'

'Yes there is: Mrs Wilson has invited us to dinner at The Moorings tomorrow night at seven o'clock.'

'How nice of her; it should be a good do.'

'I'm certain, knowing her, it will be. I'll put the car away while you make some supper. There are some pies I got from Frank Wood.'

The news was that Mr Churchill was still improving in his battle with pneumonia.

'Thank God for that,' said Richard. 'He may be an old man but I don't know what we would do without him.'

The Moorings was a very large house built of brick and stone on the Promenade at Seaton, but in the blackness, little could be seen of it when Richard drove round the semi-circular approach up to the steps at the front door. The maid admitted them, then Mrs Wilson, who was wearing a striking red evening dress, welcomed them both warmly. The maid took their top clothes and they went into a magnificent lounge which was furnished in very good taste. Joan Collinson and Terry were waiting for them, and soon they were seated in front of the good fire. Drinks were brought and a lively conversation continued until the maid announced that dinner was served.

Flora admired the dining room with its large highly polished mahogany table and Chippendale chairs. The glasses and silver shone on the white damask tablecloth, and as time passed they all enjoyed an excellent dinner. Norah Wilson explained that she had decided to serve full Christmas dinner, because the holiday was so near, and she thought it would be acceptable to them.

Flora said, 'It's been delicious, Norah, I've really enjoyed every mouthful, and I'm certain that Richard has.'

'I have, thoroughly. It was very kind of you to invite us, and we do thank you, Norah.'

'Don't thank me, its my pleasure. It was also my plan to get us together to talk about the future, but let's go into the lounge; it will be warmer there, and we can have our coffee.' Flora was the only one who did not smoke when Terry brought round the cigarettes.

Then Terry said, 'I asked mother to invite you and Flora to have dinner with us tonight because Joan and I think the scheme for a salaried partnership is excellent, but with us getting engaged the position has changed, and a partnership would be more attractive. Of course one can't plan too far ahead, but we thought you would like to consider this, because Joan has something else to tell you.'

Joan, blushing slightly, said, 'Its this, that Terry and I have decided to get married on the second Saturday in February.'

'Oh, how lovely. I'm so happy for you,' said Flora kissing Joan, and Richard said, 'Terry, congratulations, and the best of luck,' and they shook hands.'

Norah said, 'I am really happy for them too, and also I see no reason why they should wait for months on end.'

Richard, beginning to laugh, said, 'It's always said it's cheaper to live when you're married than as a single chap, so why do you need a partnership, Terry?'

'I don't believe that, it's all Tommy-rot.'

'You're right there, it's never been cheaper in my case; you see, when I asked George Duke to draft an incentive scheme, I never thought your romance would blossom as quickly as it has. But in view of what you have just told me, about the wedding and the partnership, I will ask him to draw up a rough draft for one as soon as he can, but I don't think we will get it before Christmas. In the meantime, do you want to sign these two documents?'

'Of course I do, Richard.'

'Then I'll arrange it with George, and then after they are signed they will be an earnest of our good intent, and can be operative until the partnership agreement has been drawn up and signed. So they make you permanent here, which is what I want you to be.'

'It is very nice of you to say that, Richard; I do want to stay here and so does Joan. I'm very glad that's settled, thank you so much.'

'Let's have coffee, here it comes. I'm sure we are all ready for it.'

They all agreed and then Terry asked them if they would like a drink; when the sherry, whisky and brandy had been served, the evening was spent very pleasantly.

On Sunday Keith Barrett rang and asked if he could come for an interview on Monday morning, because he was home in Seaton. Richard told him to come no later than a quarter to nine.

Flora was grumbling that she was behind with her Christmas preparations through going to London, so together they began to decorate the house. She had ordered a turkey from Frank Wood as soon as she knew that Mary and Bill would be on leave and would come to Sandhaven.

'I've also got two puddings made, Richard, a big one for Christmas day, and the other two for New Year, but I don't see how we can have a party, because the list of people is getting too big, the minimum number this year would be twenty-eight.'

'Twenty-eight, Flora! The house isn't big enough, and that would be two bottles of whisky just to give them one drink each.'

'I know, and I can't feed that lot. Would you have enough drink?'

'I haven't; and you can't be certain, because some people don't like punch, and all ask for gin one year, and the next they all want whisky. Will it be worth having it if we can't give them a drink?'

'Of course it will, and we will have to give them a drink somehow.'

'Yes, but what?'

'Go across to the Market Hotel and ask Mr Belcher what they serve at wedding lunches nowadays, and if he is no help go to the Porters.'

'I will, but when are we going to have it?'

'We can't now before Christmas, so it will have to be Boxing Day.'

Keith was early for the interview, and Joan showed him into the waiting room. Richard waited until Terry arrived, and then they went in together to interview him. He was a fresh-complexioned young man, with brown curly hair, and was about six feet tall. They agreed he could see practice with them, so Richard went and got a copy of the binding out agreement for seeing practice, and on returning found Terry and Keith getting on famously, talking about the Royal Veterinary College and members of its staff.

'Here you are, Mr Barrett, read it and if you accept it, sign both copies, keep one for yourself, and give me the other when you come tomorrow at the same time. Don't forget to bring a warehouse coat, rubber boots and a note book.'

'I won't; thank you very much, both of you.'

Richard rang Arthur at Dunthwaite and asked him to have the two foals in at ten o'clock next morning. The partners' documents being acceptable to both of them, Terry and Richard signed them in Tommy Duke's office on Monday afternoon.

At the moment Keith walked in, Joan came out of the office and said, 'Mr Holden, that was Mr Fisher from Ivy Farm at Teston; he has a cow that can't calve.'

'Thanks, Joan, I'll go there first, then to Arthur Gardner's at Dunthwaite, so you can get me there till half past eleven.'

'Na' then, who's this young fella?' asked Harry Fisher.

'Mr Barrett; he's a third year student at the Royal Veterinary College, and he's coming round with me to see practice.'

'I'll tell thee what, Mr Barrett, tha'll see a lot wi' this chap.'

'We won't if we don't have some hot water quick.' Harry strolled off to fetch some.

'Have you ever examined a cow, Keith?'

'No, I only watched everything and took notes where I saw practice in Hampshire.'

'Then you'll start now, put this overall on.'

'Who's going to do t' job?'

'I am, Harry, don't worry.'

'Am not, I only thowt there weren't room for two o'yer inside t' cow.'

Richard rolled up his sleeves, and after dressing his arms examined the cow.

'It's coming backwards, Harry.'

'It damn well would be.'

'You've washed your arms, Keith? Quick, have a feel then, tail in centre, great trochanter at each side, got it? Then give me the overall, put two ropes into the disinfectant. Harry, bring two stool legs, hurry up.'

Richard, giving an explanation of what he was doing inside the cow, soon had two feet showing at the vulva.

'The soles of its feet are pointing upwards, so the calf's on its back, or it's a breech. Put a rope on that leg. No, don't tie it, watch me fix it this way.'

'Now both of you: Harry, pull first, now you Keith, that's it, both of you pull hard; here it comes, and its tail's wagging.'

'By gum, it is wick.'

'Yes, and it's a heifer,' said Richard, looking at it lying on the straw.

'It's a real bobby dazzler wi' its four white legs.'

'It is. Let her loose, she'll soon clean it up.'

'Cum on and we'll go for us tay.'

'I am sorry, Harry, we haven't time; we're late already, we should have been docking foals by now. But thank Elsie all the same. There'll be more for you anyway.'

'Not while mi Dad's about; he lives on tay and fags. Ta'ra.'

Keith remarked, 'That was really exciting, especially the calf being alive, Mr Holden.'

'Yes, it's very rewarding to get a live calf, but don't forget if it's a breech it's got to be born quickly, or else it drowns in the amniotic fluid.'

'I won't forget that,' said Keith writing in his notebook.

'Good morning, Arthur; sorry I'm late. I've been to Teston to calve a cow. Is everything ready?'

'Aye.'

'Then will you put these docking irons in the fire, and take a dry bucket with you to bring them back in.'

'Reet.'

As soon as he returned, one of his men went into the box and the first foal was backed up to the half door, and the twitch put on its nose. Its tail was pulled over the door and clipped; a tourniquet was applied tightly to it, disinfectant poured on it and local anaesthetic injected. The animal showed its displeasure by punching the door hard.

'Give up, you noisy devil!' shouted Arthur.

'Right, let it go, and back up the other.'

The same procedure was repeated. The first foal was put back with its tail over the half door. Richard disinfected the blade of the docking knife, and found the tail was numb.

'Right, Arthur, pull it out straight; now, where do you want it cutting off?'

'Just there.'

'Move your finger.'

With a crash, the tail was chopped off.

'Quick, Keith, bring the irons in the bucket.'

'Fire's on t' reet in t' kitchen.'

He was soon back and Richard seared the stump, and after Keith had shaken powdered resin over it, it was melted to cover the raw surface.

'Come on, next one.'

The second was quickly docked and seared.

'Put those irons in the trough to cool, Keith, and don't forget them.'

'That went well, Mr Holden.'

'It did, you want plenty of help, and lots of local anaesthetic. This new chlorocain is very good; I use it all the time. Now take the tourniquets off.'

There was no bleeding, but Richard issued a warning. 'Watch them over the next couple of hours, Arthur, so they don't rub them when the anaesthetic wears off or they could bleed.'

'Aye, I'll keep mi eye on 'em.'

Mrs Gardner called from the kitchen doorway. 'Bill Rigby at Olton wants tha to call.'

'Thanks, Mrs Gardner, I'll go straight there.'

'By heck, tha's bin quick, Mr 'olden,' said Bill.

'Yes, we weren't too far away.'

'So this is this new flying machine,' he said, walking round the Rover and admiring it.

'Tha knows, young man,' said Bill, looking at Keith, 'one morning in t' summer 'e goes past 'ere like yon bloody Malcolm Campbell, 'ell 'e wore going fast, and then in 'alf an 'our, if he don't cum back going faster t' other way. I said to our Paul, "Yon silly devil 'ull kill issel yet, wi t' speed he goes."'

'Bill, you don't know, but I had four cows with milk fever that morning from half past five to nine o'clock, and I drove forty odd miles to get to them, so I had to go fast or I'd have been in trouble. Now, what's wrong?'

'I've one that's badly, and one 'olding her cleaning.' The 'badly' one was a case of pneumonia which Richard treated by giving M&B693 by stomach tube – this surprised Keith who had listened to both sides of the cow's chest.

'Oo's real bad, isn't oo?'

'Yes, Bill, her temperature is over 105°F, so I'll be back to treat her again tonight.'

Keith was allowed to examine the uterus and afterbirth of the second cow for experience, and then Richard removed the latter and put in two pessaries.

Driving home, he said to Keith, 'You've had some variety on your first morning, have you enjoyed it?'

'Yes, very much, Mr Holden; I've learnt more this morning than I have in eighteen months in Mr Clark's practice.'

'And you'll soon fill your notebook, it's a very mixed practice, so you never know what you will see next. After lunch, go with Mr Wilson. He will tell you what time he will pick you up, he lives not far from you.'

'Read that,' said Flora on Wednesday night, giving the paper to Richard. 'He could have called to see us.'

The newspaper reported that Wing Co. D.L. Oakes DSO, DFC, and Flt. Lieut. N. Robinson DFC and Bar had visited the Government factories on Dock Road. They had addressed the assembled workers in their canteen, giving a graphic account of the recent attacks on targets in Germany by Lancasters and Mosquito bombers of the RAF, and been received with great enthusiasm. The reason for the visit of the party from the Ministry of Aircraft Production and these exciting talks was to increase production of aircraft to replace the inevitable losses which took place, but the paper was proud to say that there was never a shortage of brave men to fly them.

'I don't see how he could; he couldn't just clear off and leave an official party.'

'No, I don't suppose he could, but the least he could have done was ring you.'

'Knowing Norman he would have done if he could. I'll be off now to Rigby's to treat that cow again.'

It was near closing time when Richard went across to the Market Hotel, and Ben listened to his plea for booze.

'I can't sell thee any spirits at moment, Mr Holden, it's in short supply and I need all I've got for t' next week. At weddings I gi' 'em a cocktail; tha knows tha con mek 'em real strong, but nice like, so they'll only want two drinks at most.'

'I'd never thought of that, Ben, it's a very good idea. What should I make the cocktail with?'

'Gin, whisky or brandy, and tha' con mek cheap brandy cocktails using cider. Tha puts a measure of cheap brandy in a cocktail glass and fill it up with cider. For weddings we put sugar on t' edge o' t' glass, and pop in a cherry on a cocktail stick – it looks classy like.'

'Thanks a lot, Ben, that's solved my problem; can you let me have some brandy then?'

'I con let thee 'ave 'alf a bottle, that's all, but I bet Tom Sharples at Cock Inn will 'ave some spare or Sudell at the Royal.'

'I'll pay you, Ben, and I'll want six bottles of beer, later.'

''Ere, tek 'em now while I 'ave em, they wain't last long when t' Yanks get 'ere tomorrow neet.'

Flora was very pleased with Ben's idea, and began counting how many suitable glasses they had, while Richard got all the Christmas paper decorations pinned to the walls.

'I'm glad they've lasted another year – it will look all right with holly and ivy. I must get some tomorrow, and if you see any, buy it. Oh hell, that's the phone.'

'Yes and it's half past ten.' It was John Greaves; one of his beef cows couldn't calve.

'I think he's going to be another Bob Whittaker, they always ring up at bedtime; so I'll have to leave you to check everything for the party, because it will be midnight before I am back.'

The big bull calf was dry, and its head was turned back.

'When did she start, John?'

'It could 'ave bin at dinner-time, because I saw her tail was wet, but oo asn't strained or owt.'

'Then go and get two men to help us.'

Richard spent the time he was away putting handfuls of Lux into the cow's uterus, and then pumped in slowly a lot of water, thus lubricating the calf and the uterus.

'I've getten Will and Fred frae t' next farm.'

'Thanks, now we can get on.' He firmly fixed a sharp hook into the calf's eye socket, and told John to pull steadily. Richard, holding the calf's lower jaw, easily put it in the correct position. 'That will do, stop.' He roped the head and both legs, and the three men pulled mightily for ten minutes before the dead bull calf was born. Richard drove away home in minutes and yawned – it had been a long day.

A sprightly Jean arrived on Thursday afternoon, but Mary, looking very pale and drawn, was weary when she came in the evening. Richard had met both of them at the station, but it was Flora and Jean who helped Mary into the house and fussed over her. She should not have travelled so far, having only just recovered from her illness.

When their late dinner was served, Flora made certain that she had a bowl of meat and vegetable soup, followed by braised meat with potatoes and vegetables. She could only eat a little plum tart and custard because she was full.

'Thank you, Flora, that was lovely. It is a long time since I enjoyed anything so much,' and tears ran down her cheeks.

'Don't be upset, Mary,' said Flora who gave her a kiss, and then made her sit in front of the fire.

'I am a bit, because Rosemary was killed in a low level raid the other night by Jerry bombers. We were all devastated.'

'I'm so sorry to hear that,' said Jean, 'because you had been together ever since you left school.'

'We had, I will miss her terribly, but the battery was cheered to learn that the RAF shot down three of them.'

'Have some coffee, Mary,' said Flora, changing the subject. 'I hope Bill gets here safe tomorrow.'

'What time is he coming?' asked Jean.

'I don't know, he has not rung, but he did say he would get leave.'

'Don't ask any silly questions,' said Jean who had brought a half loin of pork, 'but I am going to cook it straight away, and then we can have it cold. Have you any apples, Flora?'

'Yes. I'll go and get some, and then I'm off shopping. I must get cocktail sticks and glacé cherries.'

To Flora's relief and pleasure Frank Wood had a twelve-pound dressed turkey for her, so their traditional Christmas lunch was assured. Richard got a bottle of brandy and a quart bottle of cider from Tom Sharples; while Jack Sudell sold him two more bottles of cider, and so his preparations for Boxing Day were complete. The smell of food being cooked permeated the house on Christmas Eve; bones were being boiled to make stock for soup; Jean was busy making biscuits, having got plenty of fat from the roast pork. Richard got the job of putting the home-made stuffing into the turkey, which he sewed up and then trussed with two wooden skewers. This happy activity stopped abruptly when Bill arrived, because within minutes of their cheerful welcome they all realised that something was wrong with him. He had become very deaf. At dinner he told them that when he had returned to his unit from compassionate leave in October, he began instructing in a tank gunnery. One day on the range there was a premature bursting of the shell in the breech of the tank's gun. This killed the gunner and injured the driver. Bill, who was watching the fall of shot from the conning tower, had one ear drum burst and the other damaged. He was in the hospital at Aldershot for five days because he had the most dreadful headache, and had partly lost his sense of balance. These effects slowly disappeared, and when he was discharged from the hospital, he was given light duties.

'Why didn't you let me know?' asked Flora.

'Well, it was hardly worth it; there was nothing to see. I was kept in bed for five days and given tablets, and then I was sent back to my unit.'

'I think you were very lucky, Bill, it could have been much worse, I'm sure,' said Jean.

'It could that, if bits of the breech block had hit me I would have been a gonner; even so some of my mates thought I wasn't really deaf, until in Church I sang half a verse of a hymn when everybody else had finished. That convinced them and the Colonel, but the MO has prohibited me from going near the ranges, and I won't be going with the Unit when it moves.'

Jean secretly was relieved.

After dinner they went into the warm lounge, and had coffee. Richard brought the spare bed in then and erected it. Flora made it ready for Bill who, grinning, said, 'I won't be cold tonight for sure with that lovely fire. It's a great change from a Nissen hut – it was so cold last week we all put our greatcoats on our beds as an extra blanket.'

The church was crowded for the midnight first Communion of Christmas, and it was pleasantly warm. It was obvious that Richard's requests to both the churchwardens for more fuel had caused more to be provided for the boiler, and had mollified the vicar.

Richard and Bill with Mary between them went for a short walk that morning, a cold, bright Christmas Day, and they were all hungry. After the traditional lunch of turkey and plum pudding had been eaten they all helped with the washing up and in putting the crockery and cutlery away. By three o'clock Bill was sound asleep on the settee and Mary had gone to bed, so Richard turned on the wireless, and the three of them listened to the King's speech, which was followed by the playing of the National Anthems of the various Allies. After Jean and Flora had taken Rocky for a short walk, a pot of tea was brewed, and the rest of the afternoon was spent in looking at their presents or talking. Richard was engrossed in reading back numbers of the *Veterinary Record* and the *Tatler*. Late in the afternoon he tried both telephones to see if they were working, because neither had rung all day: something which had never happened before. About half past six Jean made pork sandwiches, and put out slices of Christmas cake and mince pies. She got them altogether to have this buffet supper, because Flora wanted plans to be finalised for the Boxing Day party.

It was decided that Mary would prepare the glasses by wetting their rims and then dipping them into sugar which would dry on. She also had to put cherries on sticks, and finally put all glasses on two trays. Bill and Richard would prepare the brandy cocktails, and then be in charge of the drinks all night. Jean was to be in charge of biscuits, and Flora was the receptionist and MC.

In the morning in the lounge the bed was quickly dismantled and put away, and the room dusted. Flora began arranging her gramophone records in the order in which she was going to play them, and then said, 'Richard, it is time we had a radiogram; you can't expect anybody to wind up your old gramophone all night. I saw a good one for £16 in the sale room the other day.'

'It will have to do for now, Flora. Anyway, how many records have you got?'

'About a couple of dozen, of old favourites and the latest hits.'

'But you won't need all those; they're not coming until after the churches' services have ended at eight o'clock, and by the time they've had a chat and a drink, it will be nine. So Bill and I will do it.'

John, who had recovered from flu, arrived and tidied up the garden, and then helped moving furniture, and bringing up coal and logs for the lounge fire. He also brought a message from Jim Lord that they would not be coming because they all had bad colds.

Soon after eight o'clock the Bishops and the Heyes arrived together, followed by all the other guests, and after the first drink the party came alive, with the two Collinson girls and their partners being the centre of attraction and congratulations. By the time the second had been drunk and the buffet supper eaten, it was literally a roaring success, with the songs being sung lustily, until the carpet was rolled back and the dancing began.

The songs ranged from the sentimental like 'Long ago and far away' and 'All the things you are,' to the catchy tunes such as 'Roll out the barrel,' 'Lili Marlene' and 'We'll meet again,' until just after ten some wanted to leave, so 'Goodnight sweetheart' was played and then 'Auld Lang Syne'. They all said how much they had enjoyed it, and one or two ladies had to be helped down the stairs, being somewhat unsteady on their legs!

Bill had 'brewed up' before the last stragglers had gone, and they all flopped down, and enjoyed the tea.

'I needed that,' said Jean.

'So did I,' said Mary, 'and hasn't it all gone off well!'

'I'd say it has,' said Bill. 'They've drunk almost all the brandy and three and a half bottles of cider, I was getting worried we might run out of drink.'

'I'm glad we didn't,' said Flora. 'It would have been dreadful if we had, with Norah and Terry and the Collinsons here. As it was, Norah said she enjoyed every minute of it, and amused me when she said it was terrific to let your hair down once in twelve months.'

'I agree with the once in twelve months bit,' said Richard. 'Now, come on Bill, and we'll put your bed up, and then we can all get some sleep.'

'I'm ready for bed,' said Flora. 'We'll wash the glasses and clean up in the morning, because though it will be the official Boxing Day, both Tom Bishop and Dick Heyes said it would be work as usual.'

'It will be,' said Jean. 'I'm off.'

'Me too,' said Mary, following her out of the room. Bill and Mary left early on Monday and soon both Richard and Terry set off on a round of visits. Joan arrived to see if she could help, and with Flora's help began to go through all the year end accounts. Later Flora left her to it, and joined Jean to help with the housework. In the late afternoon, Flora said she wanted a breath of fresh air and would take Rocky for his walk before blackout. The dog didn't show any enthusiasm for a walk. 'Come on, Rocky, what's up with you?'

Flora got his lead, but he stood still, paying no attention to anything, and then with no warning, he rolled onto his side, and began to have a fit.

'Richard!' she shouted. 'Come here quick!' and he ran in and stood watching the dog as the severity of the spasms slowly moderated.

'What's caused it?'

'I don't know, Flora, but this is what happens so often during or after distemper. Now he has had a fit, I am certain he will have more. I'll go and get a shovel, and mop this mess up.'

'But what are you going to do? Don't put him to sleep, will you?'

'Not yet, but if he has more it will be necessary; you can't leave him going from fit to fit, it's not humane.'

'But isn't there any treatment at all?'

'No, there isn't; even sedatives won't stop him getting worse.'

'Oh dear, I am disappointed, because he is such a game little beggar, and he is such a good companion. So we will have to wait and see what happens then.'

'Yes, that sums it up.'

Mr Barrett went back to London on Thursday, and thanked Richard for all the practice he had let him see, and particularly for letting him assist in the work. Richard said he expected him back at Easter, and Mr Barrett said he most definitely would come. It was on one of the evenings of that week that the news reader announced the sinking of the German battleship *Scharnhorst*.

'Hooray,' said Richard, 'they can't have many left now. Good riddance, I say, but I wish it had been ten U-Boats instead, because they're the ones that do all the damage.' When he went into the kitchen to let the dog out, he found Rocky in another severe fit, so he called Flora, and they sadly decided that this was the end. She went upstairs, tears running down her face, and Richard felt very sad as he injected the dog intraperitoneally with a lethal dose of Pentothal and watched him die. He got a sack, and was putting the body into it, when Flora shouted, 'I don't want to see his collar and lead again, throw them out, Richard,' so he put them in the sack and put it in the garage.

When, the next evening, John arrived in a cloud of cigarette smoke, Richard said, 'Hello, John, I see you're back to normal; smoking again.'

'Aye I'm mekin up for lost time. I did miss 'em when I were ill, Mr 'olden; tha sees mi sister don't let me smoke upstairs an I were too poorly to cum down til't Friday. Mr 'eyes gi mi a cigar, so I enjoyed it on Christmas Day. By the way, whers t' dog got to?'

'I've had to put him to sleep because you know that twitch he had in his leg, well, it spread all over and got to his brain, making him have fits. So don't open that sack in the garage.'

'No I won't; any road it would be the best thing for 'im, being like that.'

As he was not on duty on Friday night, New Year's Eve, Richard and Flora went to the Porter's Arms for dinner, and as it was a mild dry night they walked along arm in arm in the blackout.

'I was just thinking, Richard, it is a long time since we went out together on New Year's Eve.'

'It is that; you know, now Terry's here I feel we have turned a corner, and can begin to do what other folk do in their spare time.'

'I feel that way too, because all we've ever done is go to the pictures, and then you'd get called out or else we'd go for a chat to someone's house. It's really romantic walking along like this in the dark,' and she held his arm more firmly.

On impulse he kissed her. 'That was lovely, Richard,' and she kissed him in return.

'We're here now; in you go.' Once through the black-out curtain which hung inside the entrance, the hotel was brightly lit, and warm. Having treated his bull terrier dog, Richard knew Mr Johnson the manager, who led them to their table and called a waiter over to take their order. The dining room was full: the majority of the diners being USAAF or RAF officers; the former were noisy and obviously enjoying themselves. Though their choice of the five-shilling meal was restricted to one only of the two main courses, they enjoyed their dinner, and then went into the lounge bar where Flora ordered tea. For both of them it was a pleasant change to be able to relax and watch the world go by. Finally Richard bought Flora a large whisky and a brandy for himself; they clinked their glasses and said, 'Here's to us, and 1944.'

When they left the hotel their torch was giving a very feeble light because the battery was almost exhausted, so they linked arms to set off home. This was fortunate for Flora who, stumbling over the uneven pavement, would have fallen heavily if she had not had a firm hold of Richard's arm.

'Damn the blackout! I really caught my toe then, this pavement is bloody awful. How many more years of this will we have to put up with, I wonder?'

'I don't know, love, but I wish it could end tomorrow. I often think back to that party we had just before Christmas in 1938, with lights on everywhere and the shops full of every imaginable thing, and plenty to eat and drink. It was wonderful.'

'It was when you compare it with now, when everything you want is short. I suppose we were lucky to get a turkey. I wonder if it will ever again be like it was then.'

'Somehow I don't think it will be.'

Later after some passionate love making, sleep enveloped them both, and the old year slipped away into history.

1944

There was no lying in bed on New Year's morning 1944, both vets were out to emergencies before breakfast, and the day became very busy. Both Terry and Richard noticed that even fewer cars were on the road now that the regulations banning private motoring had come into force, but there appeared to be an increase in the number of vehicles belonging to the Services.

Dock Road was choked with them when he went to one of the stables, where he found an outbreak of strangles had begun. Four horses were ill, and one of them, a young horse, had a temperature of 105°F, so he injected it with a large dose of soluble sulphonamide. The others were dosed via the stomach tube, and the horse foreman was told to foment the horses' swollen glands three times in the day following this with the application of white liniment. To try and prevent the disease spreading to all the horses, he injected every one with strangles vaccine. The next morning the young horse was improving so the treatment was repeated; but another which was showing signs of pneumonia, he dosed with M&B693. He did this on the following two days, but its condition rapidly deteriorated and it died. By the end of the week he had lanced many parotid abscesses; the outbreak had been contained, and the horses slowly recovered over the next few weeks.

On that evening of the first day of the year, Richard asked Terry to come up into the lounge, and they began to arrange the distribution of the work that had to be done that month. When Bob Dawson had asked if they could do more work for the Ministry of Agriculture & Food and they had agreed to do so, they did not expect a list almost two pages long!

Though there were no signposts on the roads Terry had quickly found his way round the practice, but now both of them would be going well outside their own area. They decided that Terry would do the Tuberculin test at the Home Farm and Whyngate, and Richard would do Tom Priestley's and Arrowsmith's. Four mornings a week one of them would go off early to do herd inspections, and also on some evenings. Richard looked through the diary for January and told Terry that if the usual amount of work came in they would be extremely busy. Flora came in with coffee, and the two vets decided to finish trying to arrange any more work. Flora switched on the wireless, and they listened to the news while they were having their drink. When the reader said that Mosquitoes and Typhoons of the RAF had bombed Germany without loss, Richard said,

'I do hope Norman will be OK this year.' He often thought about the terrible dangers that his friend was exposed to, and because of this Richard became even more dedicated to his work. He believed that as he was in a reserved occupation and not allowed to fight, he would make his contribution to the war effort by working harder, so that more food could be produced.

The weather was mild for the time of the year, and in the first ten days of January, four TB cows had been found and slaughtered. Terry was very efficient in finding TB germs in stained specimens of milk sediment or sputum, and if Richard had slides about which he was doubtful, he began to give them to him to check. Mr Campbell Morrison called at the surgery one morning and told them they were doing a good job, and added that he was now living in Seaton, so they could phone him if they had any real difficulties, and he would deal with them. This would help Mr Dawson in Droughton, who was extremely busy. Richard said that he was disappointed that, in spite of all their efforts, the amount of TB among cattle seemed to be as great as ever. Mr Morrison told him that their work was limiting its spread until the Attested Herd Scheme could begin again in July that year. Then he was certain whole herds would be replaced by Attested cattle if the cash incentive was great enough. Even then herd inspections would have to be done regularly.

Tom Collinson of Park Hall asked Richard to examine a dry cow which had a hole in a teat which had leaked milk throughout her last lactation. It was a milk fistula in the teat of the rear hind quarter.

'When is she due, Tom?'

'In about a month.'

'Then I'll come tomorrow morning about nine and get it done. To make a good job, I'll want to cast her, so starve her and give her that dose at eight o'clock to quieten her. I'll bring Terry with me, and your John will be about, won't he?'

'Aye, an' we'll be ready for yer. Where wilta want to do it?'

'In the barn, if you'll put some clean straw down, and I'll want a table and some hot water; that's all.'

The cow was soon cast and the near hind leg drawn forward, and local anaesthetic was injected into the wall of the teat which Terry held firmly. After some minutes Richard excised the fistulous area, and then the wound was sutured with silk worm gut. After the teat had been painted over with dilute Acriflavine, it was smeared with BIPP, and the cow was allowed to rise. Later when Terry removed the sutures, the wound had healed perfectly.

It was one of those raw cold mornings, when the temperature was only just above freezing, when Richard went to Further Marsh at Ryton. In the steamy warm shippon, every nook and cranny was stuffed with straw or rags to keep in the heat, this making it the perfect incubator in which disease-producing germs could flourish and spread. Tom Walsh's cow had pneumonia.

'When did she start like this?'

'Two days sin.'
'And how long has she been calved?'
'Four week gone; yon's her calf.'
'She's in poor condition, Tom.'
'Aye, but oos milkin 'ersel away; after calf's 'ad a go, er'll still gi' a bucket full.'

After examining her chest, Richard felt her udder, and then looked at the wall in front of her. He could not find any sputum, so he dosed her with M&B693.

'Have you a box you could put her in?'
'Aye I ev, but it's a cold un.'
'That doesn't matter, wrap her up with sacks and put her in there, but leave the top half of the door open.'
'That will be a bit rough on er won't it?'
'No, it won't; it's half the battle, I'll come and see her again tonight.'

For a change the pneumonia was not tubercular and the cow recovered in four days.

The big headache for Terry and Richard, and the cause of much grumbling by their clients, was the losses from calf scour. Both dreaded the disease which quickly made a calf tucked up and hide bound, with greenish white frothy stinking diarrhoea soiling the hind quarters and running down the tail. In spite of the use of the sulpha drugs; Tinct.Opll; Brilliant Green; Catechu & Creosotum, there were widespread outbreaks with many deaths. Richard believed that treating ill calves, many of which died, was not a positive approach to the problem; they should adopt some routine preventative treatment. Terry agreed, and on problem farms they began to inject the cow with calf scour vaccine a month before she was due. When the calf was born into a clean dry disinfected area it was injected with mixed calf scour serum and immediately was put on to a teat and allowed to suck the beestings and for at least two days. Again this was not always effective, and sometimes accusations of trying to make the bill bigger were made in a jocular manner, which showed the underlying anger and frustration at the failure of the treatment and advice which had been given. It was the same with mastitis which was appearing more and more in herds which had not been infected before. George Dobson, Fred Noblett at Highgate and Stan Rainford were all having more cases. Richard advised the use of Deosan as a dairy disinfectant, and to follow his written instructions. But reports from the laboratory on milk samples showed other bacteria were causing the disease. They began to inject 12 oz of sterile Soluseptasine solution into infected quarters as a routine treatment with varying results. Fewer cows were dying of mastitis, but more and more quarters were being lost or remaining chronically infected.

Now the NFU began to inform its members that the Attested Herds Scheme would be reopened in June, and that a premium of fourpence a gallon would be paid to all Attested milk producers. This produced a number of enquiries, and soon Joan made a list in chronological order of all the farmers who would want a test to be done. Terry said that if the number grew much more they would both need two pairs of hands!

'Good morning, Mr 'olden, cum in please; Mrs Foster won't be long,' said the maid, and because he was very busy, Richard hoped this would be true. He was unprepared for Mrs Foster's appearance when she came into the room, holding her maid's arm.

Her face was twisted round to the right side, and her left eye appeared unduly prominent. She spoke with a slight impediment, and said, 'Good morning, Mr Holden; I am sorry to keep you, but as you can see I have been ill with a paralysis and I am not better yet.'

'Really, I am very sorry, Mrs Foster, to see you like this, and I do hope you recover soon.'

'Thank you; Dr Bridge says I will which is a blessing, but maybe not completely. But that's enough about me; lift Poppy up, will you, Penny.'

Richard soon announced that she was perfectly well, and her ears very clean. With Penny holding her he cut the dew claws on her hind legs. An elderly lady entered the room, carrying a tray which she placed on a side table, and her gaze took in everything.

'Thank you, Jane,' said Mrs Foster. 'Penny, put Poppy down and off you go. I can pour the coffee. That was my housekeeper, Jane Crook; she's been with me many years, and she is an angel. I don't know what I would have done without her since before Christmas when this happened.'

'Yes, it is fortunate that you have enough staff. Terry and I are so busy we really need an extra pair of hands.'

'Then you must be off; thank you for coming, Mr Holden, and I'll see you next month.'

'You will, and thank you for the coffee, Mrs Foster.'

He appreciated very much the warmth and the coffee at Wilton on this raw wet January morning, because he got very cold examining cows to see if they were pregnant, doing calving cases and removing afterbirths. This was especially true this morning, when his overall was so cold and clammy, that it made him shiver when he put it on, and to make things worse, one double sleeve had begun to leak. He was not feeling very well when he arrived at Pleasant View, Shipton.

'Hello, Eric, now what is it? Cow's not right, you say.'

'Aye, I've 'ad two cows come o'er lately, and this morning our John found this at back o' yon red un.'

This was a little foetus about two and a half inches long wrapped in its transparent membranes.

'Have you had any others pick recently?'

'Only one afore Christmas; she were a three week off, but calf were dead. Any road, oo's milking well.'

'That sounds like real pick. Is your bull new?'

'No, I got him two year sin.'

'Do you let other farmers use him?'

'Only Harold Marsden now. You'll remember that do I ed wi t' bull three or four year back; well, Bill Parkinson and one or two more fell out wi' me o'er it, and they hev their own now.'

'Has Harold had any trouble?'

'No, he said 'e asn't.'

The red cow had a white-coloured discharge, some of which Richard collected in a sterile bottle, and then he took a blood sample from the cow and the other which had aborted.

'I'll examine this mucus when I get home, but I'll examine those other two now.'

Wearing his wet overall, he was cold, but he found that though neither cow was bulling each had a discharge.

'Is it same as last time?'

'I don't think so, Eric; have you bought any cows recently?'

'Only one to keep mi milk up.'

'Has she been served?'

'Aye, a month sin, she's all reet.'

'Then I think you've got an infection here which is causing inflammation of the calf bed, so I'm going to wash these three cows out. I wouldn't serve any at the moment until I get to the bottom of this.'

That night he examined the mucus microscopically, and so did Terry, but they could not find anything abnormal.

'It's not vibrio, Richard, because they abort at five months, and he's also got some active brucella there. It could be trichomonas infection, but I don't remember much about it. I'll have to look up my lecture notes to be certain.'

'Do you think so, I've never found it in the practice yet.'

'Haven't you? Well, there's always a first time, I suppose.'

Next morning Terry brought his lecture notes in which he had written that in this disease fresh unstained material should be examined either as a hanging drop preparation, or between a slide and a coverglass, using a one-sixth lens.

'Thanks, Terry, I'll get some fresh material from Vicker's cows this morning and we can have a look at it at lunch time.'

After taking samples from Eric's cows, he went to Harold's farm. He had two cows which would not settle, one of which he had bought new calved, but she had never held to Eric's bull, so he took samples from these. They examined Eric's first, and Terry closed the iris diaphragm on the condenser of the microscope, and found the protozoon which causes the disease; then Richard also identified it. They could not find any in the samples from Harold's cows, though they must have been infected by Vicker's bull.

Terry referred to his notes and found that the organism could be very difficult to find in chronically infected animals.

'You know, Richard, with all these germs about, it's a miracle cows ever produce a live calf.'

'I agree, but you know the cow must have a very efficient immunity producing system.'

Both farmers decided that the best course of action was to sell the infected animals, and so the bull, and five cows went to Droughton Auction. Somebody else would probably buy himself an awful lot of trouble. Terry said that it was a crazy infected merry-go-round.

On the third Friday evening, Richard went with Flora to the doctor's surgery where she was given her injection. She quickly forgot about it, because Bill told them that he and Doris had decided to get married on 29th July.

'Well I never,' said Flora, 'that was the date of our wedding.'

As they left Richard said to Bill, 'You really have given Flora something to think about now, that makes two weddings in six months. I expect I won't have another clothing coupon for twelve months.'

'Me too,' said Bill, 'Doris wants all mine.'

The news that night puzzled Flora, because the BBC had said that a jet propelled aeroplane which had been invented by an officer of the RAF had flown very fast.

'I don't understand; how it can fly without a propeller.'

'I don't really know, but I think the principle must be that gas is squirted out of the back of the plane, and pushes it along. It must be the same as when you blow up a balloon hard, and let go of it, because with the air coming out, it will fly across the room.'

'What will they invent next? I suppose they won't want wings.'

'Don't be daft, it couldn't stay up without them.'

When Richard got to the junction of Mereside Road and Meatham Lane, George Bolton and his man were cleaning a ditch. George shouted, 'Wait a minute, Mr 'olden, I want thee.'

Richard lowered the car's window.

'Hello, George, now what's wrong?'

'I've gitten one wi t' skitters, and thi powders ain't stoppin it.'

'Then I'll have to have a look at her.'

The wasted hindquarters of the cow and the bubbly liquid faeces behind her were typical of Johne's disease, and so at lunchtime that day Richard was sitting at his microscope examining a stained preparation of the dung.

'Terry, have a look at this, it is Johne's disease, isn't it?'

'Yes it is; that's the third already this month; Bob Whiteside must be spending half his time in our practice.'

'I don't suppose he will worry about that as it's good for his business, but it's a bad advert for ours.'

Mr and Mrs Clewlow successfully ran the goat farm on Coach Lane in Pelham. There was a great demand for his goats' milk from tuberculosis sufferers and asthmatical children.

'Yes, Mr 'olden, I want yer to hev a look at Queenie, she's th' oldest goat we ev and er's gitten bad on her legs.'

They walked into the box which had a roof of corrugated iron, and together they lifted the very thin animal to her feet. Richard examined her mouth and found that her teeth were missing or badly worn. He was taking her temperature when the goat fell down, and then, struggling, made feeble attempts to rise.

'It is just old age, Mr Clewlow, her teeth are worn away, and her spinal cord is degenerating. You see these sores she has got on her hocks and elbows, they are caused by her lying down all the time, and they are already septic. I think she should be destroyed to end her suffering.'

'Wait a minute and I'll go and tell t' missus.'

He returned and said, 'She's upset like, but wil'ta kill her an we'll bury her.' He stroked the goat's head, and said, 'Ta-ra, Queenie, old lass,' and hurried out of the box.

Richard loaded the Greener, and shot the goat. The noise of the shot reverberated from the iron roof and deafened Richard, who said, 'Damn, that's not done my ears any good; I shouldn't have shot her in here.'

He walked outside, and the couple came out of the house to thank him after which they paid him.

Richard had a loud ringing in his ears all day, and early that evening, Flora became annoyed with him.

'What's the matter with you, Richard? Aren't you very well tonight?'

'Yes, why, what's wrong?'

'Do you realise, I have had to shout at you ever since tea, and you keep asking "What did you say?" to everything I say.'

'I'm sorry, but I am a bit deaf. I had to shoot an old goat at Clewlow's and it's made my ears buzz again.'

'So that's it; you're like you were three years ago.'

'Yes, I am, but it will soon wear off.'

'I hope it does, or I'll be hoarse at this rate.'

The cold weather, with intermittent rain, was the cause indirectly of the death of three calves at Higher Carden Hall. Big George Bamber came out of the shippon.

''ello, Richard I'm reet suited tha's cum quick, becos another un's deed sin I rang thee.'

'So that's two, where are they?'

'In t' barn, cum on.'

As they walked into it Richard said, 'I thought this was your slaughter-house for pigs and sheep.'

'It wer, but I've done wi that job.'

'Have you? Why, George?'

'Becos folks won't keep their mouths shut. Tha knows, tha' does someone a good turn on t' quiet like, and tha tells 'em to say nowt, and what do they do, but go and blab and show off to everybody. It got that one day a chap walks inta t' yard, and real brazen like asks me for some pork. That finished it. I don't want to go to jail.'

'And I don't want you to go either.' At the end of the barn a big pen had been made by tying gates together, and in it were about a dozen well grown calves, two of which were lying dead.

'These don't look right.'

'Nay they don't, they started a Tuesday.'

'How long have they been in here?'

'Sin Sunday. Wi t' weather being so bad I brought th' heifers in an tied 'em in t' small shippon where these calves have been sin t' back end. They've done well i there.'

'They have; catch one for me George.'

He walked up to a big calf and easily caught it. One or two others got up and walked about and one staggering slightly walked straight into the wall.

'That un's real badly.'

'And it's blind as well.' Richard had recognised the symptoms of lead poisoning.

'Where does the water come from to reach this tap?'

'Watter? Why from up loft, there's a tank there.'

'Let it go.' The calf stood still.

'What's med it go blind?'

'I'm not certain yet; do you often use this trough?'

'No, th' only time I use it, is if I have a cow badly or calving, an I'll fill it up then.'

'Let's go and have a look at this tank.'

There being no piped water in the early nineteenth century, the big lead-lined tank was filled with rainwater off the roof; and the overflow pipe was joined to a down spout.

Richard scratched the tank's lining with his penknife, and the metal showed bright even in the dim light.

'George they've died of lead poisoning.'

'Arta sure?'

'Yes; when did you turn the water on last?'

'A Sunday.'

'No; before then.'

'Afore then; it was after t' 'arvest. I ed an old sloppy bagged un in there to calve.'

'I think that's the reason. In four months the rain water has dissolved the lead, and those two big calves would drink the most. Turn the water off now.'

Down in the barn the trough was emptied, and the calves dosed with the antidote to lead. Richard examined a blood smear from the dead calves, and then carried out a post mortem examination, taking samples from the livers and kidneys, which he sent to the lab.

They contained very high levels of lead; another calf died but the others slowly recovered.

Flora served cut-up fresh oranges as a sweet with their meal that evening, and Richard enjoyed his immensely.

'Where did you get them?'

'At Heye's, and Dick let me have four. You know, it's months since there were any, and the queue was soon right down High Street into Queen Street.'

'I bet it was, because he usually has nothing but vegetables in the shop. You know it was the same at Jim Lord's when he got a supply of toilet rolls not long ago. I was pleased when he kept three rolls for me.'

'Yes, it is so nice the way our friends try and help us out. I did enjoy my orange, but I'll not use the other two because I've asked Terry and Joan to come for a meal tomorrow night. You see, Norah's gone to the Fosters' for the weekend, and I got a chicken off Frank Wood today.'

'That will be nice for Norah; she will be waited on hand and foot.'

'I expect she will; now, when Terry and Joan come, do you think we should give them their wedding present?'

'Why, have you got it already?'

'Yes Mr Isaacs brought it today, and I've got a card.'

'Let's have a look at it then.'

Flora unwrapped a blue presentation box which contained a pair of silver oval napkin rings; one was initialled T, and the other J.

'By jove, they're nice, love.'

'Yes, I do like them myself, though they are second-hand. Mr Isaacs put the initials on and has polished them – really, you can't tell they are not new.'

'You can't, I would not have known. Anyway I'm glad he got us something of good quality because there is so much shoddy utility stuff about.'

'So am I; they are real sterling silver; I do hope they like them.'

'Of course they will; but I think it's a bit too early to give them to them now.'

'Maybe you're right, they can have them in a week's time.'

'I think that will be better; by the way have you found out where they are going to live?'

'Yes, at the Moorings until the war ends, when Norah is going to have the house made into two flats, and she'll live downstairs, because the arthritis in her hip is getting worse.'

'They are lucky to have somewhere ready for them.'

The dinner party went well, with Flora producing a good vegetable soup, roast chicken with boiled and roasted potatoes, and vegetables, followed by the oranges and custard. Richard did not feel too well, his ears still were troubling him, and he felt tired.

Terry said, 'I'm not surprised, Richard, this month has been terribly busy, just non-stop bed and work, to the exclusion of everything else. When mother asked me if the

Allied landing south of Rome would end the fighting in Italy, I didn't know what she was talking about. I feel if it goes on like this, we will need an assistant.'

'I agree, Terry, I think we will. The work is just pouring in now. It's a long time since I've seen so many diseases as I have since Christmas, and some days to cap it all I feel a bit off with the after effects of brucellosis though I am an awful lot better than I was last year.'

'You are that,' said Flora.

'And that reminds me, Terry, you must use those elbow-length rubber gloves and plenty of disinfectant, because we really are surrounded by virulent germs.'

'I do use them now all the time, Richard, and don't you think it would be a good idea to get a locum now with a promise of permanency if he is good enough, just to help us over the spring rush?'

'I think that's a good idea, Richard,' said Flora, 'because for a week after the wedding you'll have to cope on your own.'

'He will,' said Joan, 'because we have booked a week at—'

'Be quiet, Joan,' said Terry, 'don't tell them.'

'I wasn't going to, because you said you would ring up once or twice that week, to see if you were wanted here.'

'You needn't worry about that, Joan, I'll manage; I can still do two men's work in one day when I have to, and I can't see us getting anybody at the moment with twenty-three situations vacant in the *Record* this week, and you'll have seen the letters about the shortage of assistants, haven't you, Terry?'

'Yes I have, I bet there are a lot of practices like we are just now.'

'I will put an advertisement in the *Record* for next week, but if we don't get a reply, I'll ring up the Vet School in Liverpool and ask them if they could send us somebody – you know, a chap who's failed surgery, say.'

'Yes, do that, it would be a help to get somebody just doing the laboratory work.'

On 1st February Richard received a large envelope which was marked 'Private and Confidential', and, feeling very curious, he opened it at once. It was from Mereside Greyhound Racing Company Limited, inviting him to an interview with the Board of Directors, because they had soon to appoint another official veterinary surgeon under the National Greyhound Racing Association rules.

The meeting would be held at 10 a.m. on the following Monday at the Company's offices at the Stadium at Mereside. He was asked to reply as soon as possible, or to telephone his intentions to the Company Secretary, Major Horne. He put the letter to one side, because he felt he would have to consult Terry who would have to run the practice on his own three afternoons a week if he obtained the position. The phone rang, and it was Tom Walker from Fell Top, Icken wanting to know if Richard had any lamb dysentery serum. He said that he, their Bill at Low Fell, and Waring at the Beacon would all be wanting some, and could they have bigger bottles than they had last spring.

Richard said he would have some soon, and would let him know when to come for it. On replacing the receiver he wrote out an order for vaccine and serum at once.

He drove to the garage to have his battery topped up, and his oil checked. Gordon came out, 'Hello Richard; I'm glad I've seen thee, because I'm coming to the surgery to neet; I've got an Alsatian pup to replace Blackie that I want vaccinating.'

'Don't bring it, Gordon, I'll come and do it there, because there is always distemper about now with these strays from the Camps. How old is it?'

'Nine weeks.'

'That's fine. Keep it in and isolated from other dogs. I'll get it done this week; I'll just put it in my diary.'

When he got to Park Hall to cleanse a cow, Tom Collinson said, 'I want a Tuberculin test as soon as tha con do it. Tom Priestley wore telling mi that premium on Attested milk ull be fourpence a gallon. Tha knows, Richard, I reckon that ud be £14 a week for me, it ud pay mi rent.'

'I bet it would, Tom, with all the milk you pull; I'll put it in my diary and we'll get it done soon.'

At lunchtime he went into the bank to get some money and Dick Harrison the manager said, 'Richard, can we bring Jock to the surgery tonight?'

'Yes, you can, what's the matter with him, Dick?'

'He's got toothache, his face is all swollen. Have you time to come up and have a quick look at him, because Mary's really worried?'

'Yes, lead the way.' The old dog had a discharging abscess in his face.

'The trouble may be that he's got a rotten molar tooth that will have to come out, Mary.'

'When can you do it?' asked Dick.

'Has he been fed today?'

'Not yet,' replied Mary.

'Then don't feed him and bring him about a quarter to seven tonight.'

As he left the bank, Richard said to himself, What next? everywhere I go today, I get more work to do.

That evening, with Flora's help, he gave Jock a light general anaesthetic. He extracted the rotten carnassial tooth, and syringed out the sinus. He chipped all the tartar off the others and cleaned them thoroughly. Though Jack was nine years old he soon recovered consciousness, and at nine o'clock walked out of the surgery with a very relieved Mary and Dick.

Both Flora and Terry were in favour of Richard going for the interview at the Stadium. So wearing his best suit he walked into the general office at the Greyhound Track at five minutes to ten on the following Monday morning. He was welcomed by Mr Ken Burton, the Assistant Secretary, who relieved him of his trilby and coat. The secretary, Major Horne, came into the room and introduced himself, and asked Richard to follow him. They went into the comfortable inner office, where five people were sitting around a long table smoking and talking. A tall distinguished-looking man rose to his feet and came to them.

'Mr Holden, this is the Chairman of the Board, Mr Pimlott.'

'Good morning, Mr Holden, I am pleased to meet you. I will now introduce you to the other directors.' They were the Vice Chairman who was his wife, and three other members, plus the Secretary. The Chairman briefly outlined the position: that their veterinary surgeon had become almost blind owing to illness and wished to resign his post on 31st March when his yearly contract of employment expired. Richard was the second interviewee, and the successful person would have to commence his duties on 1st April. There were three meetings held each week, on Monday, Wednesday and Saturday, all in the afternoon. He would be required to be present one hour before the time the meeting was to take place, and examine every animal which was to be raced that day, before they were locked up in the racing kennels. He would treat all injured dogs, and would be completely responsible for the health and fitness of every dog. He would have to advise the board about the purchase of new dogs and the casting of the old, useless or vicious animals. The rest of his duties and the rules of the NGR would all be detailed in his contract of employment. His fees would be paid on the last day of the month, monthly in arrears, and he would be expected to provide all dressings, drugs etc.

Mr Pimlott then asked Richard if he would like to speak about his career. He replied that he felt it to be an honour to be asked to attend the interview, and thanked them for the invitation. He said that having been qualified ten years he had considerable experience in treating dogs and performing operations on them. He now had a salaried partner, so that in the unlikely event of his being unable to perform his duties Mr Wilson would be available to deputise for him. He hoped that vaccination against distemper was carried out, and that a high standard of hygiene was maintained, and that all newly purchased animals were strictly isolated. The Chairman thanked him for his information and confirmed that every dog was vaccinated and ear-marked, and that every newcomer was strictly isolated until it was proved to be healthy. There was now a question and answer period with the other directors, after which he was informed that the Secretary would be writing to him in a few days time.

Eric Sugden at the Lodge Farm was an efficient dairy farmer, but his health was slowly deteriorating owing to attacks of asthma and paroxysms of coughing which often made him take to his bed for some days at a time. Because of this he had obtained from the Women's Land Army a land girl who helped his son Paul run the farm. Paul, an only child, had been completely spoiled and allowed all his own way in childhood. Now he was a well built young man, but a cheeky rascal, and an inveterate liar. When Terry went to the farm to see some ill calves he was met by Eric who was wheezing audibly.

'Hello, Mr Sugden, how long have they been ill?'

'Four days now.'

'How many are there?'

'Eleven.'

'Have any died?'

'No, but two of 'em look badly, an I don't want to lose any, becos they're dear to buy – they're all full pedigree tha' knows.'

'Now, don't buy any more until these get better; if you do, you might buy more trouble. What have you given them?'

'Thi powders.'

'And are they still on milk?'

'Nay, they're on replacer now.'

After examining the calves, four of which had temperatures, he injected them all with calf scour anti serum, and gave Eric a large bottle of medicine for them. He told him not to feed the milk replacer but to give them a mixture of half milk and water with a tablespoonful of salt stirred into each half a gallon. He told him that they would be seen again by Richard on Monday.

When it was all over everyone said that the wedding had been splendid on that cold dry Saturday.

Tom Collinson brought the house down when in his speech he said, 'We now ev a vet in t' family, and soon I 'ope a doctor as well. I've told our John to marry a dentist – that way we'll have no outlay to mek over our health and cows' an all. Who said farmers aren't crafty.'

Wartime shortages and restrictions had been overcome, and food rationing was in abeyance that day with so many of the bride's relatives being farmers. The church was full for the service and it was obvious that there was a black market in clothing coupons, by the number of new outfits the ladies were wearing. Joan looked radiant all in white, and was wearing her mother's veil when she joined Terry at the altar. Flora was dressed in a grey and white jacket and skirt, and Richard as usual was very proud of his lovely wife. The photographer from the local paper took two photos and rushed away, leaving Cyril Johnson from the High Street studio to take all the photographs tradition demanded for the family albums. After the excellent meal, the bride and groom changed their clothes, and when they had said their goodbyes, were given a rousing send-off from the porch of the Porter Arms. Richard had to leave early to go to a calving case at Corner Farm, Pickhill, and that evening had a very busy surgery. After he had cashed up on the Sunday he checked all the results for January, and found that the month had been the best ever for the number of visits done, and money paid in at the bank. It convinced him that they could afford either a locum or an assistant, so he wrote out an advertisement for one and sent it to the *Veterinary Record*.

He later said to Flora, 'It's unbelievable that seven years ago we thought we had made a mistake in coming to Sandhaven.'

'Yes, it is, I remember we were both very doubtful, but after the first year on our own, I told you we would do well.'

'Yes, you did, love, I was the one who took some convincing'

Though busy on the Monday, Richard made a point of going to the Lodge farm that morning. He walked across to the calf house, and saw two buckets of milk replacer in the passage. He thought, that's strange, Terry would have told Eric to use milk and water. While waiting for someone to appear, he counted the calves, there were eleven, and as their faeces were formed it was obvious they were on the mend. He walked through into the double shippon, and heard talking and giggling, so he slammed the door shut and shouted, 'Anybody home?'

After a minute Paul came out of the proven house. 'It's thee, Mr 'olden, what's ta want?'

'Hello, Paul, I've come to look at the calves Mr Wilson treated last Friday.'

'Reet, cum on then.'

'Where's your father?'

'Ee's badly and in bed.'

'I'm sorry to hear that, I hope he is soon better.'

'So do I, here they are.'

'Which were the ones that were ill?'

'That 'un, an them three in t' corner.'

As Richard examined these, the others began to suck at his clothes and to nuzzle and butt him.

'Haven't these been fed yet?'

'Oh, aye they ev.'

'But you're not feeding them that replacer in the passage.'

'Aye I am, mi dad told mi to.'

'But Mr Wilson must have told him to feed them half milk and water four times a day.'

'Nay, he didn't.'

'Look, Paul, I know I wasn't here, but we always put calves on to half milk and water because with inflamed guts they can't digest milk or starter; so don't give that to them.'

'But I'll ev to feed it now I've med it.'

'All right, then, but don't give them a lot, and give them milk and water until I come again. Here's another bottle of medicine, you'll need that, because though they have improved they are not right yet, you know. Don't buy any more until these are really better.'

'Reet, Mr 'olden, I'll do that.'

Richard doubted that his instructions would be carried out by Paul while his father was in bed, and with the distraction of the Land Girl.

He made a note to visit the eleven calves again on Thursday.

It was cold that evening when he took Flora to Dr. Bill's surgery, and after she had the injection, the doctor excused himself and hurried off to an emergency. At the surgery

John had a visit for Richard, and it was late before he finished the day's work. He had postponed all the routine work, so that this week he could deal with emergency cases, with all the new ones which came in and the surgeries. He also had two operations to do, but his determination and energy enabled him to deal with everything, though by Thursday he was getting tired and irritable.

He had the Lodge down for a visit in the afternoon of that day, but Flora rang a message through to him at Hunter's farm in Middleton that Sugden wanted a visit at once. Richard was not pleased at having to retrace his route back to Sandhaven, but soon arrived at the farm and drove up to the shippon door. But Eric opened the calf house door, and shouted, 'They're in 'ere.' As Richard walked in Eric said, 'Why didn't ta cum yesterday as tha' promised, Mr 'olden?'

'Because I told Paul it would be today.'

'Nay, tha didn't,' said Paul.

'Yes, I did, and I'll get my daily diary to show you.' Feeling angry, he went and got it, and then showed it to Eric.

'Look, it's there, on today's page eleven calves to see; I wrote it in before I drove off on Monday.'

'Any road, tha's med a mistake,' said Eric coughing loudly.

'Eric, can't you believe your eyes, I did not make the mistake.'

'Then let's git to mi calves, they're deeing now.'

Two were dead in the pen and some of the others were looking very ill with diarrhoea running down their tails.

'When did they go like this?'

'Yesterday; it would'na 'appened if tha'd cum as tha said.'

'Eric, will you listen: I bloody well said Thursday and wrote down Thursday, now do you understand?'

'Tha didn't say Thursda',' said Paul.

'You know very well that I did.'

'Shurrup Paul, what's killin 'em?'

Richard remembered his entry: eleven calves to see, but two were dead and he counted twelve alive in the pen.

'And I told you not to buy any more calves on Monday.'

'Tha did nowt o t' sort.'

'When did the other three come, then?'

'A Tuesday Tom Walsh fetched 'em.'

'And which are they?'

'That un there, an t' two dead uns.'

'Well, that's marvellous; you've undone a week's work because the eleven were getting better and now you've bought a damned germ that's killed two in two days. Can't you obey instructions?'

'Tha did'na say owt.'

'Then drag these two outside, and I'll show you why they died. Get a bucket of water.'

Richard put on his gloves, and cut open the dead calves. Both had died of an acute haemorrhagic enteritis. Eric's breathing was getting noisy, but Richard showed him the opened bowel which was red raw, and contained bloody liquid material.

'They've died from bloody dysentery, it's a real killer in calves and in us as well sometimes. I'll take a sample.' He freed a length of bowel, tied a knot at each end to keep in the contents, and wrapped it in greaseproof paper.

Eric was wheezing very noisily when he said, 'What's ta goin ta do wi' that?'

'Send it to the laboratory, so they can confirm these calves have got the germ of bloody dysentery, or you'll say I'd never told you.'

'Nay I won't; an 'ow long will it tek?'

'Till the middle of next week.'

Eric coughed, it was distressing to see him, and then he spat. He took a deep breath, and said, 'That's no damned good; what's ta goin to do for 'em now?'

'Listen carefully both of you, I'm telling you, you've brought a deadly germ into here, and you could lose the lot, and it could spread to your cows, and nobody will be able to do much for you if you get it, you could lose all these calves.'

Eric was struggling to get his breath. 'Tha'd better do summat bloody quick then; I've told yer they're all full pedigree.'

'And I'll tell you something: germs don't bother about pedigrees.'

'Tha'd better bother.'

'I'm going to; Paul, hold these calves.' Richard injected every calf with a large dose of calf scour anti serum, and then gave Eric two twenty-eight ounce bottles of scour medicine. He had sat down on a bale of straw in the passage, wheezing so noisily it was distressing to watch him.

'You have to dose them three times a day, and the bad ones four or five times, and put them all back on milk and water.'

'They've bin on it all t' time.'

'No, they haven't, Paul had two buckets of milk replacer made when I came on Monday.'

'I 'adn't, Dad; he's only saying that becos they've deed.'

'Are you calling me a liar for the third time, Paul?'

'Nay, but two ev deed.'

'Paul, they had that germ when they came. When did you first dose them?'

'Yesterday, in t' mornin.'

'Which shows they had the germ in them, and were ill when they came on Tuesday.'

'Nay, they weren't; I thought medicine would stop em ketchin t' scour.'

'It's no use talking to you. Eric, I'll come again tomorrow morning, and inject any which are still alive.' With that he walked straight to his car, got in, and drove off. Realising he was in a rage, he asked himself, 'How the hell have I kept my temper with that lad? He's got his father to believe every word he says is Gospel, and he gets his own way by getting Eric so upset he has an asthmatical attack and has to go to bed; he's a lying wicked devil.'

It was after one o'clock when he finished his morning's round of visits, on that cold day. Flora's hot soup, and real egg omelette soon warmed him up; she was able to make the latter because George Meadows had let her have half a dozen eggs on the quiet when he brought the milk, and also she had got four more oranges from Dick Heyes after queuing for ten minutes in the cold wind. She said to Richard, 'It's got to the state now that we have to be grateful for small mercies.' That evening he finished work at half past eight, then wrote up the day book, restocked his car, and said Goodnight to John.

When he walked into the lounge Flora said, 'Hello, stranger, come and sit here by the fire; you look worn out. I'll get you a drink.'

'I don't know about looking worn out, I jolly well am tonight.' She came back with a mug of tea.

'Richard, why don't you try and get a locum as Terry said.'

'Oh I have, didn't I tell you?'

'No, you didn't.'

'I'm sorry, I've forgotten, love. I wrote for one on Sunday, but I doubt we'll get one, though I've offered a high salary to a suitable applicant, in the advertisement – that may produce a reply.'

'I'm glad you've done it at last, you know you're killing yourself with all the work you do.'

'I know; but anyway Terry will be back in three days' time.'

'I for one will be glad to see him; let's listen to the news.'

At first they were both shocked to hear that the Allies had bombed the Benedictine Monastery on Monte Cassino, but when the news reader said that the Germans had turned it into a fortress, they thought the action was justified. In the same way they had approved the thousand-bomber raid on Berlin earlier that week. By the time the news ended Richard was sound asleep in his chair.

At the Lodge on Friday, three more calves had died, so he injected the nine survivors again with serum. Though he wheezed and coughed Eric was barely civil, grumbling and swearing about cattle dealers and vets, so he gave him a bottle of veterinary chlorodyne and after telling him the correct dose left the farm at once, and went on to do visits in Wyresham, Underley and then to the Launds in Wellington. Red-faced Bill Iddon was his usual cheerful self.

'Hello, Richard, ow arta?'

'Very busy, because Terry got married last Saturday, so I've been single-handed this week.'

'I thought tha would, I saw it in t' *Farmers Guardian*, he's married a Collinson. I bet Tom were pleased becos e'll ev a vet on t' shop now to deal wi all is milk fevers.'

'No, he won't; Terry will be living in Seaton.'

'E'll be all reet though wi' thee living on his doorstep. Bulls is in 'ere.'

With two men helping Richard castrated six big bull calves using his Bundizzo and then had to shorten a cow's horn. It had been broken earlier and had set pointing down, and had grown very near to the cow's eye. He put the blade in his hacksaw with the serrated edge facing up, and after the animal was securely held cut a couple of inches off the horn.

'Is she a young cow, Bill?'

'Aye, oo's just had er second calf, and er milks well.'

'Then I'll come one day next week and take the whole horn off, otherwise it will always be a nuisance.'

'That's a good idea, tha'll let mi know then.'

'I will, and I must go; cheerio for now.'

He was pleased when Mrs Foster walked into the room unaided when he got to the house in Wilton. She spoke quite well, even though her face was still twisted. After examining Poppy, he relaxed for a few minutes, talking to her about the wedding and enjoying a cup of tea.

'Thi medicines, an t' injections are no damn good,' was Eric Sugden's greeting on Saturday morning. Three more calves had died, and their owner was breathing so badly, he looked as though he could too.

'If your Paul had done as he was told, you would not have had this trouble.'

'Thee leave my Paul outa this. I believe im when he sez tha never told him about milk and water, and not to let Walsh bring any more. Then tha' forgot to cum a Wednesda.' He heaved and coughed, then he spat.

'Look, Eric, on Monday your calves were beginning to thrive again. I did not make them ill again, and I did not make the new ones die like flies; I'd never even seen them, don't you understand.'

'Aye, but tha's bin no damn good sin then.'

His breathing was very laboured when he sat down on a bale of straw.

'So that's what you think, well, let me remind you that everything I have treated for you in six years had done well, except when you didn't follow my advice when Paul didn't put your turkeys on wire floors, and blackhead killed the lot.'

'I'm sick and fed up of you blaming my Paul for everything, tha' con get out of my yard and don't cum in again.'

The smirk on his son's face said it all – I've won.

'If that's the way you feel, you can get another vet. I won't come.'

'An I've finished with thee, don't cum 'ere again, an tell yon Wilson to keep away.'

'Very well, my practice has finished with you, so good-day, Eric, and I hope your health soon improves.'

Richard was annoyed that he had lost a good client, and was furious with Paul for causing all the trouble with his lies and deceit. For Eric he still had nothing but sympathy for a man who was so sick.

The weather was turning colder on Sunday morning, so after seeing four cases he was glad to get back into the surgery. He cashed up and then wrote out the work for Terry and himself for the coming week. Planning ahead he wrote to Stan Earnshaw to inform him that he would do his TT on Tuesday 29th. At five o'clock Terry rang and, joking, asked Richard if he had had anything to do during the last week. Richard replied in the same vein, that there had been nothing to do but read the paper and drink tea. Terry laughed and said that he and Mrs Wilson would be in at quarter to nine next morning.

'Thank God,' said Richard, 'and have you had a nice time?'

'Yes, great, I'll tell you all about it tomorrow, and you and Flora will have to come and see the presents. Cheerio for now.'

At eight o'clock, a rather weary Richard went on this black cold night to Ivy Farm at Treston. Harry Fisher apologised.

'I'm sorry havin to prise thee away from t' fire on a Sunday neet, but er's a good sow, an er's bin at it sin six o'clock.'

'Don't worry, Harry, it's nice to see you; where is she?'

'In t' little farrowin shed, it's nice an warm i theer, an t' watters ready for tha.'

Though he used his kneeler, Richard's knees were painful, but he ignored this until he eventually delivered a very large dead piglet, by snaring its head with a cord on which Harry pulled hard.

'By gum, it's a whopper.'

'It is, it looks a fortnight old already.'

'Aye, it does that.' Seven piglets were delivered alive with no trouble, but Richard had to lie flat on his stomach to get the last one.

'It's lucky she is a big sow or I would never have reached that one.'

'Aye, it wor a long way in, but eight meks a nice litter an oo does do em well. Get thisen dressed, an I'll bring thee a mug of tay.'

Flora was glad to see him back, and asked him how he felt.

'Only a bit weary, love, and my knees ache. I'm glad this week is over, because it's worn me out, and convinced me that we must somehow get some help. Terry was right, you know.'

'He was, I do hope there is a reply to the advertisement soon.'

'So do I, because there is so much work waiting to be done, all the herd inspections, and testing and Panel work, and lambing will start next week but one. These last two months have fairly flown by.'

'They have, at this rate it will be Easter before you can turn round.'

'I hope it isn't; let's get to bed.'

Richard was frustrated because no herd inspections had been done for ten days, so he drove off at a quarter to seven next morning to do two. He had sent out cards informing farmers that the inspections would be done mornings and evenings that week. He had just finished his breakfast when Terry and Joan arrived and Flora welcomed the latter as though she were a long lost sister. Richard greeted them warmly, and then had them all including Mavis come into the office. He told them that owing to the row with Eric and Paul Sugden, and their slanderous remarks about his honesty and integrity, no messages had to be taken from them or medicines given to them.

'What do I tell 'em if they rings?' said Mavis.

'Just tell them to get another vet and put the receiver down at once, and Mavis, tell your John. Joan, will you send him an up to date account at once, and put a typed notice by each phone, saying that they are taboo.'

Feeling better for having got that off his chest, he opened an envelope marked 'Personal'.

It was an invitation to Bill MacDonald's wedding on Friday 3rd March in Edinburgh. He handed the invitation to Flora who was thrilled, and at once said that she would wear her blue and white floral jacket and dark blue skirt. She would borrow a large white hat from Betty Heyes; Richard could wear his dark suit. But as his wife had used all his clothing coupons, Richard had no choice!

'It means, Flora, that we will have to go on the Tuesday and stay overnight, and come back as soon as possible after the wedding. I'm sure Terry will be able to manage if I rearrange the work. I must go and get some petrol, I've a lot of work to do.'

'Hello, Gordon, fill her up. How's the pup?'

'Pup, did you say, that is Prince and he's doing all right, but you are going to have to pay me for a new back door, he's almost eaten his way through it.'

'Why don't you feed the poor little beggar, giving him the back door to eat.'

'Eat, he eats every damn thing in sight. When can I let him out?'

'You can now, Gordon, but not in town yet; wait a few more days, then you can take him anywhere. Talking of cars, is that Hillman for sale?'

'It will be, it was practically new but some fool had done a big end in. So I've rebuilt the engine, and it's in tip-top condition. Our George went to Derby in it last week, and said it went like a bird. Are you wanting another?'

'I may be, how much is it?'

'I've not put a price on it yet; I'll tell you next time you come.'

It was Terry's turn to do herd inspections on Tuesday, but Richard had to go to Jack Clough's at Leach House to calve a cow. Though they were still milking Jack shouted his noisy welcome and, helped by his two sons Dick and John, Richard soon delivered the calf but it was dead.

'It's a bad do it's dead, it's a good heifer calf.'

Jack came up. 'Aye, it's my fault, I should ev had a look at 'er afore wi started milkin, oo must ev started in t' neet. But th' engine wouldn't start, an wi messed about wi' it for 'alf an our afore we git it going, that's why we're late wi t' milk. Tha two git them churns teken down an pur 'em ont stand afore t' milk lorry comes, 'cos he won't wait.'

After a hurried breakfast Richard went to Stan Earnshaw's at Ashfield, and did the first part of the Tuberculin test on his cattle, helped by his son and Vic Dobson from Far Pasture. When he had finished he went to examine a cow on the latter's farm. The Jersey was very thin.

'I bought her at lying in time, and oo calved a good heifer calf just turned Christmas. Oo's milked real well, but oo's losing too much flesh for my liking. As oo gitten Johne's?'

'I don't think so, Vic; though she is thin all over, everything else is OK except she's a bit anaemic. Is her dung always sloppy like this?'

'Aye, an it's gitten worse.'

'Then I'll take a sample and I will let you know what I find in the morning.'

'Haemolytic B. Coli,' was the report from the laboratory on Eric Sugden's sample, and good luck to him, said Richard. There were no Johne's disease germs in the sample from the Jersey, so he examined it for Strongyle eggs. Terry came in and said that the best way to do it was to make a suspension in salt solution and centrifuge it.

'All right, professor, it's all yours. Will you do it, Terry, for me? I've a lot of writing to do in the office, and then surgery.'

Later Terry shouted for Richard to go into the dispensary. 'Look what I've found.' Richard looked down the microscope and saw a large egg.

'It is a fluke egg isn't it?'

'Yes, it is, use the fine adjustment, and you will see the operculum.'

'Yes. I can see it now; thanks, Terry, for finding it. I'll take a couple of doses of extract filicis to Dobson's tomorrow. I'll just get my Banham and Young and check the correct dose for a cow.'

That afternoon when Flora came home, she asked Richard to go upstairs with her because she had got a wedding present for Bill and Isabel. It was a Waterford cut glass bowl, eight inches in diameter, sparkling in the light as it lay on a bed of black crepe paper in a white box.

'It was cheaper than the napkin rings we got for Terry and Joan, because it's second hand. Mr Isaacs told me that he bought it at a house sale and it is perfect. Doesn't it look lovely?'

'Yes, it does, they'll like that.'

'They should, I do. It's a pity we've got to give it away when we want one ourselves.'

'Don't worry, I'll buy you a gold one.'

'Go on, you are daft side out today. Write the card, will you, and then I'll wrap it up again.'

'I will if you give me a kiss.'

She did.

'There you are, put it in the bowl. I'll take it on my way back from Earnshaw's.'

Next day Vic was a bit annoyed when Richard told him. 'Blast it, tha' knows er must ev come wi' it, I've never ed any wi' it afore ere.'

'She probably did, Vic, but she's been tied up ever since, which is lucky because she's not left eggs all over your pastures. And don't empty that midden on them, put it on your arable and plough it in. Now put her in a box, and give a dose a week apart, but if she doesn't improve, cash her, because it will mean her liver's damaged. Thanks for helping me at Stan's.'

He hadn't time to go to Southall with the present. Bill Iddon's remarks made Richard roar with laughter.

'If tha teks one 'orn off, 'er will look a cock-eyed bugger! Can't ter tek em both off?'

'Yes, I can, I did one not so long since and it's a nice looking Polly now.'

'Then git it done, Mr 'olden.' He put on a tourniquet and after injecting plenty of local anaesthetic, he sawed off both horns. Having seared the stumps with a red hot iron, he dusted them with antiseptic powder.

'That's a lot better, it can't hurt 'er eye now.'

'And she can't poke you in yours either when you are tying up.'

He was having lunch when Mac rang him from Southall to ask why a Paul Sugden had asked him for a visit, instead of ringing Richard. The latter spent ten minutes explaining what had happened at Lodge Farm, and what the laboratory report said.

'In that case I'm not going, Richard. I don't want that sort of client. Anyway, thanks for your help.'

'It's nothing, Mac, and thanks for the wedding invitation. It will be great to have a day off; we are both looking forward to it. Cheerio for now.'

Joan had not opened the envelopes which were marked 'Private & Confidential'. He opened the large one first and read in the letter that the Directors of the Mereside Greyhound Racing Company Ltd. had decided to offer the position of Official Veterinary Surgeon to him, and enclosed two copies of the conditions of employment and the rules and regulations of the National Greyhound Racing Club. He ran upstairs and showed the letter to Flora who congratulated him, and then said, 'And what's the other one?'

'I don't know, I haven't opened it yet.' He did, and as he quickly read the letter a wave of nostalgia swept over him. Mr James Craig Mortimer said that he was finishing a locum's at the practice in Holme in the North of England where he had been working owing to the death of senior partner Mr David Lewis, and that he was available at once if necessary. He enclosed copies of two recent testimonials, and if interested would the advertiser ring the Holme number, and ask to speak to him. He gave the letter to Flora to read.

'What a fantastic coincidence, isn't it Richard?'

The black male figure was suddenly there in his thoughts, blood-stained and frightening, and he shivered.

'It's upset you a bit, I can see.'

'Yes,' he lied, 'it has.' The figure faded away. 'There's no time like the present, so

I'll ring him now.'

He did, using the newly installed upstairs phone and asked for the Holme number. Mrs Steele answered, so Richard disguised his voice, and asked for Mr Mortimer, who told him that he was leaving Holme that evening. On the spur of the moment Richard said,

'Will you come straight to Sandhaven, my name is Richard Holden. You can stay the night and I'll pay your expenses.'

James said that would be great and he would try to arrive before dark.

'You heard that, love, didn't you? He'll be here about six, so pop another carrot and a spud in the pot, and will you make up the guest bed.'

'Yes, but let's have our lunch, I'm starving. I'll get it done later.'

When Terry and Joan were back from their lunch, Richard shouted,

'Come up, you two; I've got something to tell you.'

'What is it?' asked Terry.

'I've just had a reply to the advert in the *Record* from a chap who's not far away in Holme at the moment doing a locum's; his name is James Craig Mortimer.'

'Blimey, I just don't believe it. That's old Taenia, he's a great friend of mine – he was in my year, and we qualified together. I wonder why he is doing locums, he's had a good job in a Bristol practice for the last three years.'

'You can find out tonight, he's coming here for the night.'

'It will be great to see him. He's a grand chap and comes from Suffolk, all his family are farmers. You'll like him, Richard.'

'All right then, come upstairs when you've finished surgery, and we'll find out all about him.'

'We can, can't we, Joan, you have nothing else on?'

'No I haven't, but could you run me up to Park Hall first, I want clothes and things out of my wardrobe, and my writing box. Then we can come straight back here.'

'If that's all right, Richard?'

'Of course it is.'

Richard was in the office when the door bell rang, and Joan went to answer it. Grinning broadly she returned, and said in a business like manner, 'Mr Holden, there is a Mr Mortimer to see you; he says that he has an appointment.'

Richard smiled and said, 'Thank you Mrs Wilson, I'll see him now, and you will be back after seven.'

'Yes, we will, Mr Holden.'

Jim Mortimer was a very stockily built chap, about five feet eight inches tall with crinkly brown hair, and smiled often. He rose to his feet when Richard walked in.

'I'm Richard Holden; it is nice of you to come over, Mr Mortimer,' and they shook hands. 'Will you please follow me upstairs, and we can talk in the lounge.' Flora, having prepared the small bedroom for their guest, brought in a pot of tea. 'Make yourself comfortable, and you will have a cup of tea won't you?'

'Yes, thank you, I will.'

'Right, now tell me about yourself.'

'I am Suffolk born and bred, on our farm near Framlingham.'

'So you can handle heavy horses?'

'Yes, my father bred the Suffolk Punch; we had a stallion, and four breeding mares and nine geldings, because we are mainly arable. I qualified in 1939 at the RVC in London and in 1941 I went to a mainly large animal practice in Bristol with a view to a partnership in three years' time. It was a good position and I liked the area.'

'Why did you leave, then?'

'Because the boss had four girlfriends, even though he was married, and had two children as well. Things went wrong, as I found out later when the boss Mr Bosanquet had to pay a lot of money to one of his girlfriends' husband to avoid a scandal. Being hard up, he quietly sold the practice but never told me. The first I knew about it was when he gave me a month's notice late one Saturday night, so I never got my partnership, and in a month I was out of a job, and feeling damned bitter.'

'What have you done since then?'

'Long term locums, in an attempt to try and find a place with people I like, where I'd like to settle down.'

'Have you got any testimonials?'

'Yes, here they are.' They were all good, even the one from Bristol.

'They are very good, but let's go and have our meal, you must be hungry.'

Flora produced soup which was followed by fried egg and sausage with mashed potatoes, carrots and turnips. For sweet there was hot blackcurrant crumble with custard. As they ate, Flora got him to talk more about himself. He had an older sister who was married, and a brother who was a partner with his father in running the farm. He had not got a car, but had an adequate amount of equipment. When Flora went to make the coffee, Richard asked him when he would be able to come to Sandhaven. He replied that he wanted first to go home and see his family and get some more clothes, and he would be available probably by Sunday. Later Richard showed him his room, and asked him to come back into the lounge as soon as he was ready.

To save time Flora washed the pots and Richard dried them, so soon they were all back in the warm lounge. When there was a knock on the door Richard called 'Come in,' and Terry followed Joan into the room. Seeing Jim standing there, he said with a laugh, 'I'll be blest, if it isn't old Taenia, how great to see you again.'

'Terry, it is a lovely surprise; fancy you remembering my nickname.'

And the friends heartily shook hands. Once seated, the conversation quickly became general, with Joan being introduced and the wedding described, and it was at least an hour later before the future was discussed.

Richard and Terry agreed that they would like him to join the practice at once, as a locum with a view to becoming the assistant, and he was given the agreement for the latter post to read at his leisure. He then said that he was going home in the morning, but could return on Saturday to get settled in, and be shown the ropes on Sunday. Terry said that he would have to do the laboratory work, and help in any way he could until a suitable car was found for him. Jim thanked them both and said how much he appreciated their offer of an assistantship in the near future. He hoped that his work would justify the confidence they had shown in him.

Soon these two London graduates began to describe some very amusing reminiscences, thus giving Flora, Joan and Richard a very enjoyable evening.

It was freezing when Richard took Jim to the station early on Thursday morning. After the train left, Richard went to the garage, where Gordon was just opening up, and asked him if he had decided on a price for the Hillman, because he wanted to buy it. Gordon said that it was £165 and that he would guarantee it for six months.

'In that case, I'll take it now.'

'Hey, hold on, Richard, what's the blooming rush?'

'I want it for a locum we have engaged, and he's coming on Sunday.'

'Ok, you can have it by then, but it wants checking over, because our George has been all over the shop in it lately; he only got back from Liverpool in it last night. When it's ready then I'll bring it round, how does that suit?'

'Great, that will be a good help; thanks, Gordon.'

'Mind our Prince, don't run over him.'

'Sorry, I didn't see your pet lion.'

'Ger off with you.'

Back home, he had another cup of tea, and then asked Flora if she were ready to go to Mrs Clunie's, because he would take her there before he went to work.

'By jove, you are in top gear this morning; it's just like old times, all rush. Wait a tick, I must go and put my face on.'

At Meatham Guest House Mrs Clunie had a very nice bedroom for a single gentleman, which she showed to Flora. Her terms were £2 10s. a week for full board, and 3s. for laundry payable in advance, which Flora did there and then.

'All settled and paid for; away we go, Richard.'

'Good, that's another load off my mind; his digs and his car arranged.'

'You've got a car already? Crikey, you are moving this morning.'

'Yes, I've seen Gordon, and he'll bring it round when he has checked it over and cleaned it. How much were the digs? I'll give you that money; it goes on the practice expenses.'

She told him and asked, 'What make of car is it?'

'It's a second-hand Hillman, like the one I used to borrow, and Gordon guarantees it for six months because he has rebuilt it; it is like new.'

'And how much is it?'

'£165, he said.'

'That's not too dear, is it?'

'No, it isn't, and I may get it for a bit less; but anyway the practice can stand it. I think I'll let Terry drive it, it's bigger than his Morris, and he does drive carefully – that, of course, is if he wants it.'

'Knowing him, I think he will.'

When Gordon brought it after lunch, Terry did want it, and with Joan drove it round the block. He was very pleased with it, so they spent half an hour emptying the Morris and putting everything into the Hillman. Richard left them to it, did two visits and then two herd inspections. When he got back Flora told him that they were to go to the Moorings at half past seven to see the wedding presents.

John arrived, and he was given the job of washing the Morris before it got dark, and to clean it inside and polish it in the morning. He lit a fag and set to with a will.

There were only two people for surgery, so Richard spent the rest of the hour examining the samples he had taken that afternoon. One was positive for tuberculosis. He told the telephone operator to put any calls on his number through to Terry's, then he paid John and told him to lock up when he had finished. When he and Flora arrived at the Moorings, Terry welcomed them; they followed him down the hall and up the wide staircase, which divided into two branches, a left and a right, both leading onto a wide landing which ran round three sides of the stair-well. There he took their coats, and they followed Joan into the warm lounge where a big log fire was burning.

'What a lovely fire, Joan, it's perishing outside tonight.'

'Don't we know it, that's why we both brought logs up after we'd put the car away.'

'Do you like it?'

'Yes,' said Terry. 'It is larger and more comfortable than the Morris, and as we haven't many logs left, if we get some more, do you mind if we bring them back in it?'

'No, Terry, you can cover the seats, and I'm certain Harold will let us have some more, so if you're that way tomorrow ask him for both of us, will you?'

'Yes, I will. Now how about a drink? What would you like, Flora?' After they were brought they talked for a short time, and Richard explained to them all his ideas for the future for Jim, provided his work was satisfactory. They then went into what Joan called the morning room, where the presents were all displayed. There were very many: china – a lovely Aynsley coffee service decorated with flowers, and a half tea service with the Indian Tree decoration in Ford's china – both caught Flora's eye. Two wooden boxes held silver plated cutlery which shone, and in front was a Georgian silver ladle. Two silver-plated entree dishes were behind a Pyrex dish in a silver plated holder. Vases, jugs, a damask table cloth, two cream pure wool blankets, a cut glass beer tankard, and half a dozen sherry glasses filled one table. Among the silver was the present from Richard and Flora, a three piece condiment set, coffee spoons, a bonbon dish, and a Georgian sauce boat along with a Georgian cream jug.

After another drink, supper was eaten round the fire, and then Joan and Terry told them about the honeymoon. They had spent it in of all places London, and on their first night at eleven o'clock the alarm had sounded and they were all shepherded down into the basement where they remained until two o'clock. When they arrived back in their bedroom, Joan had said, 'If that damned thing goes off again, I'm not going.' Terry had cheerfully agreed! During the day they had seen the sights, and at night gone to shows, and had such a wonderful time that they had arrived back in Sandhaven on the Sunday night with less than two pounds in change between them.

The very happy and pleasant evening passed all too quickly, and as they were driving home Flora said, 'Looking at that lot, you would not think that there was a war on, would you?'

'No, you wouldn't, but I think a lot of those presents had not been bought recently, but had come out of display cabinets, and bottom drawers in the people's homes.'

'I'm sure they must have, but haven't those two got a good start on their married life in that lovely house, so beautifully furnished, and with everything they want.'

'Yes, they jolly well have; good luck to them, sez I.'

'I'll second that,' said Flora.

Stan Earnshaw was pleased with his test result. He had three doubtful reactors, and the swellings from both Tuberculins were very large and almost the same when they were measured.

'What should I do wi' 'em, Mr 'olden?'

Richard considered the question and then said, 'I'd keep them for the moment, Stan, but sell them off as soon as the time is right. When are they due?'

'That 'un's next month, but t' other two are but new served. I could sell 'em now, becos they're milking well, but price 'ull go up afore Easter, so I'll get shut of 'em then. I want to be ready for July.'

'Don't worry, you will be, Stan.'

In ten minutes he drove across the steel-works yard and up to the stables, where Tom Atherton was waiting. After Richard had rasped a horse's teeth, he cleaned and washed out the sheath of a big gelding, which had a pendulous swelling of the prepuce.

'It's a bit cold this morning for this job, Tom.'

'I bet it is, and dusta know, in spite of red hot iron in t' rolling mill, and all th'eat them converters give out, there's bin frost on t' roofs early in t' mornings.'

'Really, I wouldn't have believed it; still, we are having some lovely days. That's it, Tom; cheerio.'

He went straight to Southall with the present for Bill, and on his way home treated a cow with mastitis and left powders for her at Harry Fisher's, who said, 'I think tha'd better be bringing thi bed 'ere, Mr 'olden.'

'What! my wife would play Holy War if I did.'

'I bet her would an' so would mine!'

Then to Old Hall in Marhey, where he cleansed a new calved cow which was straining hard. A tear in the afterbirth had allowed it to loop itself around some large cotyledons – it was but a minute's job. Nevertheless it was going on for one o'clock, so he drove home, but going up the Marsh Road to Ryton he suddenly felt very cold, and filled with dread. He put his foot down hard on the accelerator, and drove on very fast.

As the month end was near, he had lunch and then went into the office and began to list all the work to be done in March, and then in detail wrote out that which would have to be done by each vet.

The March list of inspections was not as long as February's was, but Joan's list of Tuberculin tests was growing. Jim's list contained four of the latter, surgery twice a week, and one night on duty each week and one weekend in the month. He reasoned that this would break Jim in gradually, give him time to find his way round the practice and let him get to know the clients. The fact that Jim would be living in digs worried him, because, thinking about his own past, he knew he might become a nuisance to Mrs Clunie owing to his irregular hours for meals, and very early and late telephone calls.

He went across to the Coach House, climbed the stairs and was met by the smell of apples from Flora's fruit store. He turned right into the tack room, which with the fireplace at one end and two good sized windows would make a good living room, but as there was not a ceiling, one would have to be fitted. He went into the loft, and visualised it made into a large bedroom with a kitchen, bathroom and WC. As electricity, water and drainage were already installed it would make a good flat, so he would go and see Tommy Duke next week, tell him his plan, and let him find out about local authority requirements and wartime building regulations on the converting of the rooms into a flat. If it were allowed, it would be great for an assistant: he would be on the spot, there would be no difficulties about phone calls, and he could keep his eye on the patients in the hospital on the ground floor.

He would get Terry up here and find out what he thought of more expenditure having to be made.

His reverie was stopped by Joan calling up the stairs that Mr Dawson wanted him on the phone.

'Oh damn him,' he said to himself. 'Weekend again so he'll want something doing urgently.'

He did; it was suspect swine fever at John Greaves', Foxlands Farm, Waterford. Richard said he would do it on Saturday morning, and Bob said that would be great.

'What was that?' asked Flora, 'you didn't sound very pleased.'

'No, I'm not; it's a blooming swine fever as far away as possible in Waterford.'

After tea he trudged upstairs. 'I'll tell you what, love, I'll be glad to have my weekend off.'

'Yes, so will I, it does seem ages since we had one, but we are going to the Lords' on Sunday night – damn the phone, I'll get it.'

'Mr Rankin, the Reformatory School farm, it's a new-calved cow and she is staggering about. Yes, one of them will be there soon.'

'I heard it; I suppose I was tempting fate talking about a weekend off. I'll be back by nine o'clock.'

He was, because the cow's condition wasn't bad and she only went down when one of the lads grabbed her nose. After 500 c.c. of solution had been given intravenously, the big Ayrshire butted the youth who was holding the halter and rose to her feet. Richard wasted no time doing the swine fever investigation on that cold Saturday morning, quickly decided it was a possible case from the lesions he found, and wrapped all the pathological specimens in grease-proof paper, and put them in a box. After rigorously washing with disinfectant his hands, coat and wellington boots, he went to Meatham Lodge, and treated a cow for slow fever. After he had left some horse cough electuary at George Bamber's at Higher Carden Hall, he drove straight back to Sandhaven. When he had completed the form he put it into the specimen box and, after wrapping it up and sealing it, took it to the station, glad to be rid of the stink.

Terry was back after lunch completing his Ministry forms when Richard told him of his idea of a flat for Jim. Because Terry had never been there Richard took him upstairs in the Coach House to see what he was talking about. He thought it would be great for a single assistant, but suggested that in the meantime it would be more use as a laboratory. Richard said that the idea had never crossed his mind, but it would not take long to make a laboratory in the loft the next week seeing the water and a sink were already there.

Terry brought Jim and his large cabin trunk from the station at six o'clock and then went home. Richard took him to the guest-house and after introducing him to Mrs Clunie, gave him directions so that he could come to the surgery about a quarter to ten the next morning.

'Have you got Jim settled in?' asked Flora.

'Yes, he's OK there.'

'Right then, where are we going tonight?'

'We can go to the Palace.'

'I don't want to go there, I've seen *Mrs Miniver* twice already.'

'Lets go and see your heart-throb in Seaton.'

'Yes, let's; it's Gary Cooper and Ingrid Bergman in the new film *For Whom the Bell Tolls*. I'll go and get changed. I wonder if it's continuous.'

'OK; I'll fill the boiler, and put a rug in the car ready.'

They got a good seat in the circle, and soon were engrossed in the picture, with its wonderful mountain scenes in Technicolor. They both enjoyed what they considered was a wonderful picture, and were still talking about it when they were back in the lounge of the Porter's Arms enjoying their drinks. Probably because they were happy and relaxed their love-making was very intense and lasted for a long time that night.

Though Richard was the first to awaken, it was Flora who put on a dressing gown and, having made the tea, brought it, and put the tray on the bedside table. Having drunk their tea, they cuddled and went to sleep again, which resulted in them having a late breakfast.

John had cleaned the Morris inside, and then given the body such a good polishing that it shone in the sunlight, which very much impressed Jim when he arrived. He drove it round Sandhaven with Richard besides him pointing out the landmarks. Because of this he and Flora only just made it to the church on time. St. Luke's was fairly full for Mattins and they enjoyed the service, and afterwards chatted to Edna and the Reverend Tom. After lunch Richard cashed up, completed his Ministry forms, and wrote out the work for the three of them for the week ahead. He joined Flora on the settee in front of the lounge fire, and read the *Veterinary Record* and the *Farmer's Guardian* until tea time. At seven o'clock they were getting ready to go to Jim Lord's when Terry rushed in to get the strappings, because Michael Winder had a cow with a prolapsed uterus. Richard told him that the quickest way was to turn left in Pirton village, go straight on through Teston, and about two miles further on he would come to a farm with buildings on each side of the road. 'Don't forget, drive up to the buildings on the right side of the road. Have you got it?'

'Yes.'

'Good, then off you go.'

They had a pleasant evening with the Lords, most of which Flora spent holding baby Marie, and answering Thomas John's questions. Isabel said that she was content now that they had two children, who soon would be company for each other through childhood. Flora said that she envied her, but was still hopeful that she would conceive.

Jim and Richard talked about the war, trying to guess when the second front would be opened, and when the war would end. As the evening passed, Richard looked across at Flora now and then, and saw how happy and content she was nursing baby Marie. He silently asked God to make the treatment she was having effective, so that she could have a baby which would complete their happiness. They were almost reluctant to leave Jim and Isabel at ten o'clock.

On that bright Monday morning it was nice to drive to Southall where Bob Whiteside had a TB cow ready to be opened. Tommy soon eviscerated it, and then cut out the skirt and pluck. It was an advanced case from which little more than the hide and bones would be salvaged. He drove through Willington and on to Cuthbert Hall.

'Good morning, Michael, how is she?'

'All reet, she's eating and 'as fed calf; tha Mr Wilson were soon 'ere last neet an did a good job.'

'That's what I like to hear, he's a good chap. I'll take the strappings off her now, we never know when we will need them next.'

'Nay, gi' 'em to me, an I'll clean 'em for thee.'

Richard thanked him, and made his way to Welsh's at Further Marsh to see some scouring calves. After the Sugden debacle he was expecting some grumbling, but did not get any.

'Mornin, Mr 'olden. I've five wi t' scour; they're not bad yet but I don't want to lose the lot like Eric Sugden did. Tha knows I wouldna ev gone int pen if I'd a known 'is calves had skitters, but 'is Paul said nowt about it.'

'Yes, they've had a bad do losing so many calves.'

'Dusta think I brought it back 'ere frae Sugden's?'

Richard was wary in his reply. 'There is no way of telling, Tom, but when you get calves from different farms, one of them always seems to bring the scour germ. You put them altogether and it starts. Have you given these any medicine?'

'Aye they ed 'alf a bottle o' t' green un.'

'That will have helped. Just hold them while I get them injected, and give them only milk and water for two days. There's another bottle of medicine; now let me know in a couple of days if they are not doing.'

'Aye, I'll do that.'

At New Church Farm in Olton, Bill Rigby had a cow which was not eating.

'Oo's a real greedy devil, tha knows Mr Holden, oo'll eat owt.'

Richard examined her carefully but could elicit no painful response anywhere. The first stomach was as hard as a board.

'You're right, she's overeaten, Bill, that's the trouble, so I'll give you these two red drinks. Give her nothing to eat, but let her have plenty of water and give her one now. If there is no road through her by this time tomorrow, give her the other one.'

'Reet, I'll ger em down her. T.T.F.N.'

'And the same to you Bill.'

He drove to the telephone box which was beside the pub on the main road and phoned the surgery. Joan told him that there was only one call to make and it was to Harry Fisher who wanted some more mastitis powders.

'Right, I'll go and get it done.'

'Come home, Richard it's not urgent, and Flora will be home in five minutes from the WVS.'

'No, I'll do it, it will make one call less; I won't be long.'

'Very well, I'll tell Flora.'

When Richard drove into the yard at Ivy Farm he found George Duke talking to Harry.

'Hello there, I didn't know you needed an accountant.'

'Aye, I do these days, tha can't run t' farm accounts out of an old shoe box, tha knows.'

'And I'm very glad he doesn't,' said George. 'It makes my job easier, but I must go, I want to get a bit of lunch, and then go to two more farms in Ryton.'

'Right, Harry, here are your powders.'

'Gimme two packets, that 'un's better, but I ev two wi' specks in their fore milk. If this doesn't stop 'em, wilta wash 'em out next week.'

'Yes, let me know if they need it.'

'I will that, Mr 'olden, watch 'ow tha goes.'

Richard drove to the road, and, looking at his watch, saw that it was five past one.

'Blimey, Flora will have to wait for her lunch and she won't like that,' he said to himself.

Driving fast, he soon reached the main road to Sandhaven. There were a lot of Army and Air Force trucks going each way. Having put the car into overdrive, he drove very fast and soon passed those going towards the Shipton airfield. He now began to catch up with two very big Army trucks which were also moving quickly; he glanced at his rear view mirror and saw a large Air Force staff car coming up rapidly behind him. The two trucks slowed down slightly, and moved over a little to their right and Richard glimpsed a car slowing down on the left-hand side of the road. The first truck overtook it, but in the moment after the second one had drawn ahead of it, the car turned right across the road towards the café into the path of Richard's car. He swerved violently to his right, but caught the car a glancing blow, and with a tremendous crash his car ran head-on into the trunk of a big elm tree. As the first car stopped on the off side of the road, the RAF staff car squealed to a stop, and its occupants and people from the café ran to Richard's car. The Air Vice Marshal took command and he bellowed orders to his Squadron Leader to ring the police and ambulance, and as it was obvious that Richard was trapped in the wreckage, sent to the Highways Depot down the road for workmen to bring picks and crowbars. George Duke, petrified with shock, sat dazed in his car while the police, ambulance men and the workmen freed Richard who was still breathing and he was put into the ambulance which, preceded by the police car, drove at high speed to Droughton Royal Infirmary.

At half past one Flora was expecting Richard to walk in at any minute, so brewed a pot of tea, poured out a cupful and began to drink it. Fifteen minutes later dread had seized her – she knew something must be wrong because he had not phoned her. She got up and began to walk up and down the room, becoming more and more agitated. The door bell rang, and she ran down the stairs to answer it, but her heart almost stopped with fear when she saw a young-looking policeman standing there, turning his helmet round in his hands.

'Are you Mrs 'olden?'

'Yes, come in will you, what is it? where's Richard? please, please tell me.'

'I'm sorry to have to tell you, Mrs 'olden, that there's bin a car crash on the new road at Ryton, and your husband were in it, and 'as bin taken to Droughton Royal Infirmary. They want you to go and see him as soon as you can.'

A trembling Flora said, 'Oh God, I'll have to ring Terry.'

'Is there anything I can do, Mum?'

'No, thank you, I'll be OK,' and as he turned to leave a woman with a greyhound walked into the waiting room.

Flora ran into the office and phoned Terry.

'Good God, no. Oh, Flora, I'm sorry, we're on our way.'

Flora was regaining her composure a little when Joan and Terry ran in a few minutes later.

'Right, Flora, come on, let's go.'

'We can't; there's a woman in the waiting room with a dog.'

'Oh hell, is there? then I'll soon deal with her.'

He walked into the waiting room.

'Good afternoon, will you please come through.'

'Who are you? I am Mrs Bailey and I have an appointment with Mr Holden.'

'I am his partner, Mr Wilson; I am sorry Mr Holden is not available now, so I will attend to your dog. What do you want?'

'His nails cut and his eye teeth want cleaning.'

'Just hold his muzzle, and I'll tie this bandage round it.'

'Don't hurt him, that's too tight.'

'It's not, Mrs Bailey and I must have it on before I'll touch his nails.'

'Oh, all right, then.'

The nails were soon cut and the tartar scraped and chipped off the teeth.

'There you are, Mrs Bailey. That is £1 please.'

'That's a lot; Mr Holden doesn't charge me as much as that.'

'That is the correct fee; thank you, and now I must go.'

'But I want you to look at his tail.'

'I'm sorry, but I must go, Mrs Bailey; will you please ring and make another appointment.'

'Oh, of all the cheek, when I'm here with my dog. Mr Holden will hear of this.'

Terry walked to the door and opened it. 'Mrs Bailey will you please leave soon because I've got to take Mrs Holden to Droughton Royal Infirmary, to see her husband who has been injured in a car crash.'

'Oh, all right then, if that's what you want.'

The practice was forgotten as the front door was shut, and the three of them ran to the Hillman, which Terry drove very fast to Droughton Royal Infirmary. Flora was relieved as the big red brick building came into view, and Terry drove in through the main entrance, and right up to the main door. Flora gave her name at the reception desk, a nurse came at once and led them to Casualty, where they walked through the curtains into a cubicle. Silently, they all three stared at Richard lying in a semi-prone position on the bed; his head appeared flattened and was heavily bandaged, while his feet were resting against two wooden blocks. The curtains parted, and Dr Duncan entered and asked Flora if she was Mrs Holden. She quietly said 'Yes.'

'Then I am very sorry to have to tell you that your husband is dying from very severe injuries to his head, for which there is nothing I can do. I am surprised he has lived so long, we are just waiting for the end.'

Joan put her arm round Flora, and led her outside – too stunned to cry, she just flopped onto a chair. The nurse brought a cup of tea and she slowly drank it. Five minutes later on that bright cold afternoon, supporting Flora in the middle, the three of them walked slowly back to the car.

'What are you going to do, Flora?' asked Terry.

'It's not what am I going to do; it's what are you going to do, how will you manage?'

When they drove into Cross Street, Jim was sitting in his car outside No. 2. He had been completely forgotten in the tragic events of the last hour, and he had not yet got a front door key. As they walked to the front door, Terry told him what had happened, and apologised. When Flora opened the door the phone was ringing and she ran to answer it. It was a message from the hospital to say that Richard had died at ten minutes past three. Flora began to scream and wail, dropped the receiver, and ran upstairs.

The two men looked at each other and stood stock-still, shocked by the sound.

Joan rose to the occasion, she shouted, 'Quick, Terry, ring Dr Bill now, and tell him to get here fast, and then Jean her mum and tell her what's happened. Hurry up, for God's sake,' and she rushed off up the stairs after Flora whose keening could be heard all over the house. Joan flung herself down on the settee besides Flora, put her arms round her, and held her tightly until the unearthly crying subsided into a sobbing moaning.

This was how Dr Bill and Doris found the two women when they came into the room a few minutes later. Doris sat down besides Flora and held hands with Joan behind her back to hold her upright. Bill, taking both her hands in his, said, his Irish accent becoming strong with his emotion,

'Flora, I am terribly, terribly sorry for you, and we'll do all we can to help you. Are you listening to me now?'

Flora softly said, 'Yes.'

'Then I want you to take this tablet now. Doris, bring a glass of water please.'

Flora, visibly trembling – a pathetic sight with her white tear-stained face – did as Bill had told her.

When Terry had sent Jim off to do some visits, he came upstairs and kissed Flora on the cheek, and had just expressed his concern and sympathy when he had to run down to answer the door-bell. News travelled very fast in Sandhaven that afternoon. It was Jim Lord and Isabel, and on seeing them Flora began to cry again. Betty Heyes with the Revd Tom Evans and Edna came next, closely followed by Joan Bishop and Edna Duke. Betty was soon in the kitchen, brewing tea, and brought a cup at once to Flora, and asked her if she wanted anything to eat. Flora, much calmer now the sedative was taking effect, replied that she didn't. Soon the lounge was full of friends, some tearful, and all subdued.

As Jim and Isabel left with Dr Bill and Doris, Terry was talking to a policeman in the waiting room, and a reporter from the *Lancashire Daily Post* was there wanting details of Richard's life and career. Joan came down, and Terry asked her to go with him to the mortuary in Droughton to identify Richard's body; all four went their separate ways. Just before six o'clock Jean arrived in a taxi from the station, and Joan Bishop met her in the hall and told her the news. Jim came in to take evening surgery. As Jean had experienced a similar tragedy when Tom her husband had been killed in the rail crash nine years earlier, she instinctively knew how to help her daughter in her distress.

She slowly walked upstairs, and into the lounge. Flora, seeing her, began to cry and stood up, and her mother put an arm round her, and with her free hand gently stroked her hair.

'Oh Mum, I've lost Richard.'

Jean kissed her, and quietly said, 'Yes, I know you have, love, and I am dreadfully sorry for you.'

Betty Heyes and Joan Bishop tip-toed out of the room.

'Mum, whatever am I going to do?'

'Let's sit down, Flora; we'll meet that hurdle together later, but for now, my love, your life has got to go on, and I am here to help you. Now, have you had anything to eat today yet?'

'No, but I don't want anything.'

'I thought so, and neither have I, but we are going to have something to eat, my girl. I brought half a chicken and some meat pies, so I'll make some sandwiches and brew the tea. No I won't, we'll have a drink first and then I'll brew up.' She poured two whiskies and, sitting down again, gave one to Flora. As the two women drank Jean asked, 'Have you let Bill and Mary know?'

'No I haven't.'

'Then we'll have our meal now, and then I'll see what things are like downstairs.'

Flora ate some chicken sandwiches and half a pie, following this with two cups of tea, and became more composed. Jean ate a good meal, and then asked, 'What's the new man's name?'

'Jim Mortimer.'

Flora listened while Jean phoned Mary the news, and then the sisters talked for a few minutes, Mary saying she would come as fast as she could next day. Bill was devastated.

'There must be a damned curse on the men in our family, Mum, they either get badly injured or killed, let me talk to our kid.' Bill was very protective towards both his sisters, and spoke very gently and lovingly to Flora.

'I'll get compassionate leave as soon as I can, kid, God bless you, see you tomorrow.'

Jean washed the pots and then went down to see Joan and Terry. She thanked them for all they had done, and then said to Terry that as he was the surviving partner, with Richard being dead, he was in control of the practice, but it was not his. He replied that he hadn't given it a thought, with so much happening all day, and that he and Joan had only just returned from the mortuary in Droughton where they had had to identify Richard's body at the request of the Coroner's Officer.

'I am certain that we can manage. It's a godsend that Jim came on Saturday, and being old friends, I know we can work well together.'

'I am certain you will, but you must have power of attorney to pay bills, wages and things, so I think you should ring Tommy Duke, and ask him to see you in the morning.'

'Thank you very much, Mrs Dickenson, I'll do that. I've sent John and Jim home, and all incoming calls will come to me at the Moorings. I must tell you that the Coroner's Officer said that the inquest will be at 10.30 on Wednesday. Now if you will excuse us, we will go home to have a meal.'

'Yes, you must both be hungry, good night.'

Flora was pensively staring into the fire.

'Well, my girl, Terry and Jim have coped very well, and I've told Terry to ring George Duke so that he can advise us all what we should do. I expect he will come in the morning. Now who is your bank manager?'

'Dick Harrison.'

'And have you rung Richard's family?'

'No, you can do that, Mum.'

'And who's your undertaker?'

'Maurice Rawcliffe, he lives just up the road.'

'Then I'll go and ring them downstairs, and you have forty winks.'

Dr Bill and Doris came back late in the evening, and he covertly watched Flora as they talked. He gave her a sleeping table which she swallowed, and then they both left. Jean went and put a hot water bottle in each bed, and by ten o'clock both exhausted women were sound asleep.

Norah Wilson, carrying a large bunch of flowers, came with Terry and Joan on the Tuesday morning, and spent some time with Flora and Jean consoling them. Jim also expressed his sympathy to them, and then excused himself and hurried away, because Joan saw that there were already over twenty visits and revisits to be done that Tuesday. Terry and Jim lost no time in setting off to do their morning rounds.

People who had seen the announcement of the car crash in the Stop Press of the *Lancashire Evening Post* the night before had written at once to Flora, who was touched by their kindness.

When Bill and Elizabeth Meadows came in the middle of the morning, the latter said, 'Flora, love, why didn't you ring me? I'd 'ave bin 'ere before now, but we've only just found out; we're so sorry for you.' She kissed Flora, and gave her a large spray of flowers which Bill had been holding.

'Liz,' said Flora in tears, 'I don't know, I didn't know what I was doing yesterday, I was in such a state.'

'I can understand that, love, and I'm proper upset too, Flora, he were a great friend to me. Now if there's owt you want doing, we'll do it, whether it's big or small, won't we, Liz, and you will ask, won't you, Flora?'

'Yes, I will, Bill, and thank you both, but do sit down and have some coffee. Mum's making some.'

After talking for a while they left, and Flora said, 'Jean, I hope she wasn't hurt by my not letting her know, because she is such an old friend.'

'Don't worry, she won't be. When my Tom was killed, I never let Jenny Lawson know. The first thing they knew, was when they saw Tom's name in the list of those killed in the train crash in the paper next day.'

Bill MacDonald rang Flora and expressed his sympathy, and told her that he would never forget that eager young student who had gone with him on his morning round all those years ago, and that his wedding would not be quite the same with them not being there. Flora thanked him, and wished him and Isabel all happiness on Friday.

The arrival of Bill and Mary in the afternoon was a great comfort to Flora, being surrounded by her family; even so, tears came again when Tom and Edna came to see her. They both kissed Flora, and Tom said that it was a long time since anything upset him so much. Edna added that they had spent a very miserable evening after Jean had told them the news. The latter brought in tea, and asked Tom what was the position with regards to the practice and the accident. Tom quietly explained the law regarding both, and then went downstairs to talk to Terry, who had come into the surgery to get some more medicines. Tom gave him a list of all the things that must be done, and said that his brother's assistant would bring him new account books, but he would have to go and see Harrison at the bank and open a new practice account. Terry thanked Tom, but said he must go because he had a good few visits still to be done. Richard's prediction that the practice would be busy by now was proving all too true!

Flowers with cards of sympathy were coming from the 'Flower Vase' in the High Street, and on Wednesday morning a deluge of letters and cards were delivered. Two of the letters were important to Flora; the first was from Wing Commander Norman Robinson, DSO, DFC, in which he expressed his sorrow at the death of his friend, and prayed for God's blessing to rest on Flora now and always. Inexplicably his letter gave her a feeling of peace, alleviating her sense of bewilderment. She silently thanked God for that letter, and asked for his protection for Norman. The other letter was from George Duke in which he expressed his sympathy and asked for her forgiveness for being the driver of the car which was involved in the accident. He wrote that he would understand if she now decided to employ another accountant after what had happened. Flora sat looking at the letter, and then asked all her family to read it.

Bill spoke first, 'Mum, as I see it, she can't have him as her accountant, because there's bound to be a court case, and a clash of interests. Tom, being his brother, will be his lawyer at the inquest, and at any other proceedings which might arise.'

'You're right there, Bill, because after the inquest the insurance companies will be bound to contest any settlements, so, Flora, you will have to have another solicitor. Tom couldn't appear for both sides in any dispute; you see what I mean.'

'Yes, Mum, but who shall I ask? I don't know any other solicitor.'

'Then I'll soon find out. I'll ring Betty Heyes, she knows everybody for miles around, and there's Mabel Bishop at the Café.'

'Yes she'll know, ask her.' The latter did, and gave Jean the name of their solicitors in Droughton, W. Bramwell, Harrison & Co., while Hargreaves & Tanner were their accountants in Seaton.

Jim was not back from doing his afternoon visits, when Terry finished surgery that evening, but John appeared on time, carrying a large bunch of flowers. Embarrassed at showing emotion, he gave them to Flora and said, 'Our Mavis and me want yer to have these, because we're both of us proper sorry tha's lost 'im. I think it's a real shame, becos he were so good to me.'

'Thanks, John, very much, and you will thank Mavis, won't you?'

'Aye, I will that, but I must be getting on.'

At that he went downstairs, lit a fag, and began to clean the surgery.

In Droughton on Wednesday morning accompanied by her family, Flora listened while formal evidence of identification was given by Joan Wilson, and then the Coroner adjourned the inquest for a fortnight. He reiterated the police appeal for witnesses of the accident to contact them as soon as possible. After lunch the phone was busy; first, Uncle Tom Bradshaw said he and Nellie wanted to come to the funeral. Flora told them she would let them know, and rang Maurice who said that he was arranging it for eleven o'clock on Friday morning, but would come and see her in an hour or so. Thus Flora was able to give the details to Uncle Harry and Joan, but she would not speak to Mary Holden when she rang. She told Jean that she would be coming to the funeral, but would be staying for a few days with friends in Walsham, and that her father sent his apologies, because he would be unable to come because of his heart condition. Jean very politely thanked Mary, and then told Flora, who said that it didn't make a ha'porth of difference to her whether she came or not.

The bell of St. Luke's Church was being slowly tolled when on that very sunny morning 3rd March, the bearers of Richard's coffin on which was one wreath – Flora's cross of red roses – stood at the Lychgate while the mourners led by Flora and Bill made a cortège behind them. The two churchwardens, Col. Laycarte Porter and Tom Collinson, carrying their silver knobbed black wands of office led the way past the silent people lining the long path up to the church door. Behind them Frank Madden the verger preceded the Vicar, the Revd Tom Evans who in a clear resonant voice began to say the comforting opening verses of the Order for the Burial of the Dead. Flora, visibly distressed, now, was supported by Bill and Mary, one on each side of her, as they followed the coffin into the packed church. The congregation holding the order of service sheets in their hands rose to their feet, and watched as the undertaker helped to place the coffin on the two stools in front of the altar. He and the four bearers; Jim Lord, Tom Bishop, Dick Heyes and John Lamb, went and sat in the choir stalls.

When Maurice Billington had seen Flora, she had chosen three hymns, and now 'There's a friend for little children above the bright blue sky,' was sung, and was followed by the Psalm. Another hymn, 'Forth in Thy name O Lord I go' was sung before the Lesson – the 15th Chapter of the Epistle of St. Paul to the Corinthians. In his address the Vicar spoke of the universal sadness felt as the result of a life dedicated to helping their Community had been ended so tragically.

The favourite hymn of the organist, Mr Tomlinson, was also the one which was sung as the mourners followed the coffin out of Church. It was 'Onward Christian Soldiers', and he played it loudly, and with such a spirited rhythm that it uplifted the spirits of all who heard it.

When the coffin had been lowered into the grave, the words: 'Ashes to ashes, dust to dust' were said, and Flora, weeping stepped forward and threw one red rose, and a handful of earth onto it. She whispered, 'Goodbye love, till we meet again,' and quickly turned round to grab the arms of Bill and Mary because she was trembling so much. It took some time for the mourners to pay their respects, before they could leave the graveyard. They were glad soon to be out of the cold wind, and sitting in the lounge of the Porter's Arms.

Flora and Bill, each holding a large whisky in their hands, mingled with their friends and guests before the lunch. That evening Joan, Terry and Jim brought Flora a large bunch of flowers, and said that as it had been such a busy day, they had not been able to get to the service, though it had not been as bad as Tuesday when they had done thirty-three visits between them. Flora gave them a drink, and thanked them for the flowers, but was glad when they went, because she was so tired she could go straight to bed.

Though Bill and Mary left on Saturday Jean stayed on for two reasons. First, she didn't want to leave her daughter alone at night, and second, so that she could help her to have an interest again especially in answering all the letters, cards and flowers which had come. For this reason she did not put a formal 'Thank you' in the paper, but let Flora fill her days in writing her replies, and helping Joan with the monthly accounts.

It was a large piece of wedding cake which was delivered on Tuesday, and in the parcel was a letter from Bill and Isabel thanking her for the present. Ten days later the adjourned Coroner's inquest was held in Droughton. The short report in the *Evening Post* said that after other evidence had been given the pathologist said that Mr Holden had died as the result of a fractured skull. The jury returned a verdict of misadventure on the veterinary surgeon who died from injuries received in the accident which happened in Droughton New Road, Ryton on 28th February.

Many legal matters regarding the accident were unresolved by early May, but Norah Wilson had purchased the practice for Terry, and Jim had become the junior partner, having bought a quarter share in the business.

After asking Terry's permission, Flora went to the surgery one evening, and walked up the path which was bordered by the lovely spring flowers she had planted a year earlier. She stopped and looked at Richard's plate on the wall, and remembered how excited they had been five years before when he put it up. Now she was unhappy at having to take it down, and her eyes filled with tears as she took out the retaining screws, took down the plate, and put it into her shopping bag. She held it tightly against her bosom, knowing that it was a very precious piece of evidence of the wonderful life they had had together, which had ended so abruptly. Gone was her husband, who 'at all times and in all places', had worked hard to relieve pain and suffering in animals. Crying as she walked away, the lines of the Marriage Service came into her mind: 'to love, cherish and obey till death us do part.' She knew that she had.

A fortnight later Dr Bill confirmed that Flora was pregnant, and though he and Doris congratulated her, she was still sad for Richard would never know their dearest wish was coming true.

She went back to Holme, taking Ming and Bumble with her, to live with her mother Jean until her son was born on 27th November that year.